PHARMACOTHERAPEUTICS
in
Obstetrics & Gynecology

PHARMACOTHERAPEUTICS in Obstetrics & Gynecology

Ashok Kumar
MD PhD
Director Professor and Head
Department of Obstetrics and Gynecology
Atal Bihari Vajpayee Institute of Medical Sciences and
Dr Ram Manohar Lohia Hospital
New Delhi, India

Neha Pruthi Tandon
MS (Obs & Gyne) Diploma in Clinical ART FICMCH
Associate Professor
Department of Obstetrics and Gynecology
Atal Bihari Vajpayee Institute of Medical Sciences and
Dr Ram Manohar Lohia Hospital
New Delhi, India

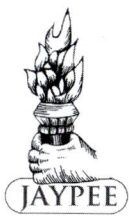

JAYPEE BROTHERS MEDICAL PUBLISHERS
The Health Sciences Publisher
New Delhi | London

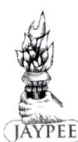 **Jaypee Brothers Medical Publishers (P) Ltd**

Headquarters
Jaypee Brothers Medical Publishers (P) Ltd
EMCA House, 23/23-B
Ansari Road, Daryaganj
New Delhi 110 002, India
Landline: +91-11-23272143, +91-11-23272703
+91-11-23282021, +91-11-23245672
Email: jaypee@jaypeebrothers.com

Corporate Office
Jaypee Brothers Medical Publishers (P) Ltd
4838/24, Ansari Road, Daryaganj
New Delhi 110 002, India
Phone: +91-11-43574357
Fax: +91-11-43574314
Email: jaypee@jaypeebrothers.com

Overseas Office
JP Medical Ltd
83, Victoria Street, London
SW1H 0HW (UK)
Phone: +44 20 3170 8910
Fax: +44 (0)20 3008 6180
Email: info@jpmedpub.com

Website: www.jaypeebrothers.com
Website: www.jaypeedigital.com

© 2024, Jaypee Brothers Medical Publishers

The views and opinions expressed in this book are solely those of the original contributor(s)/author(s) and do not necessarily represent those of editor(s) or publisher of the book.

All rights reserved. No part of this publication may be reproduced, stored or transmitted in any form or by any means, electronic, mechanical, photocopying, recording or otherwise, without the prior permission in writing of the publishers.

All brand names and product names used in this book are trade names, service marks, trademarks or registered trademarks of their respective owners. The publisher is not associated with any product or vendor mentioned in this book.

Medical knowledge and practice change constantly. This book is designed to provide accurate, authoritative information about the subject matter in question. However, readers are advised to check the most current information available on procedures included and check information from the manufacturer of each product to be administered, to verify the recommended dose, formula, method and duration of administration, adverse effects and contraindications. It is the responsibility of the practitioner to take all appropriate safety precautions. Neither the publisher nor the author(s)/editor(s) assume any liability for any injury and/or damage to persons or property arising from or related to use of material in this book.

This book is sold on the understanding that the publisher is not engaged in providing professional medical services. If such advice or services are required, the services of a competent medical professional should be sought.

Every effort has been made where necessary to contact holders of copyright to obtain permission to reproduce copyright material. If any have been inadvertently overlooked, the publisher will be pleased to make the necessary arrangements at the first opportunity.

Inquiries for bulk sales may be solicited at: jaypee@jaypeebrothers.com

Pharmacotherapeutics in Obstetrics & Gynecology

First Edition: **2024**

ISBN: 978-93-5696-582-9

Printed at: Sanat Printers

Contributors

Ajay Chauhan
MD (Internal Medicine)
Professor
Department of Medicine
Atal Bihari Vajpayee Institute of Medical Sciences
and Dr Ram Manohar Lohia Hospital
New Delhi, India

Ajit Kumar Nayak
MD (Obs & Gyne, JIPMER) DNB MNAMS FICOG FICMCH
PGDMCH Diploma in USG PDCC
Laparoscopy Infertility and Genetics
Professor and Head
Department of Obstetrics and Gynecology
FM Medical College and Hospital
Balasore, Odisha, India

Amita Suneja
MD FAMS FICOG FICMCH
Director Professor and HOD
Department of Obstetrics and Gynecology
University College of Medical Sciences and
Guru Teg Bahadur Hospital
New Delhi, India

Anjum Ara
MBBS MD MRCOG
Associate Professor
Department of Obstetrics and Gynecology
Atal Bihari Vajpayee Institute of Medical Sciences
and Dr Ram Manohar Lohia Hospital
New Delhi, India

Ankita Jain
MBBS DNB (Obs & Gyne)
Assistant Professor
Department of Obstetrics and Gynecology
Vardhman Mahavir Medical College and
Safdarjung Hospital
Gurugram, Haryana, India

Anshika Agarwal
MBBS MS (Obs & Gyne)
Senior Resident
Department of Obstetrics and Gynecology
Vardhman Mahavir Medical College and
Safdarjung Hospital
New Delhi, India

Anupma
MBBS MD DNB
Assistant Professor
Department of Obstetrics and Gynecology
University College of Medical Sciences and
Guru Teg Bahadur Hospital
New Delhi, India

Archana Chaurasia
MBBS DNB (Obs & Gyne) ECFMG Certified USA
Senior Resident
Department of Obstetrics and Gynecology
Atal Bihari Vajpayee Institute of Medical Sciences
and Dr Ram Manohar Lohia Hospital
New Delhi, India

Archana Maurya
MBBS MS (Obs & Gyne) MICOG FICOG MA
(Human Rights)
Professor and Consultant
Department of Obstetrics and Gynecology
Gajra Raja Medical College
Gwalior, Madhya Pradesh, India

Aruna Nigam
MS (Obs & Gyne)
Professor and HOD
Department of Obstetrics and Gynecology
Hamdard Institute of Medical Sciences and
Research
New Delhi, India

Ashima Taneja
MBBS MS
Professor and Head
Department of Obstetrics and Gynecology
Dayanand Medical College and Hospital
Ludhiana, Punjab, India

Ashok Kumar
MD PhD
Director Professor and Head
Department of Obstetrics and Gynecology
Atal Bihari Vajpayee Institute of
Medical Sciences and
Dr Ram Manohar Lohia Hospital
New Delhi, India

Contributors

Ashu Bhardwaj
MS DNB (Obs & Gyne)
Senior Resident
Department of Obstetrics and Gynecology
Atal Bihari Vajpayee Institute of Medical Sciences
and Dr Ram Manohar Lohia Hospital
New Delhi, India

Bharti Uppal Nayyar
MS (Obs & Gyne) Fellow in Urogynecology (AIIMS)
Chief Medical Officer (NFSG)
Department of Obstetrics and Gynecology
Atal Bihari Vajpayee Institute of
Medical Sciences and
Dr Ram Manohar Lohia Hospital
New Delhi, India

Dheerendra Kuber
MBBS MD DM (Cardiology)
Assistant Professor
Department of Cardiology
Atal Bihari Vajpayee Institute of
Medical Sciences and
Dr Ram Manohar Lohia Hospital
New Delhi, India

Durgesh
MBBS DGO DNB
Chief Medical Officer (NFSG)
Department of Obstetrics and Gynecology
Atal Bihari Vajpayee Institute of Medical Sciences
and Dr Ram Manohar Lohia Hospital
New Delhi, India

Geetanjali Nabiyal
MBBS DGO MS
Chief Medical Officer (NFSG)
Department of Obstetrics and Gynecology
Atal Bihari Vajpayee Institute of Medical Sciences
and Dr Ram Manohar Lohia Hospital
New Delhi, India

Indu Chawla
MBBS (Hons) DGO MD (Obs & Gyne)
Professor
Department of Obstetrics and Gynecology
Atal Bihari Vajpayee Institute of Medical Sciences
and Dr Ram Manohar Lohia Hospital
New Delhi, India

Jaya Chawla
MBBS MS Fellow (Maternal Fetal Medicine)
(AIIMS, New Delhi)
Associate Professor
Department of Obstetrics and Gynecology
Atal Bihari Vajpayee Institute of
Medical Sciences and
Dr Ram Manohar Lohia Hospital
New Delhi, India

JB Sharma
MD FRCOG (London) FAMS PhD FICOG MFFP DNB FIMSA
Professor
Department of Obstetrics and Gynecology
All India Institute of Medical Sciences
New Delhi, India

Juhi Bharti
MBBS MS MRCOG
Associate Professor
Department of Obstetrics and Gynecology
All India Institute of Medical Sciences
New Delhi, India

Jyoti Jaiswal
MBBS MS (Obs & Gyne) FICOG FMAS CIMP
Professor and Head
Department of Obstetrics and Gynecology
Pt JNM Medical College and
Associated Dr Bhim Rao Ambedkar Memorial
Hospital
Raipur, Chhattisgarh, India

Jyotsna Suri
MBBS MD FICOG
Professor and Consultant
Department of Obstetrics and Gynecology
Vardhman Mahavir Medical College and
Safdarjung Hospital
New Delhi, India

Kamal Chopra
MBBS MD (Chest) DTCE
Director
Department of Chest and TB
State TB Training and Demonstration Center
New Delhi, India

Kamna Datta
MBBS MS FICOG
Professor
Department of Obstetrics and Gynecology
Atal Bihari Vajpayee Institute of Medical Sciences
and Dr Ram Manohar Lohia Hospital
New Delhi, India

Kanika Kumari
MD (Obs & Gyne)
Specialist
Department of Obstetrics and Gynecology
Atal Bihari Vajpayee Institute of Medical Sciences
and Dr Ram Manohar Lohia Hospital
New Delhi, India

Kavita Kumari
MS (Obs & Gyne)
Chief Medical Officer
Department of Obstetrics and Gynecology
Atal Bihari Vajpayee Institute of Medical Sciences
and Dr Ram Manohar Lohia Hospital
New Delhi, India

Kiran Dhawan
MBBS
Postgraduate Student
Department of Obstetrics and Gynecology
Atal Bihari Vajpayee Institute of Medical Sciences
and Dr Ram Manohar Lohia Hospital
New Delhi, India

Latha Chaturvedula
MD (Obs & Gyne) DNB (Obs & Gyne) FICOG Executive MBA (Hospital Management)
Professor
Department of Obstetrics and Gynecology
Jawaharlal Institute of Postgraduate Medical
Education and Research
(An Institute of National Importance)
Puducherry, India

Madhav Bahadur
MBBS MD DM (Neurology)
Senior Resident 1st year
Neurology Department
Dr RMLIMS, Vibhuti Khand
Lucknow, Uttar Pradesh, India

Madhavi M Gupta
MBBS MS
Director-Professor
Department of Obstetrics and Gynecology
Maulana Azad Medical College and
Lok Nayak Hospital
New Delhi, India

Mamta Meena
MS (Obs & Gyne)
Senior Resident
Department of Obstetrics and Gynecology
Maulana Azad Medical College
New Delhi, India

Meghna Reddy
MS (Obs & Gyne)
Senior Consultant
Department of Obstetrics and Gynecology
Atal Bihari Vajpayee Institute of
Medical Sciences and
Dr Ram Manohar Lohia Hospital
New Delhi, India

Mousumi Das Ghosh
MD FICOG
Consultant
Department of Obstetrics and Gynecology
Tata Main Hospital
Manipal Tata Medical College
Jamshedpur, Jharkhand, India

Muskan Chaudhary
MBBS MD
Assistant Professor
Department of Obstetrics and Gynecology
Dayanand Medical College and Hospital
Ludhiana, Punjab, India

Namita Chopra
MBBS MD (Obs & Gyne) DNB MNAMS
Senior Medical Officer
Department of Obstetrics and Gynecology
Atal Bihari Vajpayee Institute of
Medical Sciences and
Dr Ram Manohar Lohia Hospital
New Delhi, India

Neelika Gupta
MD
Senior Resident
Department of Obstetrics and Gynecology
University College of Medical Sciences
New Delhi, India

Neha Pruthi Tandon
MS (Obs & Gyne) Diploma in Clinical ART FICMCH
Associate Professor
Department of Obstetrics and Gynecology
Atal Bihari Vajpayee Institute of
Medical Sciences and
Dr Ram Manohar Lohia Hospital
New Delhi, India

Niharika Dhiman
MS (Obs & Gyne)
Associate Professor
Department of Obstetrics and Gynecology
Maulana Azad Medical College
New Delhi, India

Nisha Rao
MBBS MD
Senior Resident
Department of Obstetrics and Gynecology
All India Institute of Medical Sciences
New Delhi, India

Nisha Watti
MBBS MS DNB (Obs & Gyne)
Assistant Professor
Department of Obstetrics and Gynecology
Pt JNM Medical College and
Associated Dr Bhim Rao Ambedkar Memorial Hospital
Raipur, Chhattisgarh, India

Paridhi Gupta
DNB (Obs & Gyne) MS (Obs & Gyne) MBBS (AIIMS)
Senior Resident
Department of Obstetrics and Gynecology
Atal Bihari Vajpayee Institute of
Medical Sciences and
Dr Ram Manohar Lohia Hospital
New Delhi, India

Pijush Kanti Nandi
MS (Obs & Gyne)
Assistant Professor
Department of Medicine
Maulana Azad Medical College
New Delhi, India

Pooja Verma
MS (Obs & Gyne)
Senior Resident
Department of Obstetrics and Gynecology
MGM Medical College and MTH Hospital
Indore, Madhya Pradesh, India

Pradyumna Kumar Singh
MBBS MD
Senior Resident
Department of Cardiology
Atal Bihari Vajpayee Institute of Medical Sciences
and Dr Ram Manohar Lohia Hospital
New Delhi, India

Preeti Sainia
MBBS DGO
Chief Medical Officer (NFSG)
Department of Obstetrics and Gynecology
Atal Bihari Vajpayee Institute of Medical Sciences
and Dr Ram Manohar Lohia Hospital
New Delhi, India

Priyanka Dahiya
MBBS MS (Obs & Gyne)
Associate Professor
Department of Obstetrics and Gynecology
Kalpana Chawla Government Medical College
Karnal, Haryana, India

Priyanka Shanker
MS (Obs & Gyne)
Senior Resident
Department of Obstetrics and Gynecology
University College of Medical Sciences and
Guru Teg Bahadur Hospital
New Delhi, India

Puneet Aggarwal
MBBS MD DM (Cardiology)
Assistant Professor
Department of Cardiology
Atal Bihari Vajpayee Institute of Medical Sciences
and Dr Ram Manohar Lohia Hospital
New Delhi, India

Ranjit Kumar Nath
MBBS MD DM (Cardiology)
Director Professor
Department of Cardiology
Atal Bihari Vajpayee Institute of
Medical Sciences and
Dr Ram Manohar Lohia Hospital
New Delhi, India

Reeta Bansiwal
DM (Reproductive Medicine)
Professor
Department of Obstetrics and Gynecology
Vardhman Mahavir Medical College and
Safdarjung Hospital
New Delhi, India

Rekha Bharti
MD FICOG
Professor
Department of Obstetrics and Gynecology
Vardhman Mahavir Medical College and
Safdarjung Hospital
New Delhi, India

Renu Singh
MS (Obs & Gyne)
FNB - Reproductive Medicine
Department of Obstetrics and Gynecology
Maulana Azad Medical College
New Delhi, India

Renu Tanwar
MS (Obs & Gyne)
Director, Professor and IVF Coordinator
Department of Obstetrics and Gynecology
IVF and Reproductive Biology Center
Maulana Azad Medical College
New Delhi, India

Renuka Malik
MD DGO
Professor and Senior Consultant
Department of Obstetrics and Gynecology
Atal Bihari Vajpayee Institute of
Medical Sciences and Dr Ram Manohar Lohia
Hospital
New Delhi, India

Richa Aggarwal
MD DNB
Professor
Department of Obstetrics and Gynecology
University College of Medical Sciences and
Guru Teg Bahadur Hospital
New Delhi, India

Ruchika Garg
MD Fellow – Indian College of Obstetricians and
Gynecologists Member – National Academy Medical
Sciences FIAOG FICMCH FMAS
Professor
Department of Obstetrics and Gynecology
SN Medical College
Agra, Uttar Pradesh, India

Sandhya Jain
MD DNB MRCOG (UK)
Professor
Department of Obstetrics and Gynecology
University College of Medical Sciences and
Guru Teg Bahadur Hospital
New Delhi, India

Sangeeta Kumari
MBBS MS
Postgraduate Resident
Department of Obstetrics and Gynecology
Atal Bihari Vajpayee Institute of
Medical Sciences
and Dr Ram Manohar Lohia Hospital
New Delhi, India

Seema Sheokand
MS (Obs & Gyne)
Assistant Professor
Department of Obstetrics and Gynecology
Atal Bihari Vajpayee Institute of
Medical Sciences
and Dr Ram Manohar Lohia Hospital
New Delhi, India

Shobhana Mohan Das
MD DGO FICOG Diploma in Endoscopy CIMP
Consultant Gynecologist
Institute Sun Medical Center
Thrissur, Kerala, India
Past President Indian Menopause Society

Contributors

Sumitra Yadav
MBBS MS DNB FICOG MNAMS
Professor and Head
Department of Obstetrics and Gynecology
MGM Medical College and MTH Women's Hospital
Indore, Madhya Pradesh, India

Supriya Chaubey
MS (Obs & Gyne)
Assistant Professor
Department of Obstetrics and Gynecology
Hamdard Institute of Medical Sciences and Research
New Delhi, India

Syed Habeebullah
MD MNAMS
Emeritus Professor
Department of Obstetrics and Gynecology
Mahatma Gandhi Medical College and Research Institute (Affiliated to Sri Balaji Vidyapeeth, Deemed to be University)
Puducherry, India
Former Professor and Head, JIPMER
Puducherry, India

Taru Gupta
MS DNB
Professor and Head
Department of Obstetrics and Gynecology
ESIC PGIMSR, Basaidarapur
New Delhi, India

Vaishnavi Jayaram
MBBS MS (Obs & Gyne)
Ex Senior-Resident
Department of Obstetrics and Gynecology
Maulana Azad Medical College and
Lok Nayak Hospital
New Delhi, India

Vandana Agarwal
MS DNB
Assistant Professor
Department of Obstetrics and Gynecology
Atal Bihari Vajpayee Institute of Medical Sciences and
Dr Ram Manohar Lohia Hospital
New Delhi, India

Vanshika Pundhir
MBBS MS (Obs & Gyne)
Senior Resident
Department of Obstetrics and Gynecology
University College of Medical Sciences and
Guru Teg Bahadur Hospital
New Delhi, India

Vitusha Suri
MS (Obs & Gyne)
Senior Resident
Department of Obstetrics and Gynecology
Vardhman Mahavir Medical College and
Safdarjung Hospital
New Delhi, India

Preface

"It is easy to get many prescriptions but hard to get single correct remedy"

Pharmacotherapeutics is the application of pharmacological information together with the knowledge of the disease for its prevention and treatment. It also involves selection of the most appropriate drug, dosage and duration of treatment.

Pregnancy is a special condition where drug treatment presents a special challenge because the physiology of pregnancy affects the pharmacokinetics of medications used. Certain medications can cross the placenta, reach the fetus and cause harm. From puberty to menopause, women face gynecological problems that affect the quality of life. The prolonged life expectancy of menopausal women and their higher expectations for health have encouraged new developments in hormone replacement therapy. Thus, correct knowledge of Pharmacotherapeutics is essential in obstetrics and gynecology.

Rational use of drugs requires that patients receive medications appropriate to their clinical needs, in doses that meet their own individual requirements, for an adequate period of time, and at the lowest possible cost. The essential goal of rational drug use is to minimize the cost of drug therapy, avoid preventable adverse drug reactions and drug interactions, and enhance the quality of therapeutic care while promoting patient adherence.

The book includes description of pharmacotherapeutics in obstetrics and gynecology. The book has two parts A: Obstetrics and B: Gynecology with a total of 37 chapters. We have tried to describe separately on each aspect of the disease. Medical management for liver, respiratory and heart disease in pregnancy have been elaborated in different sections. We have maintained uniformity in the book by providing the information of all drugs, which are used for a particular disease, in the form of a table.

We hope that this book would serve its purpose and help practicing obstetricians, gynecologists and both undergraduate and postgraduate students in their day-to-day practice.

We thank all the authors for their efforts, coordination and support for this endeavors.

Ashok Kumar
Neha Pruthi Tandon

Acknowledgments

We wish to express our sincere appreciation to each contributor whose profound insights and tireless dedication have significantly enriched the content of this book.

A special note of thanks goes to our esteemed institution, Atal Bihari Vajpayee Institute of Medical Sciences and Dr Ram Manohar Lohia Hospital whose cooperation and encouragement has been instrumental in the realization of this project. The collaborative spirit and support from the faculty of Department of Obstetrics and Gynecology have played a pivotal role in shaping the comprehensive nature of this work.

We especially appreciate the constant support and encouragement of Shri Jitendar P Vij (Group Chairman) and Mr Ankit Vij (Managing Director) of M/s Jaypee Brothers Medical Publishers (P) Ltd, New Delhi, India, in publishing the book and also their associates, particularly Ms Chetna Malhotra (Senior Director—Professional Publishing, Marketing, and Business Development), and Ms Charu Lata (Development Editor), who have been prompt, efficient, and most helpful.

Contents

PART A: OBSTETRICS

SECTION 1: Medical Management of Anemia in Pregnancy

1. **Iron Deficiency Anemia** 3
   JB Sharma, Neelika Gupta

2. **Megaloblastic Anemia** 9
   Kamna Datta, Sangeeta Kumari

3. **Anemia due to Other Causes** 14
   Juhi Bharti, Nisha Rao

SECTION 2: Medical Management of Hypertension in Pregnancy

4. **Gestational Hypertension and Preeclampsia** 23
   Niharika Dhiman, Mamta Meena

5. **Eclampsia** 30
   Ashok Kumar, Ashu Bhardwaj

SECTION 3: Medical Management of Heart Disease in Pregnancy

6. **Rheumatic Heart Disease** 39
   Amita Suneja, Richa Aggarwal

7. **Mechanical and Prosthetic Heart Valves: Anticoagulant Therapy** 50
   Jaya Chawla, Kiran Dhawan

8. **Heart Failure** 62
   Puneet Aggarwal, Pradyumna Kumar Singh, Dheerendra Kuber, Ranjit Kumar Nath

SECTION 4: Medical Management of Liver Disorders in Pregnancy

9. **Intrahepatic Cholestasis** 73
   Neha Pruthi Tandon, Archana Chaurasia

10. **Hepatitis and Hepatic Encephalopathy** 80
    Durgesh

SECTION 5: Medical Management of Respiratory Disorders in Pregnancy

11. **Bronchial Asthma** 93
    Ajay Chauhan

12. **Respiratory Infections** 100
    Rekha Bharti, Vitusha Suri

SECTION 6: Medical Management of Labor and Puerperium

13. **Preterm Labor** 113
    Anjum Ara

14. **Induction and Augmentation of Labor** 121
    Kanika Kumari

15. **Cesarean and Vaginal Delivery: Antibiotic Therapy** 129
    Madhavi M Gupta, Vaishnavi Jayaram

16. **Postpartum Sepsis** 135
    Jyotsna Suri, Ankita Jain

17. **Postpartum Hemorrhage** 144
    Renuka Malik, Meghna Reddy

SECTION 7: Medical Management of Infections in Pregnancy

18. **Human Immunodeficiency Viruses: Antiretroviral Drugs** 155
    Bharti Uppal Nayyar, Vandana Agarwal

19. **Tuberculosis: Antitubercular Drugs** 168
    Namita Chopra, Kamal Chopra

SECTION 8: Medical Management of Miscellaneous Disorders in Pregnancy

20. **Gestational Diabetes and Overt Diabetes Mellitus** 175
    Geetanjali Nabiyal, Madhav Bahadur

21. **Thyroid Disorders** 189
    Indu Chawla, Seema Sheokand, Paridhi Gupta

22. **Seizure Disorders** 196
    Preeti Sainia

23. **Hyperemesis Gravidarum** 206
    Kavita Kumari

24. **Constipation and Diarrhea** 215
    Sandhya Jain, Pijush Kanti Nandi, Priyanka Shanker

PART B: GYNECOLOGY

SECTION 9: Medical Management of Menstrual Disorders

25. **Abnormal Uterine Bleeding** 233
    Latha Chaturvedula, Syed Habeebullah

26. **Fibroids** 241
    Sumitra Yadav, Pooja Verma

27. **Endometriosis** 247
    Archana Maurya, Vanshika Pundhir

SECTION 10: Medical Management of Endocrine Disorders

28. **Polycystic Ovary Syndrome** 261
    Ruchika Garg, Mousumi Das Ghosh

29. **Hirsutism** 270
    Ashima Taneja, Muskan Chaudhary

30. **Primary Amenorrhea** 278
    Priyanka Dahiya

31. **Secondary Amenorrhea** 294
    Ajit Kumar Nayak

SECTION 11: Medical Management of Anovulation

32. **Ovulation Induction in Intrauterine Insemination** 305
    Reeta Bansiwal, Anshika Agarwal

33. **Ovulation Induction in IVF-ET** 318
    Renu Tanwar, Renu Singh

SECTION 12: Drugs for Postmenopausal Women

34. **Hormone Replacement Therapy** 335
    Taru Gupta, Anupma

35. **Alternatives to Hormone Replacement Therapy** 347
    Jyoti Jaiswal, Nisha Watti

36. **Drugs to Decrease Fracture Risk** 362
    Shobhana Mohan Das

SECTION 13: Medical Management of Infections in Gynecology

37. Sexually Transmitted Diseases 373
Aruna Nigam, Supriya Chaubey

Index 391

PART A: OBSTETRICS

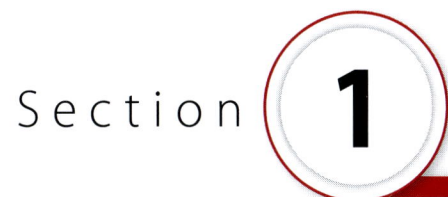

Medical Management of Anemia in Pregnancy

- **Iron Deficiency Anemia**
  JB Sharma, Neelika Gupta

- **Megaloblastic Anemia**
  Kamna Datta, Sangeeta Kumari

- **Anemia due to Other Causes**
  Juhi Bharti, Nisha Rao

Chapter 1

Iron Deficiency Anemia

JB Sharma, Neelika Gupta

■ DEFINITION

Anemia in pregnancy is defined as low hemoglobin concentration, resulting in a decrease in the oxygen-carrying capacity of the blood.
- *World Health Organization:* Hemoglobin (Hb) concentration <11 g/dL and hematocrit (Hct) <33% in antenatal period and Hb <10 g/dL in the postpartum period.
- *Centers for Disease Control and Prevention:* The cut-off point suggested is 10.5 g/dL in the second trimester and 11 g/dL in the first and third trimesters.[1]

■ SEVERITY OF ANEMIA

Iron Deficiency Anemia

The most common nutritional deficiency is anemia **(Table 1)**.

Management Options in Iron Deficiency Anemia (Table 2)
- Dietary measures
- Deworming
- Iron supplementation—oral and parenteral
- Blood transfusion.

Dietary measures:
- *Consumption of iron-rich foods*: Jaggery, spinach, pulses, eggs, liver, fish, and cereals

TABLE 1: Severity of anemia.[2,3]

Severity	ICMR	WHO
Mild	Hb: 10–10.9 g/dL	10–10.9 g/dL
Moderate	Hb: 7–9.9 g/dL	7–9.9 g/dL
Severe	Hb: 4–6.9 g/dL	<7 g/dL
Very severe	Hb: <4 g/dL	–

(ICMR: Indian Council of Medical Research; WHO: World Health Organization)

TABLE 2: Investigations in IDA.[4]

Parameter	Reference value	IDA
MCV (fL)	80–100	<75
RDW	11–14	>14
Serum ferritin (µg/L)	50–200	<15
Serum iron (µg/dL)	115 ± 50	<60
TIBC (µg/dL)	330 ± 30	>390
% transferrin saturation	35 ± 15	<15

(IDA: iron deficiency anemia; MCV: mean corpuscular volume; RDW: red blood cell distribution width; TIBC: total iron binding capacity)

- Cooking food in iron utensils
- Avoidance of excess tea and coffee intake.[5]

Under the anemia Mukt Bharat initiative by Government of India (GoI): All health facility-based programs where food is being provided are mandated to provide:
- Fortified wheat and rice (with iron, folic acid, and vitamin B_{12})

- Double fortified salt (with iodine and iron)
- Oil (with vitamin A and D).

Deworming: Increased iron loss due to hookworm infestations, schistosomiasis, and chronic malaria are important causes of anemia in pregnancy.[6]
- *Government of India, 2018:* Tablet albendazole 400 mg stat to all antenatal patients after the first trimester.
- *World Health Organization, 2017:* Where hookworm prevalence is 20% or more, one of the following anthelmintic agents can be used:
  - Tablet albendazole 400 mg stat
    Or
  - Tablet mebendazole 500 mg stat or 100 mg BD for 3 days
    Or
  - Tablet levamisole 2.5 mg/kg OD for 3 days
    Or
  - Tablet pyrantel 10 mg/kg body OD for 3 days.

If hookworm is highly endemic (prevalence 50% or more), repeat antihelminthic treatment 12 weeks after first dose.

Iron supplementation
Oral iron therapy: Oral iron is the treatment of choice as it has the following advantages:
- Easily available
- Cheap
- No anaphylaxis.

Commonly used iron preparations:
- *Ferrous sulfate, ferrous fumarate, and ferrous gluconate:* Most commonly used forms
- *Ferrous ascorbate:* Ascorbate prevents oxidation of ferrous to ferric iron; high bioavailability.[7]
- *Carbonyl iron:* Microparticles of purified elemental iron, not salt. Low toxicity, lesser gastrointestinal (GI) side effects.
- *Ferrous bisglycinate:* Amino acid chelate, absorption not decreased by phytates, high bioavailability, costly.
- *Ferric ammonium citrate:* Most commonly used ferric salt. Requires conversion to ferrous salt in the stomach, less bioavailability.

General instructions:
- Take in between meals
- Avoid consumption with tea, coffee, milk, or calcium tablets
- Start with low dose to decrease side effects
- Change brand if intolerable.

How to check compliance?
- Repeated questioning about intake
- Black color of the stool
- Symptoms such as gastritis and constipation
- Returning empty blister packs during follow-up.

Disadvantages of oral iron:
- Poor absorption
- GI side-effects:
  - Constipation
  - Heartburn
  - Epigastric pain
  - Vomiting
  - Metallic taste
  - Staining of teeth
- Poor compliance

Indicators of response to therapy:
- Improvement in symptoms, a feeling of well-being
- Improved appetite
- Increase in reticulocyte count after 7–10 days
- Rise in Hb after 2 weeks (0.8–1 g/dL/week)
- Hb reaches normal levels by 6–8 weeks.

TABLE 3: Comparison of various parenteral iron preparations.

Characteristics	Iron dextran	Iron sucrose	Ferric carboxymaltose
Type of iron complex	Type I	Type II	Type I
Concentration (mg/mL)	50 mg/mL	20 mg/mL	50 mg/mL
Route	IV/IM	IV	IV
Dosage		300 mg in 300 mL NS over 1 hour	1,000 mg in 200 mL NS over 15–20 minutes
Maximum dosage		300 mg/sitting and 600 mg/week	1,000 mg/sitting and total dose <2,500 mg
Safety profile	Category C	Category B	Category C
Disadvantage	Anaphylactic reactions	• Multiple visits • Dose limitation • Thrombophlebitis	• Hypophosphatemia • High blood pressure
Repeat dose		After 3 days	After 1 week

(IM: intramuscular; IV: intravenous; NS: normal saline)

Note: If anemia does not respond to oral iron treatment in 4 weeks (i.e., Hb concentration does not increase by 1 g/dL or Hct by 3%), further diagnostic evaluation is needed.[1]

Parenteral iron therapy:
- Indications:
  - Intolerance to oral iron
  - Mal absorption
  - Poor compliance
  - Routine supplementation to total parenteral nutrition (TPN)
  - Patients on erythropoietin
  - No response to oral iron in 2 weeks (Hb or reticulocyte count rise)
- Contraindications:
  - Anemia not attributable to iron deficiency
  - Iron overload
  - Hypersensitivity to intravenous (IV) iron
  - Liver cirrhosis
  - Acute or chronic infection
  - First trimester of pregnancy
  - Acute renal failure
- Prerequisites:
  - Correct diagnosis of IDA (rule out thalassemia)
  - Adequate supervision in the hospital setting
  - Facility for management of anaphylaxis
  - Stop oral iron at least 24 hours before therapy to avoid toxic reactions.
  - Look for reaction—chest pain, rigor chills, hypotension, dyspnea, hemolysis, and anaphylactic reaction **(Table 3)**
- Parenteral iron preparations:
  Intramuscular: Iron dextran (not recommended now)
  Intravenous:
  - Iron sucrose
  - Iron dextran
  - Ferric carboxymaltose
  - Ferumoxytol
  - Iron isomaltoside
  - Sodium ferric gluconate complex in sucrose injection

TABLE 4: Recommended dosage of iron and folic acid.[12,13]

	Prophylaxis during pregnancy	Treatment during pregnancy	Postpartum
WHO (2016)	Elemental iron: 30–60 mg daily + folic acid: 400 µg daily till term	Elemental iron: 120 mg daily + folic acid: 800 µg daily till anemia is corrected	• Elemental iron: 30–60 mg daily + folic acid: 400 µg daily • Till 3 months postpartum
GoI (2018)	Elemental iron: 60 mg daily + folic acid: 500 µg daily till term (minimum 180 days)	Mild–moderate anemia: • Two IFA tablets/day or parenteral iron • Severe anemia: Parenteral iron • Very severe anemia: Blood transfusion	• Elemental iron: 60 mg daily + folic acid: 500 µg daily • For 6 months postpartum

(GoI: Government of India; WHO: World Health Organization)
Note: As iron is absorbed in ferrous form, salts containing ferrous forms of iron, e.g., ferrous sulfate, ferrous gluconate, ferrous fumarate, or ferrous succinate should be prescribed.

Calculation of the dose (Table 4)

Ganzoni's formula:
- Iron required (mg) = (Target Hb – actual Hb) × 2.4 × prepregnancy body weight (kg)
- 1,000 mg is added to this to replenish stores
- Target Hb = 14 g/dL.

Iron dextran:
- 5% iron and 20% dextran
- It contains 50 mg/mL of elemental iron, most of which is present in the ferric state.
- Can be given intramuscular (IM), IV bolus, or IV infusion
- Test dose required (0.5 mL)
- *Prolonged use*: Staining of the skin, formation of sterile abscesses, tissue necrosis or atrophy, and sarcoma formation
- *Adverse reactions*: Fever, malaise, arthralgia, hypotension, and urticaria
- Anaphylactic reactions: 0.1–0.6%
- Z-track technique—minimizes skin staining.

Iron sucrose:
- 200–300 mg biweekly, IV infusion
- *Maximum:* 600 mg/week
- Can be given undiluted slowly at 1 mL/min or infusion of 200 mg/200 mL NS (unstable in dextrose) over 15 minutes
- *Higher dose (>300 mg/dose or 600 mg/week)*: Release of free iron from less tightly bound carbohydrate complexes, leading to infusion reactions
- *pH:* Alkaline (>10), cannot be given intramuscularly
- *Disadvantages*: Multiple visits and dose limitations
- *Life-threatening fatal reactions*: 0.002%.

Ferric carboxymaltose:
- Nondextran containing Fe complex
- Food and Drug Administration (FDA) approved in:
  • Iron deficiency anemia
  • Nondialysis-dependent chronic kidney disease
  • In pregnancy
- *Dose:* Infusion—1,000 mg in 250 mL saline, over 15 minutes
- *Do not give >1,000 mg/sitting:* It can lead to hemochromatosis.
- *Maximum dose:* 2,500 mg.

NEWER INTRAVENOUS IRON PREPARATIONS

Ferumoxytol[8]

- FDA approved in 2009
- Immunological reactivity
- *Dose*: 510 mg over >15 minutes
- Repeat after 1 week if required (3–8 days)
- Category C
- Noninferior to ferric carboxymaltose in IDA
- Not available in India
- Type I iron complex.

Iron Isomaltoside[9]

- 20 mg/kg infusion can be given in 1 hour
- Immunogenic potential
- No significant hypophosphatemia
- Category C
- Superior to ferric carboxymaltose in IDA.

JB Sharma et al. concluded that the intramuscular administration of three doses of 250 mg iron at monthly intervals appears to have good compliance and efficacy and may be used in women who cannot tolerate oral administration of iron. However, intramuscular administration of iron is appropriate only in hospital settings well equipped to treat anaphylactic crises.[10]

ROLE OF ERYTHROPOIETIN IN IRON DEFICIENCY ANEMIA

Along with parenteral iron, injection of erythropoietin in a dose of 50–150 U/kg body weight every 2–3 days subcutaneously has been used in severe anemia for a significant increase in Hb and to avoid blood transfusion.[11]

KEY POINTS

- Iron deficiency anemia is the most common nutritional deficiency anemia in pregnancy.
- Management options for IDA are dietary measures, deworming, iron supplementation (oral and parenteral) and blood transfusion.
- Daily oral iron and folic acid supplementation is recommended for pregnant women to prevent maternal anemia.

REFERENCES

1. Centers for Disease Control (CDC). CDC criteria for anemia in children and childbearing-aged women. MMWR Morb Mortal Wkly Rep. 1989;38(22):400-4.
2. Indian Council of Medical Research. Evaluation of the National Nutritional Anaemia Prophylaxis Programme. Task Force Study. New Delhi: ICMR; 1989.
3. World Health Organization (WHO, 2001). Iron deficiency anemia: assessment, prevention and control. WHO/NHD/01.3, Geneva. World Health Organization, Switzerland.
4. Letsky E. Blood volume, haematinics, anameia. In: de Swiet M (Ed). Medical Disorders in Obstetric Practice, 3rd edition. Oxford: Blackwell; 1995. pp. 33-60.
5. Sharma JB, Soni D, Murthy NS, Malhotra MJ. Effect of dietary habits on prevalence of anemia in pregnant women of Delhi. Obstet Gynaecol Res. 2003;29(2):73-8.
6. Sharma JB, Arora BS, Kumar S, Goel S, Dhamija A. Helminth and protozoal intestinal infection; an important cause for anemia in pregnant women in Delhi. J Obstet Gynecol Ind. 2001;51(6):58-61.
7. Malhotra N, Kriplani A, Pal B, Bhat V, Swami O. Ferrous ascorbate: current clinical place of therapy in the management of iron deficiency anemia. J South Asian Feder Obst Gynae. 2021;13(3):103-9.
8. Adkinson NF, Strauss WE, Macdougall IC, Bernard KE, Auerbach M, Kaper RF, et al. Comparative safety of intravenous ferumoxytol versus ferric carboxymaltose in iron deficiency anemia: A randomized trial. Am J Hematol. 2018;93(5):683-90.
9. Derman R, Roman E, Modiano MR, Achebe MM, Thomsen LL, Auerbach M. A randomized trial of iron isomaltoside

versus iron sucrose in patients with iron deficiency anemia. Am J Hematol. 2017; 92(3):286-91.
10. Sharma JB, Jain S, Mallika V, Singh T, Kumar A, Arora R, et al. A prospective, partially randomized study of pregnancy outcomes and hematologic responses to oral and intramuscular iron treatment in moderately anemic pregnant women. Am J Clin Nutr. 2004;79(1):116-22.
11. Vazenmiller D, Ponamaryova O, Muravlyova L, Molotov-Luchanskiy V, Klyuyev D, Bakirova R, et al. The Levels of Hepcidin and Erythropoietin in Pregnant Women with Anemia of Various Geneses. Open Access Maced J Med Sci. 2018;6(11):2111-4.
12. World Health Organization (2016). WHO recommendations on antenatal care for a positive pregnancy experience. Geneva, World Health Organization, Switzerland.
13. Ministry of Health and Family Welfare GoI, Office memorandum. Revised Operational strategy for oral iron for pregnant women- reg. November 2014.

Chapter 2

Megaloblastic Anemia

Kamna Datta, Sangeeta Kumari

Megaloblastic anemias are a group of disorders that are characterized by the presence of distinctive morphologic appearances of the developing red cells in the bone marrow. The marrow is mostly hypercellular, and the anemia is based on ineffective erythropoiesis. The cause is usually a deficiency of either cobalamin (vitamin B_{12}) or folate, but there are other genetic or acquired causes also. There may be defects in the metabolism of these vitamins or due to defects in deoxyribonucleic acid (DNA) synthesis not related to cobalamin or folate. This type of anemia can lead to symptoms, such as fatigue, weakness, mouth sores, tongue swelling, irritability, and shortness of breath.[1]

CAUSES OF MEGALOBLASTIC ANEMIA

- Cobalamin deficiency or abnormalities of cobalamin metabolism **(Table 1)**
- Folate deficiency or abnormalities of folate metabolism **(see Table 1)**
- Therapy with antifolate drugs (e.g., methotrexate)
- Some cases of acute myeloid leukemia and myelodysplasia
- *Other causes:*
  - Therapy with drugs interfering with the synthesis of DNA [e.g., cytosine arabinoside, hydroxyurea, 6-mercaptopurine, and azidothymidine (AZT)]
  - Orotic aciduria (responds to uridine)
  - Thiamine-responsive.

TABLE 1: Causes of folic acid and vitamin B_{12} deficiency.

Causes of folic acid deficiency[2]	Causes of vitamin B_{12} deficiency[2]
Insufficient intake of green leafy vegetables	Dietary deficiency in pure vegetarians
Malabsorption syndromes and gastrointestinal diseases, e.g., gluten-induced enteropathy	Malabsorption syndromes
Abnormally high demands are required in multiple pregnancies	Ileal disease mainly Crohn's disease
Drugs, e.g., phenytoin, pyrimethamine, and oral contraceptive pills (OCPs)	Bacterial overgrowth in small bowel
Congenital defects of folate enzymes (e.g., cyclohydrolase or methionine synthase)	

(OCPs: oral contraceptive pills)

Both folic acid and vitamin B_{12} are required for DNA synthesis. Mechanisms resulting in anemia are:
- Unbalanced cell growth
- Ineffective erythropoiesis
- Hemolysis.

There is megaloblastic erythropoiesis in bone marrow showing an asynchrony of nuclear and cytoplasmic maturation because of impaired DNA synthesis.[3]

The hematological findings in a case of megaloblastic anemia are described in **Table 2** and **Box 1**.

TABLE 2: CBC and RBC indices in megaloblastic anemia.

Complete blood with RBC indices	
Hemoglobin	<10 g%
Hematocrit	<33%
MCV	>100 fL
MCHC	Normal
Reticulocyte count	Normal or mildly increased to 2–3%
Serum unconjugated bilirubin*	Raised
Serum LDH*	Raised

*Because of ineffective erythropoiesis, there is a component of accompanying hemolysis due to which serum unconjugated bilirubin and serum LDH rises.
(CBC: complete blood count; LDH: lactate dehydrogenase; MCHC: mean corpuscular hemoglobin concentration; MCV: mean corpuscular volume; RBC: red blood cell)

BOX 1: Peripheral blood smear picture in megaloblastic anemia.

- Peripheral blood smear picture
- Macrocytes to macroovalocytes*
- Moderate to marked anisopoikilocytosis
- Nucleated RBCs
- Basophilic stippling, Cabot rings, and Howell–Jolly bodies
- Hypersegmented neutrophils**
- Pancytopenia (in 10–20% of cases)

*Diagnostic of megaloblastic anemia.
**This is the first manifestation of megaloblastic anemia. About 5% of neutrophils with five or more lobes or even a single neutrophil with six or more lobes.

Serum B_{12} levels and serum folate levels can also be measured. Red blood cell (RBC) folate levels are more specific for the diagnosis of folate deficiency than serum levels as there is no interference by the food.

Serum vitamin B_{12}:
- Normal serum levels range from 118 pmol/L (160 ng/L) to 738 pmol/L (1,000 ng/L)
- *Borderline:* It is between 74 and 148 pmol/L (100 and 200 ng/L)
- *Deficiency:* <74 pmol/L (100 ng/L)
- *Serum folate:*
  - *Normal range:* 11 nmol/L (2 µg/L) to 82 nmol/L (15 µg/L)
  - *Red cell folate:* 880–3,520 µmol/L (160–640 µg/L).

■ FOLINIC ACID

Folinic acid [5-formyl-tetrahydrofolate (THF)] (also known as leucovorin). It is a stable form of fully reduced folate. It is given orally or parenterally to overcome the toxic effects of methotrexate or other DHF reductase inhibitors, e.g., trimethoprim or cotrimoxazole. It is also given in patients with folate enzyme defect/deficiency.

Uses of Folic Acid

The uses of folic acid are as follows:
- To treat or prevent folate deficiency anemia.
- To help the fetal brain, skull, and spinal cord develop properly in pregnancy, to avoid neural tube defects such as spina bifida.
- To help reduce side effects from methotrexate (a medicine used to treat severe arthritis), Crohn's disease, or psoriasis.

Before giving large doses of folic acid, cobalamin deficiency must be excluded and, if present should be corrected; otherwise, cobalamin neuropathy may develop despite a response of the anemia of cobalamin deficiency to folate therapy. Vitamin C plays an important role in the treatment of megaloblastic anemia, as it helps in the conversion of folic acid to THF.

MECHANISM OF ACTION OF VITAMIN B_{12} AND FOLIC ACID

The mechanism of action of vitamin B_{12} and folic acid has been described earlier **(Table 3)**. Various forms of preparations available along with route, side effects, and contraindications are described in **Tables 4 and 5**.

TABLE 3: Mechanism of action of vitamin B_{12} and folic acid.

Drug	Mechanism of action	Excretion	Preparations
Vitamin B_{12}	• At the cellular level, cobalamin acts as a cofactor of two enzymatic reactions which involve methionine synthase and methylmalonyl-CoA mutase • Methionine synthase helps to convert homocysteine to methionine with the help of cobalamin. Methyl-THF converts to THF as a byproduct of this reaction, which helps in DNA synthesis. Methionine (an amino acid) converts into S-adenosylmethionine and participates in numerous methylation processes of cells. This methylation reaction is necessary for the synthesis of many molecules, such as phospholipids, and neurotransmitters, and the regulation of gene expression **(Fig. 1)**. Deficiency of cobalamin leads to folate trap leading to anemia. Vitamin B_{12} in the form of adenosylcobalamin acts as a cofactor for the enzyme methylmalonyl-CoA mutase, which converts methyl malonyl CoA to succinyl CoA. Through this reaction, it helps in metabolizing odd-chain fatty acids and branch-chain amino acids[4-6]	The main excretion route of vitamin B_{12} is through the bile, as less than 10% of the total loss of vitamin B_{12} from the body is through urine	• These drugs are usually a combination of vitamin B_{12} along with other vitamin B, folic acid with zinc, ascorbic acid, etc. • Oral as 1,500 µg, other vitamin B_{12} formulations are also available in combination with vitamins, such as pyridoxine (vitamin B_6), nicotinamide, cyanocobalamin (vitamin B_{12}), and folic acid • Injectable • Nasal spray • Nasal gel
Folic acid	• Folates (as the intracellular polyglutamate derivatives) act as coenzymes in the transfer of single-carbon units. These reactions are involved in purine and pyrimidine synthesis necessary for DNA and RNA replication. Folate is also a coenzyme for methionine synthesis, in which methylcobalamin is also involved and in which THF is regenerated • Vitamin C is also involved in the metabolism of folic acid where vitamin C in the presence of folic acid reductase converts folic acid to tetrahydrofolate	It has been shown that human excretes folic acid in the sweat as well as in the urine	• Oral • Injectable—folic acid and leucovorin

(DNA: deoxyribonucleic acid; RNA: ribonucleic acid; THF: tetrahydrofuran)

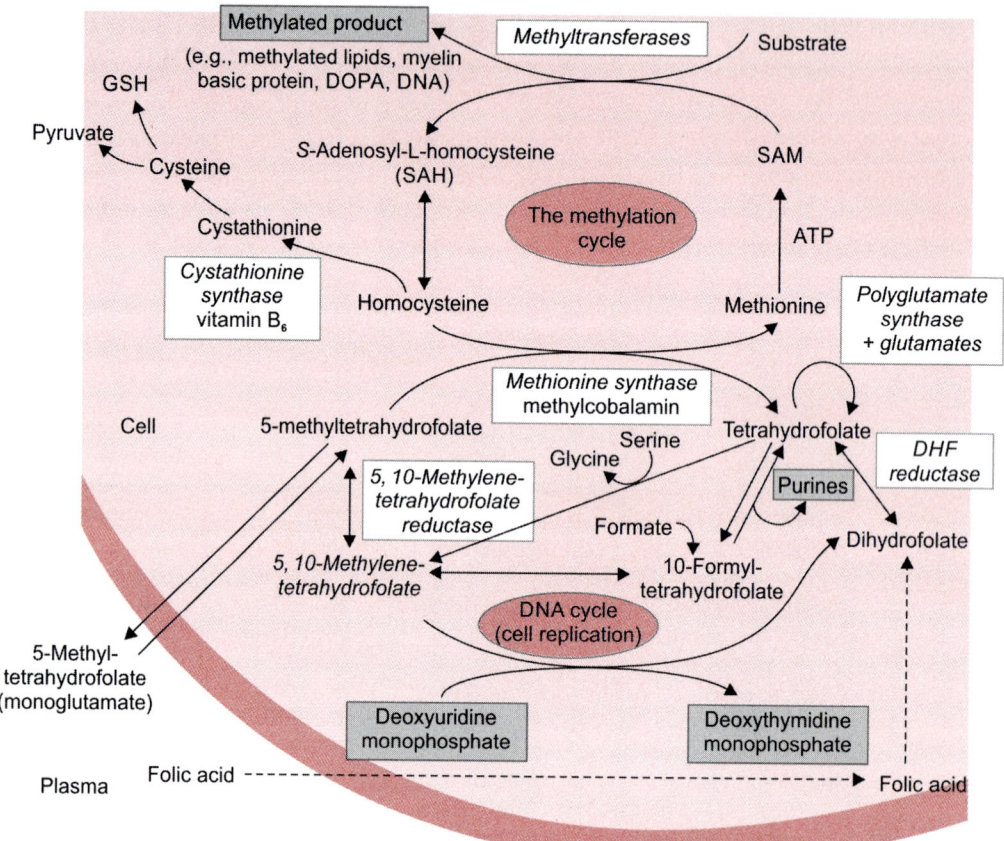

Fig. 1: The role of folates in DNA synthesis and in the formation of SAM, which is involved in numerous methylation reactions. (ATP: adenosine triphosphate; DHF: dihydrofolate; DNA: deoxyribonucleic acid; DOPA: 3, 4-dihydroxyphenylalanine; GSH: glutathione; SAM: S-adenosyl methionine)
Source: In: AV Hoffbrand, Catovsky D, Tuddenham EGD (Eds). Postgraduate Haematology, 5th edition. Oxford, UK: Blackwell Publishing; 2005.

Vitamin B$_{12}$

Mechanism of action of vitamin B$_{12}$ described in **Table 4**.

Folic Acid

Mechanism of action of folic acid described in **Table 5**.

■ MONITORING

The response to treatment should be monitored by repeating the complete blood count (CBC) and peripheral blood smear examination after two weeks of starting treatment. The hemoglobin level should be checked every two weeks until it stabilizes, and then monthly until delivery.

The choice of treatment to use depends on the underlying cause of the anemia and the specific needs of the patient. It is important to work closely with a healthcare provider to determine the most appropriate treatment plan.

TABLE 4: Formulations of vitamin B_{12}.

Name	Dosage	Route	Side effects	Contraindications
Methylcobalamin (vitamin B_{12})	1,500 µg daily	Oral	Headache, nausea, vomiting, stomach discomfort, diarrhea, and dizziness	Hypersensitivity to any of the active ingredients or excipients used in tablet
Methylcobalamin	1,000 µg (1 mg) every week for 4 weeks. Followed by 1,000 µg every month for 4–6 months	Injectable	Headache, nausea, vomiting, stomach discomfort, diarrhea, and dizziness	Hypersensitivity to any of the active ingredients or excipients used in tablet
Nasal spray or gel	250 µg in one nostril once a week	Intranasal	Headache and dizziness	Hypersensitivity to any of the active ingredients or excipients used

TABLE 5: Formulations of folic acid.

Name	Dosage	Route	Side effects	Contraindications
Folic acid and folinic acid	5 mg daily	Oral	Nausea, diarrhea, and stomach discomfort	Allergic reaction to folic acid
Leucovorin (folinic acid); folic acid	1 mg/kg	Injectable	Nausea, diarrhea, and stomach discomfort	Allergic reaction to folic acid

■ KEY POINTS

- Megaloblastic anemia mostly occurs due to a deficiency of vitamin B_{12} and folic acid.
- It is diagnosed by RBC indices and peripheral blood smear.
- It leads to symptoms, such as fatigue, weakness, mouth sores, tongue swelling, irritability, and shortness of breath.
- In patients with dimorphic anemia blood pictures of both microcytic and macrocytic anemia can be found.
- Before giving large doses of folic acid, cobalamin deficiency must be excluded and, if present should be treated.
- Both vitamin B_{12} and folic acid can be given in oral and injectable forms.
- The response to treatment should be monitored by repeating the CBC and peripheral blood smear examination after 2 weeks of initiating treatment.

■ REFERENCES

1. Hoffbrand AV. Megaloblastic anemias. In: Jameson JL, Fauci AS, Kasper DL, Hauser SL, Jameson JL, Loscalzo J (Eds). Harrison's Principles of Internal Medicine, 20th edition. New York: McGraw-Hill Education; 2018. p. 698.
2. Hiralal K. DC Dutta's Text book of Obstetrics, 8th edition. New Delhi: Jaypee Brothers Medical Publishers (P) Ltd; 2015. pp. 312-5.
3. Tripathi KD: Haematinics and Erythropoietin. Essentials of Medical Pharmacology. Seventh edition. New Delhi: Jaypee Brothers Medical Publishers (P) Ltd; 2015. pp. 606-11.
4. Oh R, Brown DL. Vitamin B_{12} deficiency. Am Fam Physician. 2003;67(5):979-86.
5. Stover PJ. Vitamin B_{12} and older adults. Curr Opin Clin Nutr Metab Care. 2010;13(1):24-7.
6. O'Leary F, Samman S. Vitamin B_{12} in health and disease. Nutrients. 2010;2(3):299-316.

Chapter 3

Anemia due to Other Causes

Juhi Bharti, Nisha Rao

Anemia is a condition in which the number of red blood cells (RBCs) and their oxygen-carrying capacity are insufficient to meet the body's physiological needs. The function of the RBCs is to deliver oxygen from the lungs to the tissues and carbon dioxide from the tissues to the lungs. This is accomplished by using hemoglobin. Anemia impairs the body's ability for gas exchange by decreasing the number of RBCs transporting oxygen and carbon dioxide.

India is one of the countries with a very high prevalence of anemia in the world. Nutritional anemia is a major public health problem in India and is primarily due to iron deficiency. This chapter pertains to drug therapy in anemia due to causes other than iron deficiency and megaloblastic.

■ ANEMIA OF CHRONIC DISEASE

- Anemia of chronic disease (ACD) is an inflammatory situation, whether acute or chronic, that induces a rise in cytokine production and hepcidin levels, which sequester iron in reticuloendothelial macrophages and prevent it from being used to form RBCs.[1]
- Low serum iron, normal to increasing iron reserves, and signs of inflammation are characteristics of ACD.

Management

The aim of treatment is not normalizing hemoglobin levels, but reducing symptoms and improving clinical outcomes.

Treat Underlying Disorder

Most important:
- Other causes of anemia should be identified and treated if possible.
  - *Iron:* Supplemental iron is often only given to people who already have an iron deficit.[2]
  - Erythropoiesis-stimulating agents (ESAs)[3] **(Box 1)**.
    - *Mechanism of action of ESA:* The mechanism of action of ESAs is shown in **Flowchart 1**. The doses,

Flowchart 1: Mechanism of action of erythropoiesis-stimulating agents.

The erythropoietin receptor (EPO-R), also known as exogenous epoetin alfa, binds to erythropoietin and stimulates intracellular signal transduction pathways

↓

A conformational shift is brought about when a molecule of the Janus family tyrosine-protein kinase 2 (JAK2) binds to the EPO-R on the surface of erythroid progenitor cells

↓

Final step: Inhibition of apoptosis during erythroid differentiation via the EPO-activated JAK2/STAT5/Bcl-x pathways

CHAPTER 3: Anemia due to Other Causes

> **BOX 1:** Erythropoiesis-stimulating agents—doses, adverse effects, contraindications, pharmacokinetics, and pharmacodynamics.
>
> *Dosing:*
> - *Epoetin*: 50–100 units/kg/week
> - *Darbepoetin*: 40–100 µg subcutaneously every 2–4 weeks
>
> *Route of administration:*
> *Drugs:* Epoetin or darbepoetin
> - Administered subcutaneously/intravenously
> - The amount of epoetin that must be administered subcutaneously to reach a specific Hb is roughly 30% less than what must be administered intravenously
> - Darbepoetin can be administered intravenously or subcutaneously, and both methods are equally effective
>
> *Target hemoglobin value:* Hb concentrations between 10 and 11.5 g/dL with the least amount of ESA
>
> *Adverse effects:*
> - Chest pain
> - Thrombosis
> - Stroke
> - Headache
> - Unusual tiredness
> - Seizure
> - Deranged blood sugar
> - Low potassium
> - Constipation
> - Increased blood pressure
> - Muscle pain
> - Fever
> - Pain or redness at the injection site
>
> *Contraindications:*
> - Active malignancy
> - History of stroke
> - Uncontrolled hypertension
>
> *Pharmacokinetics:*
> *Absorption:*
> - It takes longer for the subcutaneous route to reach peak concentration than the intravenous method, which takes 20–25 hours, and the peak is always much lower (5–10% of the peak seen with intravenous administration)
> - Subcutaneous injectable erythropoietin has a bioavailability of 20–40%, which is substantially lower than that of the intravenously injected medication
>
> *The volume of distribution:* The intravenous epoetin alfa distribution volume (40–63.80 mL/kg) was frequently comparable to the plasma volume
>
> *Metabolism:*
> - When erythropoietin and epoetin alfa bind to EPO-R, the ligand is internally processed by the cell and degraded
> - The lymphatic system or the reticuloendothelial scavenging pathway may also break down erythropoietin and epoetin alfa
>
> *Half-life:* About 6 hours in intravenous injection
>
> *Pharmacodynamics:*
> - Boost the reticulocyte count within ten days of treatment, then the RBC count, hemoglobin level, and hematocrit, typically between 2 and 6 weeks
> - Depending on the dose administered, the rate of hemoglobin rise may vary
> - Patients receiving hemodialysis at dosages >300 units/kg three times per week do not have a larger biological response
>
> (EPO-R: erythropoietin receptor; ESA: erythropoiesis-stimulating agent; RBC: red blood cell)

pharmacokinetics and safety profile of ESA is discussed in **Box 1**.

Indications

When the ferritin level is >200 ng/mL and the transferrin saturation is >20% in patients with hemoglobin (Hb) 10 g/dL.

We often offer iron before administering an ESA to individuals with transferrin saturation (TSAT) of 20% and ferritin 500 ng/mL because they may respond to iron with an increase in Hb. We do not utilize ESA in such patients if the response to iron supplementation is sufficient.

Transfusion

Only people with severe, life-threatening, and symptomatic anemia, for whom it is impossible to wait for a response to previous treatments, should have RBC transfusions.[1]

■ THALASSEMIA

Group of inherited blood disorders with abnormal formation of red blood cells:
- Iron chelators should be reviewed; deferasirox and deferiprone ideally have to be discontinued 3 months before conception.
- All chelation therapies are potentially teratogenic in the first trimester. *Desferrioxamine* is the only chelation agent that can be used in the second and third trimesters (category-C)
- *In labor and delivery*: For the duration of labor, massive intravenous (IV) desferrioxamine 2 g over 24 hours should be given to thalassemia-affected women.[4]

Desferrioxamine[5] (Box 2)

Mechanism of Action

Binds iron in the tissues and circulation, and the iron-bound form is effectively eliminated in the urine and bile.

BOX 2: Desferrioxamine—doses, adverse effects, contraindications, pharmacokinetics, and pharmacodynamics.

Dose: 60 mg/kg/day

Route:

Parenterally: Slow subcutaneous infusion of a 10% solution over 8–12 hours for a minimum of 5 days/week

Monitoring:

Audiology:
- Before initiation
- Audiogram every 12 months

Ophthalmology: Children every 6 months and annually in adults

Kidney: Every 3 months, serum electrolytes, urine protein, and creatinine/blood urea levels should be checked

Liver function: In every 3 months, hepatic enzymes need to be checked

Side effects:
- Acute therapy complications:
  - Abdominal discomfort/pain
  - Diarrhea
  - Nausea
  - Vomiting
  - Hypotension
  - Anaphylaxis
  - Mucormycosis
- Chronic therapy complications:
  - Visual and auditory neurotoxicity

Pharmacokinetics

Absorption: After being administered intramuscularly or subcutaneously, deferoxamine is promptly absorbed, but it is only ineffectively absorbed from the digestive tract when the mucosa is intact

The volume of distribution: Not available

Metabolism: There is a little hepatic metabolism of deferoxamine, which is primarily metabolized in the plasma

Route of elimination:
- Mainly via plasma enzymes; however, the metabolic pathways are not yet known
- Some are also passed through the bile into the feces

Half-life: A biphasic elimination pattern was seen in healthy volunteers, with a first rapid phase half-life of 1 hour and a second slow phase half-life of 6 hours

Pharmacodynamics:
- Works by boosting the removal of free iron from the body through the urine
- The agent lessens the harm done to numerous organs and tissues, including the liver, by eliminating excess iron

- The reticuloendothelial system's macrophages release iron generated from senescent RBC, chelate it with deferoxamine, and then quickly excrete it in the urine.
- Hepatic cells take in iron-free deferoxamine, which they then internalize, interact, bind, and expel iron in bile from the chelatable intracellular iron pool.
- Remove iron directly from myocardial cells.

Indications

- *Transfusion-dependent beta-thalassemia (previously beta-thalassemia major)*:
    - After 10 units of packed red blood cells (PRBC), or >100 cc/kg/year (PRBC hematocrit 60)
    - Ferritin is >1,000 ug/L
    - A cardiac T2* <20 milliseconds, or a magnetic resonance imaging (MRI) with a liver iron content >3 mg/g dry weight.
- *Nontransfusion-dependent thalassemia*:
    - Ferritin alone underestimates the iron load
    - Liver iron concentration (LIC): It is used to determine iron stores and the initiation of chelation

Magnetic resonance imaging measurement of the LIC ≥5 mg/g dry weight.

Review Transfusion Requirements

- If regularly transfused, the frequency may increase in the later stage of pregnancy.
- Pretransfusion aims >10 g/dL may not be possible due to the physiology of pregnancy.
- If not regularly transfused, inform women of the probable need for blood transfusion during pregnancy. Perform red cell phenotyping if not previously done.[6]

SICKLE CELL DISEASE

- Inherited blood disorders characterized by sickling of red blood cells during physiological stress leading to vasoocclusion.[7]
- Increased red cell turnover and chronic hemolytic anemia which will also be affected by the physiological changes of pregnancy.[7]

Management

- Hydroxycarbamide should be discontinued in both men and women planning pregnancy, at least 3 months before conception.
- Routine prophylactic transfusion is not currently recommended but all patients should be assessed for the potential benefit based on disease severity.

Blood Transfusion

Routine prophylactic transfusion is not recommended but if required blood should be matched for extended red cell phenotype, Kell, and be *Cytomegalovirus* and sickle negative (see local transfusion policy).[7,8]

Prophylactic transfusion should be considered in women with:

- Medical, obstetric, or fetal issues associated with sickle cell disease (SCD) in the past or present.
- Women who had been on hydroxycarbamide because of a serious illness.
- Multiple pregnancies
- Patients on prepregnancy transfusion programs should continue throughout the pregnancy.
- Transfusions may be required if the hemoglobin falls below the patient baseline [usually 60–80 g/L in Hank's balanced salt solution (HbSS)] due to aplastic or hemolytic crisis and acute SCD complications.

Sickle Cell Crisis

This is the most common reason for admission and occurs in 7–20% of pregnancies. Pain is the prominent feature and prompt analgesia is required.[7,9]

Immediate Measures

- *Give appropriate analgesia:* This should be within 30 minutes of presentation as per National Institute for Health and Care Excellence (NICE) guidelines. This may include Paracetamol and diclofenac, but often opiate analgesia is required.
- If opiates are required, morphine should be dosed based on booking weight:
  - If <50 kg, give 5 mg morphine sulfate subcutaneous (SC)/IV
  - If ≥50 kg, give 10 mg morphine sulfate SC/IV
- *Assess response:* Review after 30 minutes and give a second dose of morphine if required (provided there is no evidence of opioid toxicity). Ongoing monitoring should continue at least every 4 hours.

Note: Respiratory rate and consciousness level should be monitored every 15–30 minutes initially then every 4 hours unless specific concerns.

- *Monitor oxygen levels:* If oxygen saturations are <95% on air, offer oxygen at 5 L/min and escalate to the medical team. Inform hematology on-call.
- Keep warm
- *Ensure adequate hydration:* Aim for 60 mL/kg/24 hours and monitor fluid balance. Give IV fluids if required.
- Fetal monitoring
- *Consider antibiotics:* If features of infection (such as fever, unexplained tachycardia, and focal symptoms).

PAROXYSMAL NOCTURNAL HEMOGLOBINURIA

The treatment of paroxysmal nocturnal hemoglobinuria (PNH) and postpartum care is briefly summarized in **Table 1**.

ECULIZUMAB[10] (BOX 3)

Mechanism of Action

Complement protein C5—targeting monoclonal antibody that blocks cleavage into C5a and C5b and the development of the final complement complex C5b-9.

TABLE 1: Paroxysmal nocturnal hemoglobinuria (PNH)—treatment and postpartum care.

Treatment	Postpartum care
• Folic acid supplements • Eculizumab (monoclonal antibody against complement C5) • Role of anticoagulation: continue prophylactic Low molecular weight heparin throughout pregnancy and up to 6 weeks to 6 months postpartum • Both ravulizumab and eculizumab are acceptable choices • Patients who become pregnant while taking a C5 complement inhibitor, continue therapy throughout pregnancy and while breastfeeding	• Treat with low molecular weight heparin during the last trimester and continue treatment for 8–12 weeks postpartum as pregnancy increases the already-high thromboembolic risk • Oral contraceptives increase thromboembolic risk in women with PNH • Nonhormonal forms of contraception are preferred for sexually active women with PNH

CHAPTER 3: Anemia due to Other Causes

> **BOX 3:** Eculizumab—doses, adverse effects, contraindications, pharmacokinetics, and pharmacodynamics.
>
> *Administration:*
> - Given as a fixed dose (based on weight or body surface area)
> - 600 mg intravenous (IV) once/week for the first 4 weeks, followed by 900 mg IV 1 week later, followed by 900 mg IV once every 2 weeks thereafter
>
> *Adverse effects:*
> - Risk for *Neisseria meningitidis* infection and other encapsulated organisms
> - Extravascular hemolysis
> - Breakthrough symptoms
> - Headache
> - Nasopharyngitis
> - Back pain
> - Nausea
>
> *Contraindications:*
> - Hypersensitive reaction to eculizumab
> - Unresolved *N. meningitidis* infection or not vaccinated for infection
>
> *Pharmacokinetics:*
> - Absorption: Intravenous infusion: Bioavailability is 100%
>
> *The volume of distribution:* 5–8 L
>
> *Metabolism:* Metabolized to small peptides and amino acids
>
> *Route of elimination:* Most monoclonal antibodies are catabolized in lysosomes to amino acids, and only a small proportion is expelled in bile. Monoclonal antibodies are not removed in the urine
>
> *Half-life:* $T_{1/2}$: 270–375 hours
>
> *Pharmacodynamics:*
> - A monoclonal antibody that treats certain autoimmune diseases by preventing the activation of terminal complement
> - Because severe meningococcal infections have occurred in the past, patients taking this drug should have a vaccination against *N. meningitis*

In paroxysmal nocturnal hemoglobinuria, inhibition of this complex impairs complement-mediated intravascular hemolysis.

■ HEREDITARY SPHEROCYTOSIS[8]

Splenectomy—beneficial:
- *Mild disease:* Avoid splenectomy or do partial splenectomy.
- *Moderate:* Till puberty
- *Severe disease:* At 4–6 years of age.

■ PYRUVATE KINASE DEFICIENCY[8]

- Supportive treatment
- Blood transfusion.

■ GLUCOSE-6-PHOSPHATE DEHYDROGENASE DEFICIENCY

- Acute hemolytic anemia (AHA) is preventable
- *In case of severe anemia:* Blood transfusion
- *In case of renal failure:* Dialysis
- *In pregnancy:* Avoid drugs and chemicals known to exacerbate hemolysis in glucose-6-phosphate dehydrogenase (G6PD) deficiency.

■ IMMUNE HEMOLYTIC ANEMIA

First Line

Glucocorticoids—prednisone—1 mg/kg/day.

Second Line

Low-dose prednisone, rituximab, azathioprine, cyclosporine, cyclophosphamide, and IV immunoglobulins.

The chapter navigates the complexities of anemia during pregnancy, focusing on drug therapy in anemia in pregnancy due to other causes. It requires multidisciplinary approach involving primary treating clinicians, obstetricians, hematologists, fostering evidence-based and patient-centered care.

■ KEY POINTS

- In ACD, the treatment of choice is ESA, such as epoetin or darbepoetin.
- Indications of ESA in ACD is when Hb <10 g/dL with transferrin saturation >20% and ferritin >200 ng/mL.
- *Thalassemia in pregnancy:* The drug of choice for iron chelation is desferrioxamine, safe in the second and third trimesters only.
- In thalassemia—target Hb should be kept at 10 g/dL.
- *SCD:* Hydroxycarbamide must be stopped at least 3 months before conception. Routine prophylactic transfusion is not recommended.
- *PNH:* The drug of choice is eculizumab (C5 monoclonal antibody). Prophylactic anticoagulation should be considered.
- *G6PD deficiency:* It is important to avoid drugs known to exacerbate hemolysis in G6PD deficiency.
- Autoimmune hemolytic anemia—treatment of choice is steroids.

■ REFERENCES

1. Williams D, Davison J. Chronic kidney disease in pregnancy. BMJ. 2008;336(7637):211-5.
2. Amstad Bencaiova G, Krafft A, Zimmermann R, Burkhardt T. Treatment of anemia of chronic disease with true iron deficiency in pregnancy. J Pregnancy. 2017;2017:1-7.
3. Morton A, Burke M, Morton A, Kumar S. Anaemia in chronic kidney disease pregnancy. Obstet Med. 2021;14(2):116-20.
4. Royal College of Obstetricians and Gynaecologists. (2014). Management of Beta Thalassaemia in Pregnancy (Green-top Guideline No. 66). [online] Available from: https://www.rcog.org.uk/guidance/browse-all-guidance/green-top-guidelines/management-of-beta-thalassaemia-in-pregnancy-green-top-guideline-no-66/ [Last accessed December, 2023].
5. Piccioni MG, Capone C, Vena F, Del Negro V, Schiavi MC, D'Ambrosio V, et al. Use of deferoxamine (DFO) in transfusion-dependent β-thalassemia during pregnancy: a retrospective study. Taiwan J Obstet Gynecol. 2020;59(1):120-2.
6. Origa R, Comitini F. Pregnancy in thalassemia. Mediterr J Hematol Infect Dis. 2019;11(1):e2019019.
7. Oteng-Ntim E, Pavord S, Howard R, Robinson S, Oakley L, Mackillop L, et al. Management of sickle cell disease in pregnancy. A British Society for Haematology Guideline. Br J Haematol. 2021;194(6):980-95.
8. American College of Obstetricians and Gynaecologists. (2023). Hemoglobinopathies in pregnancy. [online] Available from: https://www.acog.org/clinical/clinical-guidance/practice-advisory/articles/2022/08/hemoglobinopathies-in-pregnancy [Last accessed December, 2023].
9. Shi H, Chen L, Wang Y, Sun M, Guo Y, Ma S, et al. Severity of Anemia During Pregnancy and Adverse Maternal and Fetal Outcomes. JAMA Netw Open. 2022;5(2):e2147046.
10. Stefanovic V. The Extended Use of Eculizumab in Pregnancy and Complement Activation-Associated Diseases Affecting Maternal, Fetal and Neonatal Kidneys-The Future is Now? J Clin Med. 2019;8(3):407.

Section 2

Medical Management of Hypertension in Pregnancy

▲ **Gestational Hypertension and Preeclampsia**
Niharika Dhiman, Mamta Meena

▲ **Eclampsia**
Ashok Kumar, Ashu Bhardwaj

Chapter 4

Gestational Hypertension and Preeclampsia

Niharika Dhiman, Mamta Meena

Hypertension (HT) is a complex pregnancy-associated disorder with unknown pathogenesis. During pregnancy, preeclampsia (PE) appears after 20 weeks of gestation in two possible scenarios: (1) Early or (2) late preeclampsia onset.[1] The worst maternal and fetal prognosis is during the early manifestation of the disease, which frequently leads to pregnancy termination or premature delivery. Currently, preeclampsia is the leading cause of fetal and maternal mortality during pregnancy. This is why not only better diagnosis strategies (early diagnosis) but also exploration of new drugs for preeclampsia management are needed. Preeclampsia is associated with 4.6% (95% uncertainty range 2.7–8.2) of pregnancies globally and contributes major cause of adverse pregnancy outcomes. Of the global 830 maternal deaths that occurred daily in 2015, hypertensive disorders of pregnancy particularly preeclampsia accounted for 14% of the mortalities.[1]

■ MANAGEMENT

In gestational hypertension and preeclampsia without severe features, the goal should be of continued monitoring until delivery at 37 weeks of gestation (in the absence of abnormal antepartum testing, preterm labor, preterm prelabor rupture of membranes, or vaginal bleeding). The target of therapy is to lower the mean arterial blood pressure (BP) by no >15–25%, with a target systolic BP in severe hypertension due to preeclampsia, the aim is to control blood pressure to 160/110 mm Hg within hours, followed by a target BP of 110–140/70–85 mm Hg.[2]

Aim of Antihypertensive Therapy

Target BP ≤135/85 mm Hg [National Institute for Health and Care Excellence (NICE) 2019].

Prophylaxis

Low-dose aspirin (75 mg/day): Aspirin is responsible for inhibiting the synthesis of prostaglandins by the irreversible acetylation and inactivation of cyclooxygenase. Aspirin inhibits the biosynthesis of platelet thromboxane A2, and it has been hypothesized that preeclampsia could be prevented by preventing the imbalance in the thromboxane-to-prostacyclin ratio.[3]

The American College of Obstetricians and Gynecologists (ACOG) advises daily low-dose aspirin, starting in the *late first trimester*, specifically for women with a history of preeclampsia leading to prior preterm delivery before 34 weeks gestation,

SECTION 2: Medical Management of Hypertension in Pregnancy

TABLE 1: ACOG recommendation for emergent hypertension.

Labetalol	Hydralazine	Nifedipine
• If BP is *160/110 mm Hg* • 20 mg IV, ↓ BP in 10 minutes • BP ≥ threshold *(160/110 mm Hg)* give 40 mg IV, ↓ BP in 10 min • BP ≥ threshold *(160/110 mm Hg)* give 80 mg IV, ↓ BP in 10 minutes • BP ≥ threshold *(160/110 mm Hg)* give 10 mg IV hydralazine	• 5–10 mg IV, ↓ BP in 20 minutes • BP ≥ threshold *(160/110 mm Hg)* give 10 mg IV, ↓ BP in 20 minutes • BP ≥ threshold *(160/110 mm Hg)* give 20 mg IV labetalol, ↓ BP in 10 minutes • BP ≥ threshold *(160/110 mm Hg)* labetalol 40 mg IV	• 10 mg oral (immediate release), ↓ BP in 20 minutes • BP ≥ threshold *(160/110 mm Hg)* give 20 mg oral, ↓ BP in 20 minutes • BP ≥ threshold *(160/110 mm Hg)* give 20 mg oral, ↓ BP in 20 minutes • BP ≥ threshold *(160/110 mm Hg)* labetalol 40 mg IV

(ACOG: American College of Obstetricians and Gynecologists; BP: blood pressure; IV: intravenous)

or preeclampsia in more than one prior pregnancy **(Table 1)**.[3]

The *ACOG* and the Society for Maternal-Fetal Medicine make the following recommendations:

- Low-dose aspirin (81 mg/day) prophylaxis is suggested in women at a high risk of preeclampsia and should be started between 12 and 28 weeks period of gestation (optimally before 16 weeks) and continued daily until delivery.[3]
- Low-dose aspirin prophylaxis should be advised for women with more than one of several moderate risk factors for preeclampsia.[3]

Calcium supplementation: It has been studied for preeclampsia prophylaxis depending on observations that dietary calcium intake is inversely related to the incidence of preeclampsia.[4]

A 2010 meta-analysis of available randomized controlled clinical trial data results showed that calcium supplementation decreased the risk for preeclampsia by approximately 50%. However, the ACOG does not consider calcium supplementation to inhibit preeclampsia for women with normal dietary calcium intake.

According to World Health Organization (WHO) guidelines, in a population where calcium intake is low, calcium supplementation as part of antenatal care is recommended for the prevention of preeclampsia, particularly among those at higher risk of hypertension. Guidelines recommend daily of calcium is 1.5–2.0 g from 20 weeks of the gestation.[5]

Indian National guidelines for calcium supplements during pregnancy recommend 500 mg of calcium twice daily for all pregnant women.

Antioxidant supplementation: Numerous studies have been done to investigate a possible prophylactic or therapeutic role for antioxidant supplementation in the hypertensive disorders of pregnancy.[4,6]

In randomized controlled clinical trials, supplementation with 1,000 mg of vitamin C and 400 IU of vitamin E did not reduce the incidence of preeclampsia in healthy nulliparous women or in women at increased risk for preeclampsia.[4,6]

One of these trials even showed evidence of harm, with a greater incidence of low birth weight, unexplained fetal loss after 24 weeks' period gestation, and umbilical cord blood acidemia in patients randomized to the antioxidant group. The ACOG does not consider the administration of vitamin C or vitamin E to inhibit preeclampsia.

Fluid management: Volume expansion is not advised, and fluids should be limited to 80 mL/h or 1 mL/kg/h. In the case of hemorrhage, losses should be replaced appropriately. Administration of additional fluid may be considered before intravenous hydralazine, neuraxial anesthesia, or immediate delivery.

According to a 2011 ACOG Committee Opinion considers labetalol or hydralazine as the first-line treatment for acute-onset, severe preeclampsia in pregnant or postpartum patients.

Drug Therapy (Table 2)

Labetalol:[7]
- *Mechanism of action:* Combined alpha- and beta-blocker labetalol nonselectively antagonize β-adrenergic receptors, and selectively antagonize α-1 adrenergic receptors. For oral administration, labetalol has three times the β-blocking ability than α-blocking ability.
- *Dose:* 100 mg two times, increase 100 mg every 2 days; 100–400 mg TDS. Labetalol is the most commonly used drug with an initial dose of 100 mg tablets orally twice a day. This dose may be increased according to patients' response. The maintenance dose is started from 100 mg twice and can be given to a maximum dose of 2,400 mg/day.
- *Max dose:* 2,400 mg
- *Onset of action:* 2 hours. Better uteroplacental perfusion than β-blockers
- *Side-effects/caution:* Side-effects of beta blockers include headache, vomiting, taste distortion, rashes, bradycardia, nausea, difficulty in micturition, postural hypotension, and dizziness.

It was associated with ↓ peripheral resistance without significantly reducing cardiac output (CO) and heart rate (HR), maintains placental perfusion and fetal oxygenation, ensures better and quicker control of BP, is better tolerated, ensures safe prolongation of pregnancy and maternal and fetal outcome better in Labetalol group than methyldopa.

Nifedipine:[7]
- *Mechanism of action:* Calcium channel blocker
- *Dose and route:* 30 mg OD as extended-release (ER) tablet; increase the dose for 7–14 days, 10–20 mg BD, repeated after 30 minutes, if needed.
- *Onset of action:* 30–45 minutes
- *Max dose:* 120 mg
- *Caution:* Sublingual not recommended. Interactions with $MgSO_4$—severe hypotension, neuromuscular blockade, ankle edema, and headache.

Hydralazine:
- *Mechanism of action:* Hydralazine is responsible for acting on a direct vasodilator and leading to a vasodilator with a direct relaxing effect on smooth muscle in the blood vessels, most commonly acting on in the arterioles.
- *Dose and route:* 25–30 mg OD—TDS, orally.
- *Onset of action:* 10–20 minutes and persists for 10–12 hours
- *Side-effects:* The most commonly reported adverse effects are tachycardia and palpitations. Other adverse effects, such as headache, gastrointestinal disturbance, hypotension, diarrhea, flushing, nausea, vomiting, arthralgia, joint swelling, myalgia, and anorexia. Prolonged use of hydralazine is responsible for lupus erythematosus or rheumatoid arthritis-like

TABLE 2: Drug therapy.

Name	Labetalol	Nifedipine	Hydralazine	Esmolol	Methyldopa
Mechanism of action	Peripheral α-1 and (nonselective) β-1 and 2 receptor antagonist	Direct-acting vasodilator, cerebral, and coronary vasodilation	Calcium channel blocker (vasodilator)	Selective B1 antagonist	Alpha-methyl analog of dopa. Central sympatholytic, stimulation of presynaptic of α-2 receptors in the nucleus tractus solitarius decreases noradrenaline release
Dosage	100 mg, increased according to patients' response	30 mg stat followed by 20 mg BD	20–40 mg	500–1,000 µg/kg loading dose over 1 minute, followed by an infusion starting at 50 µg/kg/min and increasing up to 300 µg/kg/min	• Oral dose: 250–1,000 mg/day • IV: 250–1,000 mg infusion over 30–60 minutes
Route	Oral	Oral	IV	IV	Oral/IV
Maximum dose	2,400 mg/day	120 mg/day	30 mg/day, repeated if needed	500–1,000 µg/kg loading dose over 1 min, followed by an infusion starting at 50 µg/kg/min and increasing up to 300 µg/kg/min	4 g/day
Side-effects	Headache, vomiting, taste distortion, rashes, bradycardia, nausea, difficulty in micturition, and postural hypotension	Severe hypotension, neuromuscular blockade, ankle edema, headache, and flushing	Palpitation, vasodilation, and nasal stiffness	A-V heart blocks, congestive heart failure (CHF), and bradycardia	Sedation, postural hypotension, dry mouth, liver toxicity, and autoimmune disease

Contd...

Contd...

Name	Labetalol	Nifedipine	Hydralazine	Esmolol	Methyldopa
Contraindications	Bronchial asthma, cardiogenic shock, and cardiac failure	Second- and third-degree heart block, lactation	Dissecting aneurysms and raised intracranial pressure	Concomitant use of B-antagonist	Active hepatic disease and direct Coombs-positive hemolytic anemia
Pharmacokinetics	1–2 hours	~2 hours	15–17 minutes, duration can be up to 10 hours	4–8 hours	Onset 4–6 hours, up to 24 hours

symptoms develop on prolonged use (>100 mg/day).

Methyl dopa:[7]
- *Mechanism of action:* Centrally acting α-agonist
- *Dose:* 250 mg 2–3 times, increase every 2 days
- *Maximum dose:* 3,000 mg
- *Onset of action:* 6 hours
- *Side-effects:* Sedation, lethargy, and reduced mental capacity are common. Other including dryness of mouth, nasal stuffiness, headache, fluid retention, weight gain, hemolytic anemia, and flu-like illness.

Clonidine:
- *Mechanism of action:* Centrally acting alpha-agonist
- *Indication:* It is used in chronic hypertension patients during pregnancy which was associated with complications including fetal growth restriction, prematurity birth, preeclampsia, placental abruption, and hypertension crisis.
- *Peak:* 2–4 hours
- *Duration:* 6–24 hours
- *Dose:* 100 μg OD or BD
- *Max dose:* 300 μg TDS
- *Sise-effects:* Sedation, mental depression, dryness of mouth, constipation, and rebound hypertension if the dose is missing for 1–2 days.

Esmolol
- *Indication:* There are no adequate and well-controlled studies in pregnant women. Esmolol is a category C drug in pregnancy. Esmolol is associated with fetal bradycardia.
- *Mechanism of action:* β1-blocker
- *Onset:* 1 minute
- *Duration:* 10–20 minutes
- *Dose:* Low dose (LD) 0.5–1 mg/kg over 1 minute followed by 50 μg/kg/min infusion.
- *Preferred use:* Cardioselective
- *Side-effects:* Perioperative hypertension, myocardial infarction (MI)/ischemia, fetal bradycardia, and decompensated heart failure (DHF).

Sodium nitroprusside:
- *Mechanism of action:* Smooth muscle vasodilator
- *Dose and route:* Dose—0.3–0.5 μg/kg/min maximum of 2 μg/kg/min, IV
- *Onset of action:* 0.5–1 minute
- *Preferred use:* Reserved for extreme emergencies and for the shortest time

- *Side-effects/caution:* Hypotension and bradycardia. Risk of fetal cyanide toxicity. Used for a limited period only, continuous intra-art monitoring is mandatory.

Nitroglycerin:
- *Mechanism of action:* Direct vasodilators affect veins more than arterioles.
- *Indication:* It is an ideal agent for severe pregnancy-induced hypertension complicated by cardiogenic pulmonary edema. Nitroglycerin infusion effectively reduces preload by venous dilatation and, at higher doses, results in arterial vasodilation.
- *Onset:* 2–5 minutes
- *Duration:* 5–10 minutes
- *Dose:* 5 µg/min IV infusion, ↑ by 5 µg/min every 3–5 minutes (maximum 200 µg/min)
- *Preferred use:* Hypertension emergencies with acute coronary syndromes or acute pulmonary edema
- *Side-effects:* Headache and tachycardia; methemoglobinuria if given >24 hours

Ketanserin: It is a selective serotonin S2-receptor antagonist. Ketanserin decreases BP significantly in patients with severe preeclampsia. It is effective as dihydralazine with fewer side effects. It is also comparable with alpha-methyldopa. Administration of ketanserin to patients with hemolysis, elevated liver enzymes, and low platelets (HELLP) syndrome allowed delivery to be postponed for 5.3 days. According to a randomized trial ketanserin with aspirin used in patients with mild to moderate hypertension which was associated with a significant decrease number of cases of preeclampsia and severe hypertension, less perinatal mortality, lower rates of abruptio placentae, and early-onset preeclampsia.[8]
- *Indication:* Severe hypertension in pregnancy
- *Mechanism of action:* Selective serotonin receptor antagonist with weak adrenergic receptor blocking properties. The drug is responsible for lowering BP in essential hypertension. It is also responsible for inhibiting platelet aggregation.
- *Side effects:* Headache, dizziness, fatigue, sedation, light-headedness, lack of concentration, drowsiness, dry mouth, and gastrointestinal disturbances. Rare but serious adverse effects of ventricular tachycardia.

Phosphodiesterase inhibitors:
- *Sildenafil:* This is a phosphodiesterase type 5 inhibitor that is responsible for increasing intracellular cyclic guanosine monophosphate (cGMP) in the vascular smooth muscle, leading to vasodilation.[9]
- *Side-effects:* Headache, dyspepsia, flushing, nasal congestion, back pain, myalgia, nausea, dizziness, and rash.

■ KEY POINTS

- Aim of antihypertensive therapy—target BP ≤135/85 mm Hg (NICE).
- According to ACOG daily low-dose aspirin, starting in the late first trimester, specifically for women with a history of preeclampsia leading to prior preterm delivery before 34 weeks' gestation, or preeclampsia in more than one prior pregnancy.[3]
- Low-dose aspirin prophylaxis should be advised for women with more than one of several moderate risk factors for preeclampsia.
- Labetalol is one of the most commonly used antihypertensive drugs for hypertension during pregnancy.
- ACOG recommends antihypertensive medication when BP is >160/110 mm Hg, whereas the NICE recommends antihypertensive when the BP is 140/90 mm Hg, on the other hand, the European Society of Cardiology recommends antihypertensive to be administered when the BP is >150/95 mm Hg.[10]

REFERENCES

1. Roberts JM, Hubel CA. The Two-stage model of preeclampsia: variations on the theme. Placenta. 2009;30(Suppl A):S32-7.
2. Gestational hypertension and preeclampsia. ACOG practice bulletin No. 202. American College of Obstetricians and Gynecologists. Obstet Gynecol. 2019;133:el-25.
3. ACOG Committee Opinion No. 743: low-dose aspirin use during pregnancy. Obstet Gynecol. 2018;132(1):e44-52.
4. Hofmeyr G, Lawrie TA, Atallah ÁN, Duley L, Torloni MR. Calcium supplementation during pregnancy for preventing hypertensive disorders and related problems. Cochrane Database Syst Rev. 2014; 6:CD001059.
5. Hofmeyr GJ, Lawrie TA, Atallah ÁN, Torloni MR. Calcium supplementation during pregnancy for preventing hypertensive disorders and related problems. Cochrane Database Syst Rev. 2018;10(10):CD001059.
6. Rumbled A, Duley L, Crowther CA, Haslam RR. Antioxidants for preventing pre-eclampsia. Cochrane Database Syst Rev. 2008;2008(1):CD004227.
7. Ward K, Taylor RN. Genetic factors in the etiology of preeclampsia/eclapsia. In: Taylor RN, Robert JM, Cunninggham FG (Eds). Chesley's Hypertensive Disorders in Pregnancy, 4th edition. Amsterdam: Academic Press; 2014. pp. 57-80.
8. Gumusoglu SB, Schickling BM, Vignato JA, Santillan DA, Santillan MK. Selective serotonin reuptake inhibitors and preeclampsia: A quality assessment and meta-analysis. Pregnancy Hypertens. 2022;30:36-43.
9. Trapni A Jr, Goncalves LF, Trapani TF, Vieira S, Pires M, Pires MMS. Perinatal and hemodynamic evaluation of sildenafil citrate for preeclampsia treatment: a randomized controlled trial. Obstet Gynecol. 2016;128(2):253-9.
10. Awaludin A, Rahayu C, Daud NAA, Zakiyah N. Antihypertensive Medications for Severe Hypertension in Pregnancy: A Systematic Review and Meta-Analysis. Healthcare (Basel). 2022;10(2):325.

Chapter 5

Eclampsia

Ashok Kumar, Ashu Bhardwaj

Eclampsia is defined as new-onset tonic-clonic, focal, or multifocal seizures in the absence of other causative conditions such as epilepsy, cerebral vascular accident, or drug use, during pregnancy or in postpartum period. Eclampsia is mostly associated with preeclampsia, often with severe features. The results of few randomized placebo controlled trials indicate that seizures occur in about 1.9% of patients with preeclampsia[1] and in about 3.2% patients with severe preeclampsia.[2] Eclampsia is a significant cause of maternal morbidity and mortality, particularly in low-resource settings.

In addition to appropriate management of labor and delivery, the two main goals of management of women with preeclampsia during labor and delivery are:[3]
- Prevention of seizures and
- Control of hypertension.

The initial steps in the management of a woman with eclampsia remain basic supportive measures, such as calling for help, prevention of injury to mother due to jerky, often violent, involuntary movements, placement in lateral decubitus position, prevention of tongue bite by using mouth gag, prevention of injury by using side rails of bed, prevention of aspiration, administration of oxygen, and monitoring vitals including oxygen saturation. Magnesium sulfate is administered to treat and prevent recurrent seizures.[4]

■ PATHOPHYSIOLOGY

Convulsions in eclampsia are caused by excessive release of excitatory neurotransmitters, especially glutamate. This causes massive simultaneous depolarization of neurons resulting in bursts of action potential.

Two general theories have been proposed to explain underlying cerebrovascular pathology.
1. Hypoxia in brain due to vasospasm in cerebral vasculature, in response to acute and severe hypertension.
2. Vasogenic edema in brain due to sudden elevations in systemic blood pressure exceeds normal cerebrovascular auto regulatory capacity.

■ ROLE OF MAGNESIUM SULFATE

It is now clearly proven that magnesium sulfate is the best drug to prevent convulsions in women with preeclampsia with severe features and to stop them in those with eclampsia.

Mechanism of Action

The mechanism of action of magnesium sulfate is likely multi-factorial, encompassing both vascular and neurological mechanisms.[5,6]

- It is a calcium antagonist, hence results in vascular smooth muscle relaxation and vasodilation. This helps in lowering total peripheral vascular resistance.
- In addition, $MgSO_4$ also has an effect on the cerebral endothelium. It decreases smooth muscle contraction and paracellular permeability via calcium-dependent second messenger systems such as myosin light chain kinase. This helps in reducing vasogenic edema.
- $MgSO_4$ also acts centrally to inhibit N-methyl-D-aspartate (NMDA) receptors, providing anticonvulsant activity. It also increases seizure threshold.

Dosage (Box 1)

When magnesium sulfate is given to arrest eclamptic seizures, 10–15% of women may have a subsequent convulsion. In such a case, an additional 2-g dose of magnesium sulfate in a 20% solution is slowly administered intravenously.[7]

Pharmacology

After administration, about 40% of plasma magnesium is protein bound. The unbound magnesium ions the active form, which diffuses into the extravascular-extracellular space. The clinical effect and toxicity of $MgSO_4$ are linked to its concentration in plasma.

Parenterally administered magnesium is cleared almost totally by renal excretion, with 90% of the dose excreted during the first 24 hours after an intravenous infusion of $MgSO_4$. The pharmacokinetic profile of $MgSO_4$ after intravenous administration can be described by a two-compartment

---

BOX 1: Dosage regimens of magnesium sulfate for severe preeclampsia and eclampsia.

Continuous intravenous infusion:
- Zuspan regimen
  - *Loading dose:* 4 g of magnesium sulfate (20%) diluted in 100 mL of IV fluid, given over 15–20 minutes
  - *Maintenance dose:* 1 g/hour IV infusion (50%)
- Assess deep tendon reflexes, urinary output, and respiratory rate periodically
- Measure serum magnesium levels if serum creatinine >or equal to 1.0 mg/dL
- Magnesium sulfate is discontinued 24 hours after delivery
- *Sibai regimen*
  - *Loading dose:* 4–6 g of magnesium sulfate (20%) diluted in 100 mL of IV fluid, given over 15–20 minutes
  - *Maintenance dose:* 2 g/hour IV infusion (50%)

For women requiring cesarean delivery (before onset of labor), the infusion should ideally begin before surgery and continue during surgery, as well as for 24 hours afterward

Intermittent intramuscular injections:
- Pritchard regimen
  - *Loading dose:* 4 g of magnesium sulfate (20%) given intravenously at a rate not exceeding 1 g/minute, and 5 g deep IM (50% solution) in each buttock (total 14 g)
  - *Maintenance dose:* 5 g IM (50% solution) every 4 hours in alternate buttock; only after ensuring that patellar reflex is present, RR >14, urine output in previous 4 hours is >100 mL
  - Magnesium sulfate is discontinued 24 hours after delivery
- Dhaka (low dose) regimen
  - *Loading dose:* 4 g of magnesium sulfate (20%) given IV, and 3-g deep IM (50% solution) in each buttock (total 10 g)
  - *Maintenance dose:* 2.5 g IM (50% solution) every 4 hours in alternate buttock; Magnesium sulfate is discontinued 24 hours after delivery

TABLE 1: Serum magnesium concentration and toxicities.

mmol/L	mEq/L	mg/dL	Effect
2–3.5	4–7	5–9	Therapeutic range
>3.5	>7	>9	Loss of patellar reflexes
>5	>10	>12	Respiratory paralysis
>12.5	>25	>30	Cardiac arrest

model with a rapid distribution alpha phase, followed by a relative slow beta phase of elimination.[7]

In pregnant women, apparent volumes of distribution usually reach constant values 3–4 hours after administration. Hence, the initial 4-g loading dose of magnesium sulfate can be safely administered of renal function owing to its volume of distribution. Whenever plasma creatinine levels are >1.0 mg/mL, serum magnesium levels are determined to guide the infusion rate.

The adverse effects of magnesium sulfate (respiratory depression and cardiac arrest) come largely from its action as a smooth muscle relaxant. The serum concentration of magnesium is related to its adverse effects and toxicities **(Table 1)**. In cases with renal dysfunction, determination of serum magnesium levels is done every 4 hours. If the serum level exceeds 9.6 mg/dL (8 mEq/L), the infusion should be stopped and serum magnesium levels should be determined at 2-hour intervals. The infusion can be restarted at a lower rate when the serum level decreases to <8.4 mg/dL (7 mEq/L). Patients at risk of impending respiratory depression may require tracheal intubation and emergency correction with calcium gluconate 10% solution, 10 mL IV over 3 minutes, along with furosemide intravenously to accelerate the rate of urinary excretion.[4]

PLAN FOR TERMINATION OF PREGNANCY

Eclampsia is one of the conditions that preclude conservative management in women with severe preeclampsia even at gestation <34 weeks. Immediate delivery is advised. A simultaneous course of corticosteroids can be administered. The route of delivery is individualized based of cervical condition, however chances of cesarean delivery increase with decreasing gestation.[4]

ANTIHYPERTENSIVE DRUGS (TABLE 2)

The treatment of severe hypertension is done promptly to prevent damage to vital organs and complications such as congestive heart failure, myocardial ischemia, renal injury or failure, and ischemic or hemorrhagic stroke.[3] Antihypertensive treatment should be initiated expeditiously for acute-onset severe hypertension (blood pressure of 160/110 mm Hg or more) that is confirmed as persistent (15 minutes or more). Intravenous hydralazine or labetalol and oral nifedipine are the three agents most commonly used.[8]

Labetalol

Labetalol is a selective alpha-1 and nonselective beta-blocker. Hence, it lowers blood pressure by blocking both alpha and beta adrenergic receptors.

Pharmacokinetics: Labetalol is given intravenously to treat acute severe hypertension. After intravenous administration, the onset of action is 2–3 minutes, peak effect is seen in 15 minutes and half-life is 5–6 hours.

It is recommends to start with a 20-mg intravenous bolus dose in severe hypertension. If not effective within

TABLE 2: Antihypertensive drugs.

Name	Mechanism of action	Dosage[8]	Side effects	Contraindications/precautions	Onset of action
Labetalol	Alpha-1 and nonselective beta-blocker	• 10–20 mg IV, then 20–40–80 mg every 10–30 minutes to a maximum cumulative dosage of 300 mg; or constant infusion 1–2 mg/minute IV • Orally-start with 100 mg thrice a day, up to a maximum of 2,400 mg/day	Postural hypotension, tremors	Avoid in women with asthma, preexisting myocardial disease, decompensated cardiac function, and heart block and bradycardia	1–2 minutes
Nifedipine	Calcium channel blocker	10–20 mg orally, repeat in 20 minutes if needed; then 10–20 mg every 2–6 hours; maximum daily dose is 180 mg	May observe reflex tachycardia and headaches	Myocardial infarction[8]	5–10 minutes
Hydralazine	Direct arteriolar vasodilator	5 mg IV or IM, then 5–10 mg IV every 20–40 minutes to a maximum cumulative dosage of 20 mg; or constant infusion of 0.5–10 mg/hour	Higher or frequent dosage associated with maternal hypotension, headaches, and abnormal fetal heart rate tracings	• Avoid in coronary artery disease, aortic dissection • Cautious use in lactation, excretion in human milk is unknown	10–20 minutes
Nitroglycerine	Direct vasodilator (arteries and veins)	Start with IV 5 µg/min and titrate (maximum 100 µg/minute)	Headache, palpitations, flushing, and dizziness	Used for acute hypertension	

10 minutes, this is followed by 40 mg, then 80 mg every 10 minutes. If hypertension persists, hydralazine is then given.[9]

Hydralazine

Hydralazine causes peripheral vasodilation by its direct effect on arterial smooth muscle.

Pharmacokinetics: When administered by IV bolus, hydralazine has an onset of action of 5–20 minutes, peak effect at 10–80 minutes and a duration of action of 2–6 hours.

The initial dose is 5–10 mg given intravenously, and a 10-mg dose is repeated after 15- to 20-minute intervals, until a systolic pressure to <160 mm Hg and diastolic blood pressure to 90–110 mm Hg is achieved. Hydralazine decreases diastolic blood pressure more than systolic blood pressure.[8]

Nifedipine

Nifedipine is given orally, and belongs to class of calcium-channel blockers.

Pharmacokinetics: After oral administration, bioavailability is 30–60%, a half-life is 2 hours.[8]

Nifedipine is given in 10 mg initial immediate-release oral dose to be followed by 10–20 mg dose after 20–30 minutes if necessary. Nifedipine given sublingually is no longer recommended as this route is associated with dangerously rapid and extensive effects.

Role of Diuretics

Diuretics like furosemide are used in antenatal period solely to treat pulmonary edema. Potent loop diuretics are not used in antenatal period, as they can further compromise placental perfusion by redistributing intravascular volume, which most often is already reduced in severe preeclampsia.

■ KEY POINTS

- Eclampsia is a significant cause of maternal morbidity and mortality. Magnesium sulfate is the best drug to prevent convulsions in women with preeclampsia with severe features and to stop them in those with eclampsia.
- Magnesium sulfate is usually given by either the intramuscular or intravenous routes. The intramuscular regimen (Pritchard regimen) is given as 4-g intravenous loading dose, immediately followed by 10 g intramuscularly and then by 5 g intramuscularly every 4 hours in alternating buttocks.
- The intravenous regimen (Zuspan regimen) is given as a 4-g dose, followed by a maintenance infusion of 1–2 g/hour by controlled infusion pump.
- The initial 4-g loading dose of magnesium sulfate can be safely administered regardless of renal function, owing to its volume of distribution.
- Antihypertensive treatment should be initiated expeditiously for acute-onset severe hypertension along with administration of magnesium sulfate. Intravenous hydralazine or labetalol and oral nifedipine are the three agents most commonly used.

■ REFERENCES

1. Altman D, Carroli G, Duley L, Farrell B, Moodley J, Neilson J, et al. Do women with preeclampsia, and their babies, benefit from magnesium sulphate? The Magpie Trial: a randomised placebo-controlled trial. Lancet. 2002;359(9321):1877-90.
2. Coetzee EJ, Dommisse J, Anthony J. A randomised controlled trial of intravenous magnesium sulphate versus placebo in the management of women with severe preeclampsia. Br J Obstet Gynaecol. 1998; 105:300-3.
3. Cunningham FG, Leveno KJ, Bloom SL, Dashe JS, Hoffman BL, Casey BM, et al. Hypertensive disorders. In: Dashe JS, Bloom SL, Spong CY, Hoffman BL (Eds). Williams Obstetrics. 25th edition. New York, NY: McGraw Hill Medical; 2018. pp. 710-45.

4. Gestational hypertension and preeclampsia. ACOG Practice Bulletin No. 222. American College of Obstetricians and Gynecologists. Obstet Gynecol. 2020;135:e237-60.
5. Nelson SH, Suresh MS. Magnesium sulfate-induced relaxation of uterine arteries from pregnant and non-pregnant patients. Am J Obstet Gynecol. 1991;164:1344-50.
6. Belfort MA, Saade GR, Moise KJ Jr. The effect of magnesium sulfate on maternal and fetal blood flow in pregnancy-induced hypertension. Acta Obstet Gynecol Scand. 1993;72:526-30.
7. Lu JF, Nightingale CH. Magnesium sulfate in eclampsia and pre-eclampsia: pharmacokinetic principles. Clin Pharmacokinet. 2000;38(4):305-14.
8. Benowitz NL. Antihypertensive agents. In: Katzung BG, Masters SB, Trevor AJ (Eds). Basic and Clinical Pharmacology. 12th edition. New York: McGraw Hill; 2012.
9. Committee on Obstetric Practice. Committee opinion no. 692: emergent therapy for acute-onset, severe hypertension during pregnancy and the postpartum period. Obstet Gynecol. 2017;129(4):e90-5.

Section 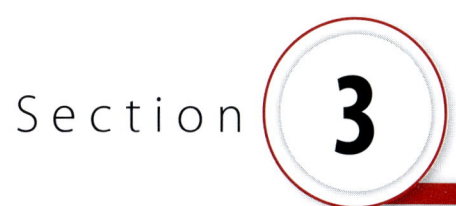 3

Medical Management of Heart Disease in Pregnancy

- **Rheumatic Heart Disease**
  Amita Suneja, Richa Aggarwal

- **Mechanical and Prosthetic Heart Valves: Anticoagulant Therapy**
  Jaya Chawla, Kiran Dhawan

- **Heart Failure**
  Puneet Aggarwal, Pradyumna Kumar Singh, Dheerendra Kuber, Ranjit Kumar Nath

Chapter 6

Rheumatic Heart Disease

Amita Suneja, Richa Aggarwal

Cardiovascular diseases complicate around 1–3% of all pregnancies but account for 10–15% of maternal mortality. Although congenital heart disease is the leading cardiac disease in pregnancy in the developed world, rheumatic heart disease (RHD) is still responsible for 50–90% of all maternal cardiac complications in low- and middle-income countries.

The hallmark of RHD is damage to the cardiac valves leading to valvular heart disease and left ventricular (LV) dysfunction. The physiological hemodynamic changes during pregnancy **(Box 1)** can unmask previously silent maternal cardiac dysfunction or worsen the previously controlled cardiac condition.[1]

MANAGEMENT OF RHEUMATIC HEART DISEASE IN PREGNANCY

The management of RHD during pregnancy will be discussed under the following headings:
- General principles of management
- Management of specific lesions
- Labor and delivery considerations
- Contraception in women with RHD

General Principles of Management
- Optimize oral healthcare, including routine dentistry checkups

---

BOX 1: Hemodynamic changes during pregnancy.

- *During pregnancy:*
  – 30–50% increase in cardiac output
    - 30% increase in stroke volume
    - 10–20% in heart rate
  – 35–40% fall in systemic vascular resistance
    - Systemic vasodilation
    - Low-resistance uteroplacental circulation
  – 40–50% increase in plasma volume
    - Preload reduction due to compression of IVC by the gravid uterus
- *During labor and delivery:*
  – 30% increase in cardiac output during the first stage of labor
    - Increase in heart rate (due to pain and anxiety)
    - Increased stroke volume (300–500 mL of blood is "autotransfused" into the systemic circulation with each uterine contraction)
  – 60–80% increase in cardiac output immediately after postdelivery
    - Relief of IVC compression—rapid increase in preload
    - Massive autotransfusion from the uterine blood volume
    - Mobilization of dependent edema and interstitial fluid
    - Relative increase in systemic vascular resistance
- *Hypercoagulable state:*
  – Increased concentration of clotting factors—20% reduction in prothrombin time and aPTT
  – Increased platelet adhesiveness
  – Decreased fibrinolysis

(aPTT: activated partial thromboplastin time; IVC: inferior vena cava)

- Secondary prevention with penicillin prophylaxis
- Infective endocarditis prophylaxis.

Secondary Prevention with Penicillin Prophylaxis

Secondary prophylaxis of RHD comprises long-term antibiotic prophylaxis to prevent the development of RHD or worsening of preexisting RHD triggered by recurrent acute rheumatic fever (ARF) episodes caused by group A streptococcal (GAS) infection.[2]

The standard secondary prophylaxis regimen is benzathine penicillin G (BPG) administered deep intramuscularly in a dose of 1.2 million units, after a sensitivity test every 3 weeks.[3] *It is very important that the correct form of penicillin must be prescribed: Long-acting intramuscular BPG, and should not be confused with short-acting intramuscular procaine penicillin G.*

Benzathine penicillin G is a fusion of two penicillin G molecules and is characterized by low solubility and low hydrolysis which is responsible for its slow absorption from a depot intramuscular injection, producing low but adequate serum concentrations for streptococcal prophylaxis, for a long duration.[2]

In cases of allergy to penicillin, oral erythromycin in a dose of 500 mg twice daily is the drug of choice for secondary prophylaxis.

As per Indian guidelines,[4] secondary prophylaxis should continue:
- Lifelong in patients with severe disease or in postintervention patients, one may opt for secondary prophylaxis until the age of 40 years
- ARF with healed, mild, or moderate carditis: until age 25 or for 10 years after the last ARF (whichever is longer)
- ARF without carditis: until age 18 or for 5 years after the last ARF (whichever is longer).

Infective Endocarditis Prophylaxis

Infective endocarditis (IE) is a well-recognized complication of RHD which is more commonly seen in patients following valve repair or replacement surgery but may also occur in individuals with native rheumatic valves. Many authorities no longer recommend infective endocarditis prophylaxis in pregnant women with valvular heart disease.[5]

However, considering the high risk of mortality or major morbidity, some guidelines do recommend antibiotic prophylaxis for RHD patients.[6,7] Prophylaxis is recommended for women with chronic RHD of any severity, those with prosthetic heart valves (bioprosthetic or mechanical), and those with a history of previous endocarditis. In these patients, antibiotics should be given 30–60 minutes before the estimated time of delivery and should continue for at least 24–48 hours after delivery[8] **(Table 1)**. Infective endocarditis prophylaxis should also be given

TABLE 1: Infective endocarditis antibiotic prophylaxis regimens.

Treatment	Antibiotic	Dosage
Intravenous therapy	Ampicillin or cefazolin or ceftriaxone	2 g 1 g
Allergic to penicillin or ampicillin (intravenous)	Cefazolin/ ceftriaxone/ clindamycin	1 g 600 mg
Oral	Amoxicillin	2 g
Allergic to penicillin or ampicillin (oral)	Cephalexin Clindamycin Azithromycin	2 g 600 mg 500 mg

in case of prolonged labor or in the event of premature rupture of the membranes.

Management of Specific Lesions

The increased cardiac output during pregnancy causes an increase in transvalvular gradient by 50%, which increases the risk of maternal and fetal complications in stenotic valve diseases. Regurgitant lesions are generally better during pregnancy because the placental circulation leads to a reduction in systemic vascular resistance, which reduces afterload and helps increase forward flow.

Mitral Stenosis

Mitral stenosis (MS) is the most common valvular lesion seen in pregnant women with RHD. It is characterized by the "fish mouth" appearance of the mitral valve as the anterior and posterior leaflets become scarred at the commissures.[9]

Medical management:
- Limitation of activity
- Beta-blockers
- Use of diuretics.

Beta-adrenergic blocking agents or β-blockers are the mainstay of medical therapy in women with MS with heart failure (HF) symptoms or clinically significant pulmonary hypertension (pulmonary artery systolic pressure >50 mm Hg on echocardiography). They slow the heart rate and lengthen the diastolic filling time of the left ventricle, thus reducing the transvalvular gradient, lowering left atrial pressure, and reducing pulmonary venous pressure.[10,11] β-1 selective agents, such as metoprolol, and bisoprolol are preferred as they do not interfere with β-2 mediated uterine relaxation and peripheral vasodilation and, thus are associated with lower rates of fetal growth restriction. The dosage and safety of commonly used β-blockers during pregnancy are summarized in **Table 2**. The former Food and Drug Administration's (FDA's) A to X categorial system has been replaced by the Pregnancy and Lactation Labeling Rule (PLLR), which provides detailed information on animal and clinical data of the drug with a descriptive risk summary.[12]

Diuretics should be added in patients with pulmonary edema or ongoing symptoms despite β-blockers, however, high doses

TABLE 2: Safety profile of commonly used β-blockers during pregnancy.

Drug	Dose	Former FDA category	Placenta permeable	Use during lactation	Potential adverse effects
Metoprolol	IV 2.5–5 mg bolus over 2 minutes, up to three doses followed by oral 25–100 mg twice daily	C	Yes	Compatible	Fetal bradycardia and hypoglycemia
Bisoprolol	2.5–10 mg once daily	C	Yes	Compatible	Fetal bradycardia and hypoglycemia
Carvedilol	3.125–25 mg twice daily, may use carvedilol sustained release 10–80 mg once daily	C	Yes	No human data	• Inadequate human data • Fetal bradycardia and hypoglycemia

(FDA: Food and Drug Administration; IV: intravenous)

should be avoided as they may compromise placental circulation.[11] Intravenous (IV) loop diuretics (furosemide and bumetanide) are usually preferred, the initial diuretic dose is dependent on the severity of congestion. For moderate congestion: 20–40 mg IV 12 hourly is given, for severe congestion: 40–80 mg IV 12 hourly or bolus 60 mg IV along with continuous infusion at 10–20 mg/h is given. The maximum total daily dose is 400–600 mg.[7]

Digoxin is indicated in patients where β-blockers are contraindicated or are not tolerated, or is added along with β-blockers in patients where adequate rate control is not achieved.[10]

For HF, a loading dose to initiate digoxin therapy is not necessary and digoxin is usually initiated and maintained at 0.125–0.25 mg daily dose. Plasma levels of 0.5–0.9 ng/mL are suggested to be efficacious, and serum levels >2 ng/mL indicate drug toxicity. Management of HF is discussed in detail in a later section.

Patients with atrial fibrillation (AF), left atrial thrombus, and/or a history of embolism should receive therapeutic anticoagulation. Anticoagulation should also be given in women with severe MS at risk of stroke, such as large left atrium (≥60 mL/m^2), or congestive HF.[11,12] Anticoagulation is discussed in detail in the next section.

Vaginal delivery is generally preferred, cesarean section is reserved only for obstetric indications or in patients who are in New York Heart Association (NYHA) class III/IV or have pulmonary hypertension (PH), or in whom percutaneous mitral commissurotomy cannot be performed or has failed.

Aortic Stenosis

Aortic stenosis (AS) is characterized by a fixed stroke volume, therefore, increasing the heart rate is the only mechanism by which these patients can increase their cardiac output which is required to accommodate the demands of pregnancy and the increased blood volume. Increased heart rate leads to reduced diastolic ventricular filling and hence reduced coronary perfusion resulting in ischemia of the coronary arteries, hypotension, and syncope.[9] In contrast to MS, in which β-blockers are useful to decrease heart rate and improve filling time, *β-blockers are not recommended in patients with AS*, unless treating an arrhythmia, because increased heart rate is an important compensatory mechanism for fixed stroke volume.

There is no optimal medical treatment for AS, therefore it is important to have preconception evaluation and valve intervention is recommended in women with severe AS, who have LV dysfunction with left ventricular ejection fraction (LVEF) <50%, or in cases who become symptomatic on exercise testing.[10]

Women who become symptomatic during pregnancy should be managed with activity restriction and cautious use of diuretics, avoiding a sudden drop in preload.

To prevent hemodynamic decompensation in patients with AS, it is preferable to maintain normal to high preload and normal or low afterload. Reduction of preload (e.g., large blood loss, hypotension) or increased afterload (vasopressors) should be avoided with maintenance of euvolemia or positive fluid balance.[9]

In mild and moderate AS, vaginal delivery is preferable. The second stage of labor should be cut short as Valsalva increases intrathoracic pressure and decreases preload. Cesarean section is recommended in women with severe symptomatic AS. General anesthesia is generally preferred as epidural anesthesia poses a high risk of hypotension which can precipitate poor coronary perfusion.[10]

Mitral Regurgitation and Aortic Regurgitation

Mild regurgitation is usually well tolerated in pregnancy. However, it is important to monitor mitral regurgitation (MR), which can worsen as the pregnancy progresses owing to physiological LV dilatation.

The mainstay of treatment includes activity restriction, reducing dietary sodium intake, and medical therapy for HF including diuretics, β-blockers, and/or vasodilators. Vasodilators should be used cautiously in the pregnancy as they may lead to uteroplacental hypoperfusion.[11] Commonly used vasodilators such as angiotensin-converting enzyme inhibitors and angiotensin receptor blockers are contraindicated during pregnancy due to their teratogenicity; preload and afterload reducing effects can be obtained using hydralazine and nitrates in combination, which are safe during pregnancy.[1]

Beta-blockers are recommended with an MR but should be avoided in AR, as heart rate reduction prolongs the diastolic filling time during which AR occurs. Vaginal delivery is preferred for both MR and AR, with epidural analgesia as it reduces the systemic vascular resistance, along with the addition of diuretics postdelivery.[9]

Women with severe aortic regurgitation (AR) with symptoms or reduced LV function are at significant risk of HF and arrhythmias.[10]

Tricuspid Regurgitation

Isolated tricuspid regurgitation (TR) is generally not seen with RHD and maternal risk is usually determined primarily by the severity of left-sided valve lesions or the presence of pulmonary HT. TR is often well-tolerated during pregnancy and managed medically with diuretics.[10]

Multiple Valve Diseases

In multiple valve disease, risk and management should be based on the most hemodynamically significant lesion.[10]

Lesions are additive using the modified World Health Organization (mWHO) risk index. In combined lesions, valvular heart disease is considered severe even if both stenosis and regurgitation are only of moderate severity, and assessment is based on pressure gradients.

Assessment of each valve lesion should be done taking into account the interaction between the different valve lesions, for example, associated MR may lead to underestimation of the severity of aortic stenosis, since reduced stroke volume due to MR lowers the flow across the aortic valve and, hence the aortic gradient.[13]

Arrythmias Associated with Rheumatic Heart Disease

AF: Atrial fibrillation is a common complication of RHD. The prevalence of AF depends upon the type of valvular involvement with the highest frequency seen in patients with a combination of mixed mitral valve disease and tricuspid regurgitation (70%) as compared to isolated MS (29%) or isolated MR (16%).[3] Complications of AF include HF, stroke, peripheral thromboembolism, and sudden death.

Treatment of AF in pregnant women includes prompt initiation of anticoagulation and rhythm control to prevent thromboembolic episodes and the risk of pulmonary edema. For sustained AF, rate control with β-blockers or digoxin is the initial strategy.[14] Beta blockers are more effective at heart rate control than digoxin during pregnancy. Since an elevated heart rate is crucial to maintain the augmented cardiac output in pregnancy, the goal of ventricular rate control should be at 70–90 bpm rather than <60 bpm as in a nonpregnant state. Metoprolol is the preferred β-blocker. For use in AF, a loading dose of digoxin should be given followed by a maintenance dose:

Rapid digitalizing (loading-dose) regimen:[15]
- An initial intravenous dose of 0.25–0.5 mg of digoxin is given over 10–15 minutes, followed by 0.25 mg every 6 hours for a total loading dose of 0.75–1.5 mg. Intravenous digoxin begins to act in 15–30 minutes with a peak effect in 1–5 hours.
- PO: 0.5 mg initially followed by 0.25 mg every 6 hours for a total loading dose of 0.75–1.5 mg.

Maintenance: PO: 0.125–0.25 mg/day; may increase dose every 2 weeks based on clinical response, serum drug levels, and toxicity.

Digoxin has been used for both fetal and maternal cardiac indications as it readily crosses the placenta without any fetal harm or teratogenicity and is considered safe during pregnancy and lactation.

In the case of refractory or recurrent AF, a rhythm control strategy with antiarrhythmic drugs (AAD) is reasonable.[16] Sotalol or flecainide is the preferred AAD in this setting **(Table 3)**. Dronedarone is contraindicated and amiodarone should only be used in the setting of life-threatening arrhythmias because of the risk of fetal harm. Electrical cardioversion should be considered if the patient is hemodynamically unstable.

Paroxysmal supraventricular tachycardia (PSVT): PSVT is a tachyarrhythmia with an abrupt onset and cessation that involves atrial tissue or atrioventricular junctional tissues. It should be treated promptly to prevent deleterious effects on uteroplacental perfusion.

Vagal maneuvers including carotid sinus massage, Valsalva, and facial ice immersion are considered the first line of nonpharmacological treatment for supraventricular tachycardia (SVT) in all trimesters.[17] Adenosine is the first-line pharmacological treatment for SVTs in all trimesters. Intravenous adenosine does not enter fetal circulation because it has an extremely short half-life of 10 seconds, and hence, is indicated for only acute treatment. It is intravenously in a dose of 6–12 mg and the maximum amount of IV adenosine that can be administered is 24 mg (*see* **Table 3**). It has a higher conversion rate (84%) than β-adrenergic and calcium channel blockers.[18] It has been linked to preterm labor during the third trimester.

Supraventricular tachycardias which are refractory to IV adenosine should be treated with β-adrenergic blockers such as propranolol, sotalol, and metoprolol, which can be prescribed not only acutely but also in a chronic setting. Verapamil is considered a third-line agent.[17] It is a nondihydropyridines calcium channel blocker that should be avoided in the first trimester of the pregnancy because of its association with fetal arrhythmias, such as fetal bradycardia and heart block. Rapid IV administration of verapamil can lead to maternal hypotension.

For patients with frequent symptomatic episodes, β-blockers are considered the first-line treatment for the prevention of SVT.[16] Although digoxin is safe in pregnancy, it is generally ineffective when used alone but has been effective when used in combination with β-blockers.[19] Calcium channel blockers such as verapamil and diltiazem are used as second-line agents. Pharmacologic

TABLE 3: Safety profile of antiarrhythmic drugs used in pregnancy.

Drug	VW class	Dose	Former FDA category	Placenta permeable	Use during lactation	Potential adverse effects
Adenosine	V	IV 6–12 mg, maximum dose 24 mg	C	No	Yes	No fetal adverse effects reported
Verapamil	IV	• IV 0.075–0.15 mg/kg over 2 minutes. Second bolus in 15–30 minutes if needed • Oral 120–480 mg/day	C	Yes	Yes	Well tolerated
Diltiazem	IV	• IV 0.25 mg/kg over 2 minutes. A second bolus can be given if HR >100 bpm • Oral 120–480 mg/day	C	No	Yes	Possible teratogenic effects use only when the benefit outweighs the risk
Sotalol	III	Oral 80–160 mg, maximum of 320 mg every 12 hours, based on renal function	B	Yes	Yes	Bradycardia and hypoglycemia
Flecainide	IC	• Acute conversion • Oral 200–300 mg, single dose • IV 1.5–2 mg/kg, maximum 150 mg infused over 10 minutes • Chronic prevention • 50–200 mg BD	C	Yes	Yes	Inadequate human data

(VW class: Vaughan–Williams classification of antiarrhythmic drugs, IV: intravenous)

prophylaxis with flecainide can be used for long-term suppression of SVTs.

Atenolol is a cardioselective β-1-adrenergic blocker which is a class D drug and must be avoided in the first trimester of the pregnancy. It has been linked to fetal growth restriction. In addition to atenolol, amiodarone should also be reserved for life-threatening circumstances. It is also a class D medication and is used only in conjunction with electric cardioversion.

If the patient is hemodynamically unstable or the arrhythmia is drug-refractory, electric cardioversion should be used to terminate SVT.

Labor and Delivery Considerations

An individualized delivery plan should be made in consultation with the obstetrician, cardiologist, and anesthetist and should include information on preferred timing and mode of delivery, method of induction, type of analgesia/anesthesia, hemodynamic monitoring during labor and postpartum, infective endocarditis prophylaxis and switching over of anticoagulants (if the patient is on anticoagulants). Delivery in women with cardiac disease is best accomplished in a tertiary care hospital under the care of a multidisciplinary team.

Vaginal delivery is preferred for most women with RHD unless indicated for obstetric indications, as it poses less cardiac risks. It is associated with less blood loss, more rapid recovery, and less thrombogenic and infectious risk.

European Society of Cardiology (ESC) guidelines recommend considering induction of labor at 40 weeks of gestation in all women with cardiac disease; this reduces the risk of emergency cesarean section by 12% and the risk of stillbirth by 50% in women without heart disease, and the benefit is likely to be greater for women with heart disease.[12]

For induction of labor, misoprostol 25 μg or dinoprostone 1–3 mg can be used safely. Mechanical methods such as cervical ripening balloons, artificial rupture of membranes, and oxytocin infusions can be used safely in these women.[12]

Adequate pain relief with epidural anesthesia during vaginal delivery is advisable as it reduces the catecholamine release associated with sudden increases in heart rate and stroke volume and also allows for a controlled descent of the fetus to the pelvic floor, diminishing the frequency and intensity of the Valsalva maneuver. Epidural is preferred over spinal anesthesia due to lower rates of hypotension.[10]

An assisted second stage of delivery using forceps or vacuum, which shortens the time to delivery should be considered as it minimizes the frequency and intensity of maternal effort with the Valsalva maneuver, which transiently drops cardiac output.

Cesarean delivery should be considered in women with RHD presenting with preterm labor on oral anticoagulants, in patients with symptomatic lesions (AS and MS), severe pulmonary hypertension, or presenting with signs of acute HF.

Ergometrine is relatively contraindicated because of its propensity to cause coronary artery spasms and increasing blood pressure. Oxytocin induces vasodilatation in the subcutaneous vessels, and vasoconstriction in the splanchnic bed and coronary arteries, leading to hypotension, tachycardia, and myocardial ischemia. Low-dose oxytocin infusion is generally preferred. In the event of PPH, oxytocin and prostaglandins are generally well tolerated.[10] However, the use of mechanical approaches including intrauterine balloon and uterine compression sutures should be emphasized. Although high-dose (600 μg) misoprostol for PPH prophylaxis has not been found to have an effect on cardiac parameters in women without cardiac disease, but the theoretical risk of coronary vasospasm and arrhythmias exists.

Contraception in Women with Rheumatic Heart Disease

The risk of using a particular type of contraception should be balanced against the risk of pregnancy in a woman with RHD who runs a risk of severe morbidity and mortality in case of unplanned pregnancy.

The estrogen component of combined oral contraceptives increases the risk of venous thromboembolism by 2–7-fold. Additional risks associated include arterial and cardiac thrombosis, atherosclerosis, hyperlipidemia, and hypertension. The risks of ischemic stroke and ischemic heart disease are also increased.[10] Little evidence suggests that both estrogen and progestins interact with warfarin, hence frequent monitoring of international normalized ratio (INR) is important when starting any hormonal contraceptives in women already on warfarin.

Progestogen-only methods are the contraceptives of choice for women with severe cardiac disease, as they are not associated with an increased risk of arterial or venous thrombosis. Additional anticoagulation monitoring is required if a woman is on warfarin because of drug-drug interaction.[12]

Levonorgestrel-based long-acting reversible intrauterine devices or contraceptive implants are the safest and most effective contraceptives. However, pain during insertion may cause a vasovagal response, especially in patients with pulmonary HT, hence in these patients, intrauterine device (IUD) insertion should be done in a hospital setting. Women at risk of infective endocarditis must be given prophylactic antibiotics before insertion.[10,12]

Depo-Provera is an effective contraception with the advantage of 12-weekly injections and a quick return to fertility when its use is stopped. The risk of hematoma formation at the injection site for women on anticoagulants is worrisome.

Copper IUDs are popular in low-resource settings because of their cost-effectiveness and low thrombogenic potential.[1]

Barrier methods have high failure rates but reduce the risk of pelvic inflammatory disease. They are prescribed in combination with long-acting reversible progestin contraception.[12]

Valvular heart disease due to RHD remains an important cause of cardiac decompensation during pregnancy, especially in LMICs where it accounts for 50–90% of maternal cardiac complications. The associated mortality is high as a large proportion of cases in LMICs are first diagnosed during pregnancy. However, with early recognition and good antenatal care, good maternal outcomes can be achieved. All women with valvular heart disease should be managed by a multidisciplinary Pregnancy Heart Team before and during pregnancy. Preconceptional comprehensive evaluation is essential to provide guidance to women regarding her risk during pregnancy. Pregnancy is often well-tolerated in cases of mild-to-moderate valvular heart disease. Women with severe mitral stenosis and symptomatic severe aortic stenosis are at high risk of poor outcomes and should be considered for valvular intervention before conception. Contraception should also be discussed with women who have valvular disease.

■ KEY POINTS

- The standard secondary prophylaxis regimen is 1.2 million units of BPG administered deep intramuscularly after a sensitivity test every 3 weeks.
- Beta-1 selective adrenergic blocking agents are the mainstay of medical therapy in women with MS with HF symptoms or clinically significant pulmonary hypertension.
- Diuretics should be added in patients with pulmonary edema or ongoing symptoms despite β-blockers, however, high doses should be avoided as they may compromise placental circulation.
- Digoxin is indicated in patients where β-blockers are contraindicated or are not tolerated or is added along with β-blockers in patients where adequate rate control is not achieved.
- Treatment of AF in pregnant women includes prompt initiation of anticoagulation and rhythm control to prevent thromboembolic episodes and the risk of pulmonary edema.

- Adenosine is the first-line pharmacological treatment for SVTs in all the trimesters.
- Progestogen-only methods are the contraceptives of choice for women with severe cardiac disease, as they are not associated with an increased risk of arterial or venous thrombosis.

■ REFERENCES

1. Nanna M, Stergiopoulos K. Pregnancy complicated by valvular heart disease: an update. J Am Heart Assoc. 2014;3(3):e000712.
2. de Dassel JL, Lennon D, Dougherty S, Ralph AP. Secondary Prevention of Acute Rheumatic Fever and Rheumatic Heart Disease. In: Dougherty S, Carapetis J, Zuhlke L, Wilson N (Eds). Acute Rheumatic Fever and Rheumatic Heart Disease, 1st edition. St Louis, MO: Elsevier Science Ltd; 2020. pp. 207-34.
3. Kumar RK, Antunes MJ, Beaton A, Mirabel M, Nkomo VT, Okello E, et al. Contemporary Diagnosis and Management of Rheumatic Heart Disease: Implications for Closing the Gap: A Scientific Statement From the American Heart Association. Circulation. 2020;142(20):e337-57.
4. Working Group on Pediatric Acute Rheumatic Fever and Cardiology Chapter of Indian Academy of Pediatrics; Saxena A, Kumar RK, Gera RP, Radhakrishnan S, Mishra S, et al. Consensus guidelines on pediatric acute rheumatic fever and rheumatic heart disease. Indian Pediatr. 2008;45(7):565-73.
5. Thornhill MH, Lockhart PB, Prendergast B, Chambers JB, Shanson D. NICE, and antibiotic prophylaxis to prevent endocarditis. Br Dent J. 2015;218(11):619-21.
6. Ralph AP, Noonan S, Wade V, Currie BJ. The 2020 Australian Guideline for prevention, diagnosis and management of acute rheumatic fever and rheumatic heart disease. Med J Aust. 2021;214(5):220-7.
7. Dougherty S, Essop MR, Webb R, Price S, Wilson N. Complications of rheumatic heart disease and acute emergencies. In: Dougherty S, Carapetis J, Zuhlke L, Wilson N (Eds). Acute Rheumatic Fever and Rheumatic Heart Disease, 1st edition. St Louis, MO: Elsevier Science Ltd; 2021. pp. 301-36.
8. Committee on Practice Bulletins-Obstetrics. ACOG Practice Bulletin No. 199: Use of Prophylactic Antibiotics in Labor and Delivery. Obstet Gynecol. 2018;132(3):e103-19.
9. Bortnick AE, Levine LD. Valvular heart disease in pregnancy. Clin Obstet Gynecol. 2020;63(4):910-22.
10. Mocumbi A, Beaton A, Soma-Pillay P, Dougherty Scott, Sliwa K. Rheumatic Heart Disease in Pregnancy. In: Dougherty S, Carapetis J, Zuhlke L, Wilson N (Eds). Acute Rheumatic Fever and Rheumatic Heart Disease, 1st edition. St Louis, MO: Elsevier Science Ltd; 2021. pp. 171-93.
11. Lewey J, Andrade L, Levine LD. Valvular heart disease in pregnancy. Cardiol Clin. 2021;39(1):151-61.
12. Regitz-Zagrosek V, Roos-Hesselink JW, Bauersachs J, Blomström-Lundqvist C, Cífková R, De Bonis M, et al. 2018 ESC Guidelines for the management of cardiovascular diseases during pregnancy. Eur Heart J. 2018;39(34):3165-241.
13. Bonis MD, Lancellotti P. Combined and multiple valve diseases. In: Camm AJ, Luscher TF, Maurer G, Serruys PW (Eds). The ESC Textbook of Cardiovascular Medicine, 3rd edition. The European Society of Cardiology Series. New Delhi: ESC Publications; 2018.
14. Enriquez AD, Economy KE, Tedrow UB. Contemporary management of arrhythmias during pregnancy. Circ Arrhythm Electrophysiol. 2014;7(5):961-7.
15. Mooradian AD. Digitalis. An update of clinical pharmacokinetics, therapeutic monitoring techniques and treatment recommendations. Clin Pharmacokinet. 1988;15(3):165-79.
16. Tamirisa KP, Elkayam U, Briller JE, Mason PK, Pillarisetti J, Merchant FM, et al. Arrhythmias in pregnancy. JACC Clin Electrophysiol. 2022;8(1):120-35.

17. Ibetoh CN, Stratulat E, Liu F, Wuni GY, Bahuva R, Shafiq MA, et al. Supraventricular Tachycardia in Pregnancy: Gestational and Labor Differences in Treatment. Cureus. 2021;13(10):e18479.
18. Page RL, Joglar JA, Caldwell MA, Calkins H, Conti JB, Deal BJ, et al. 2015 ACC/AHA/HRS guideline for the management of adult patients with supraventricular tachycardia: a report of the American College of Cardiology/American Heart Association Task Force on Clinical Practice Guidelines and the Heart Rhythm Society. J Am Coll Cardiol. 2016; 67(13):e27-115.
19. Okello E, Mordi I, Lang C, Sable C, Dougherty S, Wilson N. Medical Management of Rheumatic Heart Disease. In: Dougherty S, Carapetis J, Zuhlke L, Wilson N (Eds). Acute Rheumatic Fever and Rheumatic Heart Disease, 1st edition. St Louis, MO: Elsevier Science Ltd; 2021. pp. 107-32.

Chapter 7

Mechanical and Prosthetic Heart Valves: Anticoagulant Therapy

Jaya Chawla, Kiran Dhawan

■ MAGNITUDE OF THE PROBLEM

Heart disease complicates pregnancy in about 1.46% of cases, as per most recently published data on Southeast Asia.[1] The European Society of Cardiology (ESC) Registry of Pregnancy and Cardiac disease (ROPAC) estimates 29% cases of heart disease in pregnancy to be accounted for by valvular heart disease and the likelihood of facing a pregnancy complication with mechanical valve prosthesis is astronomically high at 42%.[2]

Since, being on anticoagulation is an independent risk factor for heart failure and maternal mortality, this chapter has been dedicated to a focused discussion on the options of anticoagulant therapy in pregnant women with mechanical valve prosthesis.[2]

Mechanical valve prosthesis merits lifelong anticoagulation to mitigate the risks of thromboembolism which are potentially lethal to both the mother and the fetus. This risk is amplified during pregnancy and puerperium owing to the hypercoagulable state and owing to physiological changes of pregnancy that alter the pharmacokinetics of the drugs used. The risk is further modified based on the site of the prosthesis with right-sided lesions faring worse than the left-sided ones and mitral valve prosthesis having a graver prognosis compared to aortic in terms of thromboembolic sequelae. The ROPAC data suggests that the risk of valve thrombosis during pregnancy overall is nearly 4.7% with mortality rates as high as 20%.[2]

This risk varies with the anticoagulant medication. The two most appropriate drugs to keep the maternal risks of thromboembolism in check are the vitamin K antagonists and heparin.

Vitamin K antagonists: They are one of the two most important categories of drugs used in anticoagulation. The prototype drug in this category is warfarin, others being acenocoumarol and phenprocoumon.

Vitamin K taken from diet is reduced by the enzyme vitamin K reductase to vitamin KH2 (reduced vitamin K). This reduced vitamin K is the substrate for the carboxylation of glutamate to carboxyglutamate in tissues. This conversion is necessary for the biological activity of coagulation factors II, VII, XI, and X. This carboxylation is coupled to another reaction that oxidizes reduced vitamin K to vitamin K epoxide. The enzyme vitamin KO reductase is needed to reduce vitamin K epoxide to K1. Warfarin blocks this step thereby reducing the bioavailability of these clotting factors.[3]

In addition, as is understood, supplementing vitamin K_1 in any form oral or parenteral can circumvent this block. Also, the step of carboxylation of glutamate also takes place in bones. Placental transfer of warfarin in the first trimester affects this step leading to features of warfarin embryopathy, discussed later in this chapter.

■ PHARMACOKINETICS

Warfarin, administered orally, is completely absorbed through the gastrointestinal tract. It is 99% protein bound in circulation. Its half-life on an average is 40 hours (20–60 hours range). It is a racemic mixture of two optically active isomers S-warfarin and R-warfarin. The former being 5 times more potent than the latter and the half-life of the former being slightly shorter than the latter (37–89 hours vs. 21–43 hours).[4] It is metabolized in the liver via the cytochrome P450 enzyme pathway. Therefore, enzyme-inducing agents are likely to have a drug–drug interaction (DDI) with warfarin **(Table 1)**.

TABLE 1: Warfarin: Drug interactions.[5]

S. no.	Bioavailability		Mechanism
	Increased by	**Decreased by**	
1.		Cholestyramine	Decreases absorption
2.		Barbiturates	Decrease clearance
3.		Rifampicin	Induces cytochrome P450
4.		Carbamazepine	Decrease clearance
5.		Phenytoin prolonged use	Induces cytochrome P450
6.	Phenytoin initially		Displaces warfarin from protein binding sites
7.	Trimethoprim-sulfamethoxazole		Decreased clearance
8.	Sulfonamides		Decrease absorption of vitamin K by altering gut flora
9.	Metronidazole		Decreased clearance
10.	2nd/3rd-generation cephalosporins		Interrupt the vitamin K cycle **(Fig. 1)**
11.	Phenylbutazone		Decreased clearance
12.	Sulfinpyrazone		Decreased clearance
13.	Salicylates in doses >1.5 g/d		Anticoagulant properties
14.	Aspirin, NSAIDs, penicillins, moxalactam		Decrease platelet function
15.	Cimetidine and omeprazole		Decrease clearance*
16.	Thyroxine		Accelerates metabolism of clotting factors
17.	Amiodarone		Decrease clearance

*Warfarin is made up of a racemic mixture of two optically active isomers warfarin-S and warfarin-R. These drugs decrease clearance of the less potent R isomer. Therefore, effect is not very significant clinically.
(NSAID: nonsteroidal anti-inflammatory drug)

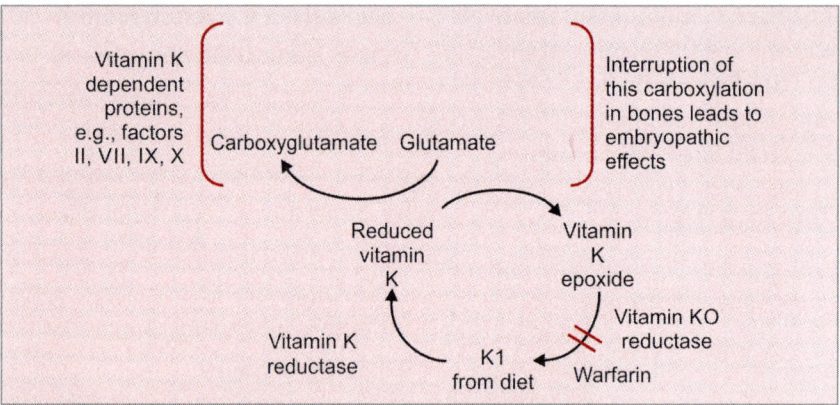

Fig. 1: Mechanism of action of warfarin.

MONITORING OF ANTICOAGULANT EFFECT: WARFARIN

The anticoagulant effect of warfarin is measured using prothrombin time (PT) international normalized ratio (INR). It reflects changes in three out of the four clotting factors that are dependent on vitamin K for their biological activity. The rate of curtailment of their activity by warfarin is proportionate to their corresponding half-lives. Hence, for the initial few days of therapy alteration in PT is a result of reduction in factor VII activity, whose half-life is 6 hours. Thereafter, further increase in PT is related to ameliorated activity of factors II and X.

Optimum anticoagulant effect is expected within 2–7 days after initiation of therapy, depending upon the dose. It usually takes 3 days to stabilize.[5] Since anticoagulation achieved with warfarin would take time, it is prudent to initiate simultaneous therapy with low molecular weight heparin (which has a shorter peak) when rapid therapeutic action is desired. The initial dose of warfarin is usually 2–3 mg once a day which is later titrated to achieve an INR between 2 and 3 **(Table 2)**.[3]

ADVANTAGES

The risk of valve thrombosis in a regime using VKA throughout pregnancy is between 0.4 and 4%,[7] which is the minimum risk when compared with all other choices as discussed later. Acknowledging the lack of robust evidence, in the form of randomized controlled trials, the ESC recommends that VKA throughout regimes are the safest regime to prevent valvular thrombosis during pregnancy, when administered under stringent INR monitoring.[8]

DISADVANTAGES

Vitamin K antagonists cross the placenta and are therefore associated with embryopathy in the first trimester between weeks 6 and 12. The risk is dose dependent. With low dose VKAs (implying warfarin <5 mg per day, acenocoumarol <2 mg per day, and phenprocoumon <3 mg per day), the risk is between 0.45 and 0.9%.[7,9,10]

Warfarin embryopathy is characterized by skeletal defects such as epiphysial stippling of long bones, nasal bridge hypoplasia, central nervous system anomalies such as ventriculomegaly and agenesis of corpus callosum and congenital cardiac defects.[6]

TABLE 2: Anticoagulant drugs in pregnancy with mitral valve replacement: Clinical considerations.

S. no.	Name	Dosage	Maximum dose	Route/ frequency of administration	Pharmacokinetics	Adverse effects	Contraindications	Cost*
1.	**Vitamin K antagonist**							
a.	Warfarin	1/2/5 mg tablets	10 mg/d	Per oral once a day	• T½: 40 hours • Metabolism in liver by CYP450	• Warfarin embryopathy, fetopathy, miscarriage, intrauterine demise • Hemorrhage	Malignant hypertension	Varies from 11 to 20 INR for a pack of 10 tablets
b.	Acenocoumarol	1/2/3/4 mg tablets	5 mg/d	Per oral once a day	• T½: 8–11 hours • Metabolism in liver by CYP450	Hemorrhage		Varies from 31 to 64 INR for a pack of 10 tablets depending on strength
c.	Phenprocoumon	50/100/200/ 300/400 mg tablets	5 mg/d	Per oral once a day	• T½: 6 days • Metabolism in liver by CYP2C9, CYP3A4	Hemorrhage	Hypersensitivity, hypotension, left ventricular outflow tract obstruction, cardiogenic shock	
2.	**Heparin**						• Active hemorrhage (antepartum or postpartum) DIC, thrombocytopenia (platelet count <75,000/cc), uncontrolled hypertension defined as diastolic BP >120 mm Hg or systolic BP >200 mm Hg, medical renal disease with GFR <30 mL/min/1.73 m², severe hepatic dysfunction with increased prothrombin time, history of stroke within last 4 weeks • Bleeding disorders like von Willebrand's disease or hemophilia	

Contd...

SECTION 3: Medical Management of Heart Disease in Pregnancy

Contd...

S. no.	Name	Dosage	Maximum dose	Route/ frequency of administration	Pharmacokinetics	Adverse effects	Contraindications	Cost*
a.	UFH	25,000 IU in 5 mL vial	5,000 units for every single dose		• T½: 1–2 hours • Hepatic metabolism	Hemorrhage, heparin-induced thrombocytopenia, heparin-induced osteopenia	• The platelet count is 100,000/mm or lower • The patient cannot have routine monitoring tests performed to monitor therapeutic heparin • The patient has an active, uncontrollable bleed except for DIC • Patients with a history of heparin-induced thrombocytopenia should also avoid heparin use • Patients with known case of bleeding disorders	204–305 INR
b.	LMWH	• 40 mg/ 0.4 mL • 60 mg/ 0.6 mL	120 mg BD or 180 mg OD of enoxaparin		• T½: 2–7 hours • Renal metabolism	Hemorrhage	• The platelet count is 100,000/mm or lower • The patient cannot have routine monitoring tests performed to monitor therapeutic heparin • The patient has an active, uncontrollable bleed except for DIC • Patients with known case of bleeding disorders	• 385–427 INR • 355–577 INR

*From Med India

(DIC: disseminated intravascular coagulation; LMWH: low molecular weight heparin; UFH: unfractionated heparin)

Source: Royal College of Obstetricians and Gynaecologists. Reducing the risk of venous thromboembolism during pregnancy and the puerperium. Green Top Guideline No. 37a. London (UK): RCOG; 2015.[6]

In addition, with use in the second and third trimesters, there is a risk of fetopathy involving the fetal central nervous system (CNS) and eyes. The estimated risk is 0.7–2%. Warfarin is also associated with a dose-dependent risk of miscarriage and fetal demise. Owing to the risk of fetal intracranial hemorrhage, vaginal birth is contraindicated when the mother is on warfarin.[8]

The rate of postpartum hemorrhage increases with all anticoagulant drugs. Keeping this in mind, it is prudent to delay the overlap of warfarin with low molecular weight heparin (LMWH) by 5–7 days post-delivery irrespective of the route of birth.[6]

Warfarin toxicity: The most clinically relevant side effect is bleeding which could manifest as postpartum hemorrhage besides bleeding from other sites, such as hematemesis, melena, epistaxis, and hematuria.

How to treat bleeding due to warfarin: Four-factor prothrombin complex concentrate (4f-PCC) should ideally be administered for reversal. In case 4f-PCC is not available, fresh frozen plasma can be used.[11] If there is no bleeding but the INR is close to 10, warfarin should be stopped and oral vitamin K started 1–5 mg a day. The oral route will take at least 24 hours to reverse warfarin-induced coagulopathy, so in case of bleeding or when a more rapid response is desired, intravenous vitamin K, 1–10 mg as guided by the severity should be administered. This route is expected to reverse the pathology in 4–6 hours.

In case a more rapid response is warranted, 4f-PCC can reverse coagulopathy in 15–30 minutes and with much less volume transfused than FFP.[12,13]

HEPARIN STRUCTURE AND BIOSYNTHESIS

Heparin is a biomolecule belonging to the class of glycosaminoglycans (GAGs) that are large linear polysaccharide structures, composed of repeated structural motifs. Heparin synthesis occurs through a complex process that involves many enzymatic steps.[14] The discovery that heparins' anticoagulant effects toward coagulation factor Xa (FXa) and thrombin could be separated, led to the production of shorter heparin subtypes with optimized anticoagulant activity and reduced risk of bleeding as compared with UFH. These heparins are obtained by fragmentation of UFH and are commonly known as LMWHs. The size of UFH molecules ranges from 6 to 60 kDa; while LMWHs vary between 1 and 10 kDa.[15,16]

Pharmacokinetics

Heparin is a large, highly ionized molecule which is not absorbed orally. When injected intravenously (IV) it acts immediately, but after subcutaneous (SC) injection anticoagulant action takes approximately 60 minutes. Heparin does not cross the blood–brain barrier or placenta thus, making it a safe option for the fetus during pregnancy. It is metabolized in liver by the enzyme heparinase and excreted in urine. Heparin is released endogenously from mast cells and is degraded by tissue macrophages. After administering IV injection of doses <100 U/kg, the half life averages 1 hour. Beyond this period, dose-dependent inactivation is seen and t½ is prolonged to 1–4 hours. Half life is longer in patients with cirrhosis and renal failure, and is shorter in patients suffering from pulmonary embolism.[17]

Mechanism of Action

Heparin is an immediately acting anti-coagulant which is effective both in vivo and in vitro. It acts by indirectly activating plasma antithrombin III (AT III, a serine proteinase inhibitor) **(Fig. 2)**. This heparin-AT III complex then binds to clotting factors of the

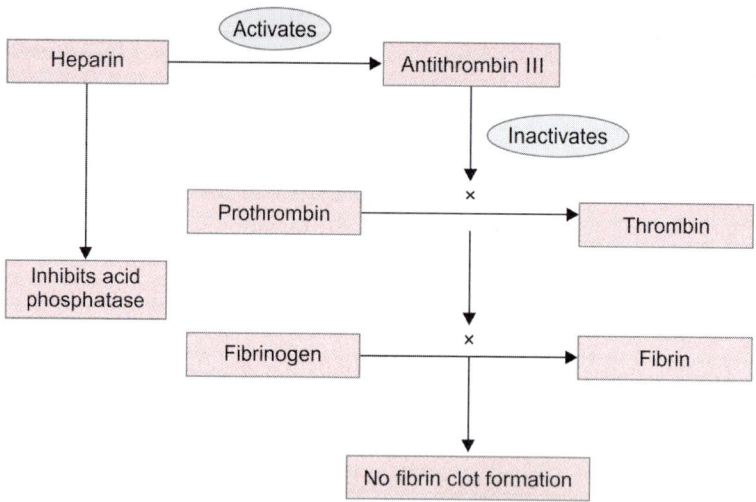

Fig. 2: Mechanism of action of heparin.

intrinsic and common pathways (Xa, IIa, IXa, XIa, XIIa, and XIIIa) which then inactivate them. At low concentrations of heparin, factor Xa-mediated conversion of prothrombin to thrombin is selectively affected. The anticoagulant mechanism of heparin is exerted mainly by inhibition of factor Xa as well as thrombin (IIa) mediated conversion of fibrinogen to fibrin.[17]

The LMWH has several advantages over UFH as it has a higher bioavailability, has a better predictable dosing, and is associated with less adverse reactions. Thus, LMWH has become the heparin of choice for many clinical conditions such as venous thromboembolism (VTE), major surgery, and acute coronary syndrome.[18,19] UFH, however, is usually preferred in patients with renal failure due to less dependence on the kidneys for clearance and also improved reversibility with protamine.[20]

Unfractionated Heparin

Unfractionated heparin (UFH) is administered parenterally, used subcutaneously when given for prophylaxis and as a continuous intravenous infusion when administered therapeutically as it assures fast and potent anticoagulation when given intravenously. UFH has a faster onset of action when compared to warfarin. Therapeutic efficacy of UFH is achieved within 20–60 minutes when administered subcutaneously. The half-life of UFH is shorter than LMWH, being 1.5 hours when administered subcutaneously and 30 minutes via intravenous route **(Table 3)**.[8]

Side Effects and Reversal Agents

- Hemorrhage is the main adverse reaction in patients receiving UFH. The incidence of major bleeding depends on the indication of its use, dosage, and route of administration. Usually, UFH when used for therapeutic purposes is associated with a 2.0% incidence of major bleeding event.[9]
- Effect of UFH can be reversed with protamine sulfate. The dose depends on the amount of UFH administered. One milligram of protamine sulfate neutralizes 100 units of UFH.
- Another important adverse reaction associated with UFH use is heparin-induced thrombocytopenia (HIT).

TABLE 3: Heparin and its derivatives.

	UFH	LMWH
Mechanism	Enhances AT effect on factor Xa and thrombin	Enhances AT effect more specifically on factor Xa than thrombin
Plasma protein binding	Nonspecific	Less binding
Dose response curve	Unpredictable	More predictable
Half life	1–2 hours	2–7 hours
Dosing frequency	Continuous IV drip, subcutaneous twice or thrice daily	Subcutaneous BD or once daily
Clearance	Hepatic and reticuloendothelial system. No renal clearance	Renal clearance. Dose adjustment required in renal impairment
Ability to cause HIT	Yes	Yes
Routine monitoring	aPTT	Factor Xa

(aPTT: activated partial thromboplastin time; AT: antithrombin; LMWH: low molecular weight heparin; UFH: unfractionated heparin)

It occurs in 0.1–5% of patients who receive therapeutic doses of heparin.[10] There are two types of HIT, with the first type, which is rare in clinical practice, is associated with the exposure of patients to UFH or high heparin doses for the first time. This is due to a nonimmune thrombocytopenic response caused by binding of heparin to platelet factor 4, which results in ultra-large complexes (ULCs) that trigger platelet activation or via a fibrinogen receptor modulated lowering of platelet counts. HIT type 2 is an immune-mediated response where antibodies are generated against ULCs. It causes life-threatening thrombosis and thrombocytopenia and is seen usually 5–10 days after the initiation of heparin therapy. Immediate stopping of heparin is important to allow increase of platelet counts. American Society of Hematology recommends the use of nonheparin anticoagulants (such as danaparoid, fondaparinux) for treatment of acute HIT.[7] However, data supporting their use in pregnancy is very limited.

Low Molecular Weight Heparin

These are parenterally administered drugs, and include dalteparin, enoxaparin, and tinzaparin. Compared with UFH, the LMWHs have the advantage of having a more predictable dose-response curve.[11] Thus, the LMWHs are administered at a fixed dose, which is based on total body weight, and do not require tight regulation and monitoring as is with the use of warfarin and UFH.[11] These drugs have nearly 100% bioavailability and reach peak levels within 2–4 hours after subcutaneous administration.[8,11] Their half-life is of 3–4 hours and these drugs are eliminated majorly (80%) via renal clearance, thus requiring dose reduction in patients with renal insufficiency.[8] Additionally, since dose is based on total body weight, dosing complications arise in obese patients.[11] Although therapeutic monitoring is not routinely indicated, in cases of patients with renal insufficiency, obesity, or in an iatrogenic overdose, anti-factor Xa levels can be used to monitor LMWH.[8,11] Ideally, the anti-factor

Xa level should be obtained 4 hours after the administration of LMWH. Certain studies though recommend routine monitoring with a combination of trough and peak anti-Xa levels in high-risk patients (i.e., women with MHV), and only peak anti-Xa levels in patients with low-risk pregnancies (i.e., women with acute VTE during pregnancy). Generally, LMWH is administered every 12 hours, and the dose is adjusted to maintain anti-Xa levels based on the specific indication for anticoagulation (i.e., for patients with MHV: target trough anti-Xa level is 0.6 U/mL, and peak anti-Xa level 1.0–1.2 U/mL; and for patients with acute VTE: target peak anti-Xa level is 0.5–1.0 U/mL).[12-14]

Side Effects and Reversal Agents

- Acute bleeding is the major risk associated with LMWH. When used in prophylactic doses the incidence of major bleeding is 1.5–1.7%.[15]
- When given in therapeutic dosage, risk of acute bleeding is slightly raised at 2%, with even higher incidences observed when it is used to treat acute coronary syndrome (ACS).[15] In the event of major bleeding, protamine sulfate can be used as a partial reversal agent and can neutralize up to 60% of the anticoagulation effect of LMWH.[15] Initial doses of 1 mg per 100 units of antifactor Xa should be administered within 8 hours of LMWH administration.[16] A second dose of 0.5 mg per 100 units anti-factor Xa can also be repeated. In case of major bleeding associated with LMWH, cryoprecipitate and FFP are also recommended.[15,17]

Data on other adverse or side effects of heparin use is scarce. These include the association of heparin with osteoporosis[18] and skin lesions.[19] It is usually seen that long-term use of UFH is associated with a 2.2–5% incidence of heparin-induced osteoporotic fracture, which is far less associated with LMWH. The molecular mechanism of heparin-induced osteoporosis usually involves the resorption of bone by osteoclasts. In addition, there is also suppression of osteoblast function.[19] Very little data is available on the incidence of heparin-induced skin lesions, but a study from 2009 found that 7.5% of patients receiving subcutaneous heparin developed skin lesions. In all these patients, a delayed-type hypersensitivity reaction was the reason for the lesion which occurred after prolonged heparin use.

ANTICOAGULATION IN PREGNANCY: TRIMESTER-WISE RECOMMENDED PROTOCOLS

As per the ESC guidelines,[8] women on VKAs should be counseled regarding the dose-related risk of embryopathy and offered the choice of:

- Continuing with VKAs throughout pregnancy
- Switching over to heparin from 6 to 12 weeks to mitigate this risk and switch back to VKAs from 12 weeks onward

In both circumstances, at 36 weeks of gestation, they should be admitted for switch over to heparin, to prevent going in labor on a VKA as this has the potential risk of intracranial hemorrhage for the fetus.

After 6 hours of birth, women should be started on unfractionated heparin for anticoagulation and their aPTT monitored **(Fig. 3)**.

In case of cesarean birth, therapeutic dose of LMWH should be stopped 24 hours of elective surgery and women shifted to unfractionated heparin which is monitored using aPTT. Unfractionated heparin is stopped 6 hours prior to surgery and spinal

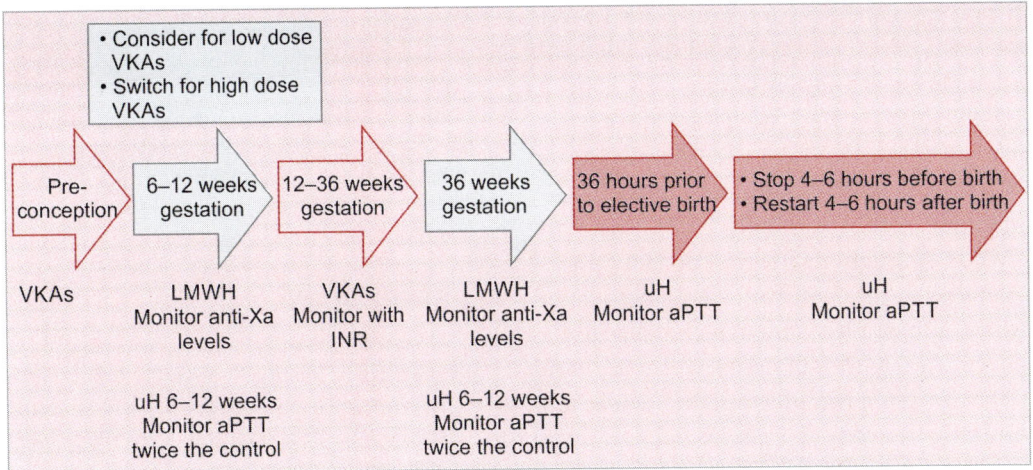

Fig. 3: Recommended timeline for anticoagulants in pregnancy. (VKA: vitamin K antagonists; LMWH: low molecular weight heparin; uH: unfractionated heparin; aPTT: activated partial thromboplastin time; INR: international normalized ratio)
Source: ESC guidelines[8]

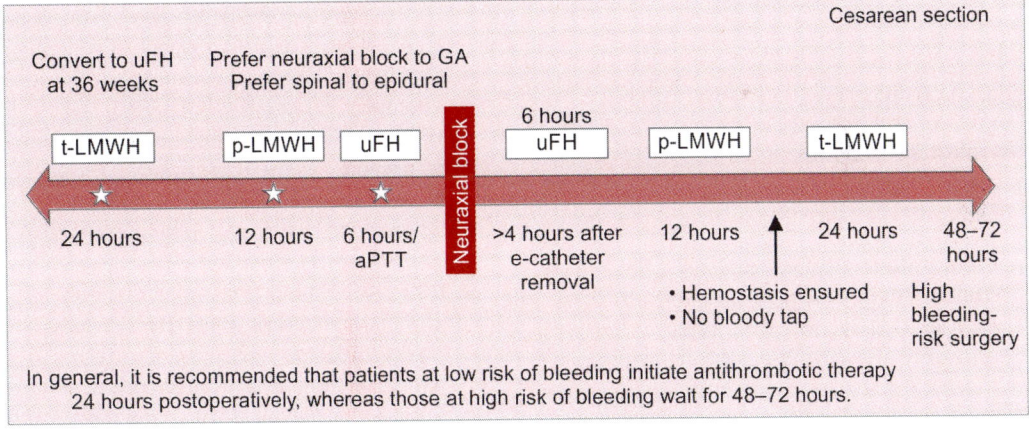

Fig. 4: Timeline of anticoagulant therapy immediately prior to and following a cesarean section. (t-LMWH: therapeutic dose low molecular weight heparin; p-LMWH: prophylactic dose low molecular weight heparin; GA: general anesthesia; e-catheter: epidural catheter)

anesthesia is preferred. If there is no risk of hemorrhage, UFH may be restarted 6 hours later (taking care that epidural catheter, if inserted, has been removed at least 4 hours prior). Therapeutic dose of LMWH can be started after 24 hours provided there is no risk of hemorrhage. In case of high risk of bleeding, this should be delayed for until 48 hours **(Fig. 4)**.[8]

All anticoagulants carry an increased risk of miscarriage. VKAs during the first trimester are associated with an increased risk of miscarriage compared with LMWH or UFH (28.6% vs. 9.2%), and the live birth rate is lower.[20] The risk of fetal loss is dose-related (13.4–19.2% with low dose VKA; overall risk with VKA is 32.5%). Incidence of fetal loss with a combined heparin/VKA regimen is approximately 22.7% and with LMWH throughout pregnancy is 12.2%.[7,21] VKA use in the first trimester is associated with embryopathy (limb defects, nasal hypoplasia) in 0.6–10% of cases; in second and third trimester, risk of fetopathy (ocular and central nervous system abnormalities, intracranial hemorrhage) is around 0.7–2%.[7,22-26] Hemorrhagic complications (including retroplacental bleeding leading to premature birth and fetal demise) and postpartum hemorrhage in the mother occur with all anticoagulants, but the incidence is lower with VKA throughout pregnancy than with LMWH/UFH.[7]

■ KEY POINTS

- Unfractionated heparin (UFH) and LMWH do not cross the placenta, thus substitution of VKA with UFH or LMWH in weeks 6–12 almost eliminates the risk of embryopathy.
- The risk of embryopathy is also dose-dependent (0.45–0.9% with low-dose warfarin).[7,21]
- During the second and third trimesters and until the 36th week, VKAs are recommended in women who require low-dose anticoagulation.
- It is ideal to discontinue VKA and start adjusted-dose intravenous UFH (maintaining aPTT ≥2 control) or adjusted-dose LMWH at the 36th week of gestation because of their lower half lives.
- If the woman delivers while on VKA or in less than 2 weeks after discontinuation of a VKA, cesarean section is indicated to prevent intracranial hemorrhage in the fetus.
- It is recommended to anticipate the timing of delivery to ensure safe and effective peripartum anticoagulation.
- Immediate echocardiography is recommended in women with mechanical valves presenting with dyspnea and/or an embolic event.
- Addition of low-dose aspirin to VKA or heparin has no proven advantage in preventing valve thrombosis but is associated with significantly more maternal bleeding complications, including fatal events.[8]

■ REFERENCES

1. Shrestha P, Kuikel S, Bajracharya S, Ghimire A, Shrestha R, Mishra A, et al. Pregnancy with heart disease in South Asia: a systematic review and meta-analysis of prevalence and outcome. Ann Med Surg. 2022;80:25-36.
2. Roos-Hesselink J, Baris L, Johnson M, De Backer J, Otto C, Marelli A, et al. Pregnancy outcomes in women with cardiovascular disease: evolving trends over 10 years in the ESC Registry of Pregnancy And Cardiac disease (ROPAC). Eur Heart J. 2019;40(47):3848-55.
3. Hirsh J, Fuster V, Ansell J, Halperin J. American Heart Association/American College of Cardiology Foundation Guide to Warfarin Therapy. Circulation. 2003;107(12):1692-711.
4. Walfisch A, Koren G. The "warfarin window" in pregnancy: the importance of half-life. J Obstet Gynaecol Can. 2010;32(10):988-9.
5. Holford NH. Clinical pharmacokinetics and pharmacodynamics of warfarin. Understanding the dose-effect relationship. Clin Pharmacokinet. 1986;11(6):483-504.
6. Royal College of Obstetricians and Gynaecologists. Reducing the risk of venous thromboembolism during pregnancy and the puerperium. Green Top Guideline No. 37a. London (UK): RCOG; 2015.
7. Xu Z, Fan J, Luo X, Zhang WB, Ma J, Lin YB, et al. Anticoagulation regimens during pregnancy in patients with mechanical heart valves: A systematic review and meta-analysis. Can J Cardiol. 2016;32:1248.e1-e9.
8. Regitz-Zagrosek V, Roos-Hesselink JW, Bauersachs J, Blomström-Lundqvist C, Cífková R, De Bonis M, et al. ESC Guidelines for the management of cardiovascular diseases during pregnancy: The Task Force

for the Management of Cardiovascular Diseases during Pregnancy of the European Society of Cardiology (ESC). Eur Heart J. 2018;39(34):3165-241.
9. Zagrosek-Regitz V, Pieper PG, Iung B. Valvular heart disease. In: Camm AJ, Lüscher TF, Maurer G, Serruys PW (Eds). The ESC Textbook of Cardiovascular Medicine, 3 edition. London: OUP Oxford; 2018.
10. Hassouna A, Allam H. Limited dose warfarin throughout pregnancy in patients with mechanical heart valve prosthesis: a meta-analysis. Interact Cardiovasc Thorac Surg. 2014;18:797-806.
11. Tomaselli GF, Mahaffey KW, Cuker A, Dobesh PP, Doherty JU, Eikelboom JW, et al. 2020 ACC expert consensus decision pathway on management of bleeding in patients on oral anticoagulants. J Am Coll Cardiol. 2020;76(5):594-622.
12. Holbrook A, Schulman S, Witt DM, Vandvik PO, Fish J, Kovacs MJ, et al. Evidence-based management of anticoagulant therapy: Antithrombotic therapy and prevention of thrombosis, 9th edition: American College of Chest Physicians Evidence-Based Clinical Practice Guidelines. Chest. 2012;141(2 Suppl):e152S-84S.
13. Yates SG, Sarode R. New strategies for effective treatment of vitamin K antagonist-associated bleeding. J Thromb Haemost. 2015;13 Suppl 1:S180-6.
14. Shriver Z, Capila I, Venkataraman G, Sasisekharan R. Heparin and heparan sulfate: analyzing structure and microheterogeneity. Handb Exp Pharmacol. 2012;(207):159-76.
15. Bertini S, Bisio A, Torri G, Bensi D, Terbojevich M. Molecular weight determination of heparin and dermatan sulfate by size exclusion chromatography with a triple detector array. Biomacromolecules. 2005; 6(01):168-73.
16. Bertini S, Fareed J, Madaschi L, Risi G, Torri G, Naggi A. Characterization of PF4-heparin complexes by photon correlation spectroscopy and zeta potential. Clin Appl Thromb Hemost. 2017;23(07):725-34.
17. Tripathi KD. Drugs affecting Coagulation, Bleeding and Thrombosis. In: Essentials of Medical Pharmacology. New Delhi: Jaypee Brothers Medical Publishers; 2015.
18. Walenga JM, Lyman GH. Evolution of heparin anticoagulants to ultra-low-molecular-weight heparins: a review of pharmacologic and clinical differences and applications in patients with cancer. Crit Rev Oncol Hematol. 2013;88(01):1-18.
19. Laporte S, Liotier J, Bertoletti L, Kleber FX, Pineo GF, Chapelle C, et al. Individual patient data meta-analysis of enoxaparin vs unfractionated heparin for venous thromboembolism prevention in medical patients. J Thromb Haemost. 2011;9(03):464-72.
20. Hirsh J, Warkentin TE, Shaughnessy SG, Anand SS, Halperin JL, Raschke R, et al. Heparin and low molecular-weight heparin: mechanisms of action, pharmacokinetics, dosing, monitoring, efficacy, and safety. Chest. 2001;119(Suppl 1):64S-94S.
21. Alshawabkeh L, Economy K, Valente AM. Anticoagulation During Pregnancy. J Am Coll Cardiol. 2016;68(16):1804-13.
22. Sillesen M, Hjortdal V, Vejlstrup N, Sorensen K. Pregnancy with prosthetic heart valves—30 years' nationwide experience in Denmark. Eur J Cardiothorac Surg. 2011;40:448-54.
23. Chan WS, Anand S, Ginsberg JS. Anticoagulation of pregnant women with mechanical heart valves: A systematic review of the literature. Arch Intern Med. 2000;160:191-6.
24. van Driel D, Wesseling J, Sauer PJ, Touwen BC, van der Veer E, Heymans HS. Teratogen update: Fetal effects after in utero exposure to coumarins overview of cases, follow-up findings, and pathogenesis. Teratology. 2002;66:127-40.
25. Vitale N, De Feo M, De Santo LS, Pollice A, Tedesco N, Cotrufo M. Dose-dependent fetal complications of warfarin in pregnant women with mechanical heart valves. J Am Coll Cardiol. 1999;33:1637-41.
26. Wesseling J, Van Driel D, Heymans HS, Rosendaal FR, Geven-Boere LM, Smrkovsky M, et al. Coumarins during pregnancy: Long-term effects on growth and development of school-age children. Thromb Haemost. 2001;85:609-13.

Chapter 8

Heart Failure

Puneet Aggarwal, Pradyumna Kumar Singh, Dheerendra Kuber, Ranjit Kumar Nath

The most common cause of morbidity and mortality observed during pregnancy is heart failure (HF) where its prevalence ranges from 13[1] to 33%[2] (in women with preexisting cardiac disease vs. with cardiomyopathy respectively) and it is the most frequent complication of cardiovascular disease observed in pregnancy. Congenital heart disease (CHD) in western countries and rheumatic heart disease (RHD) in low- and middle-income countries are most common cause, accounting for up to 88–90% of cases.[3]

Multiple hemodynamic changes occur within the maternal cardiovascular system, supporting the safety along with health of the mother and her fetus during pregnancy **(Fig. 1)**. These continuous adaptions create physiologic stress which can risk the balance especially in previously compromised patients and in others it may result in development of new cardiovascular condition or precipitate heart failure.

In the postpartum period around 60% cases of heart failure are observed whereas during delivery it accounts to be 27% cases and during the gestation period the heart failure cases numbered to be 13%.[4] In mothers with known cases of cardiac disease, the timing of heart failure displays a bimodal distribution with the peaks both at 20–30 weeks of gestation and postpartum.[1] The onset of HF is experienced at the weeks before and after delivery by the patients with known cardiomyopathy while those with valvular heart disease develop HF throughout their gestation period. An earlier onset of HF, i.e., at about 25 weeks of pregnancy is experienced by the women with shunt lesions.[1]

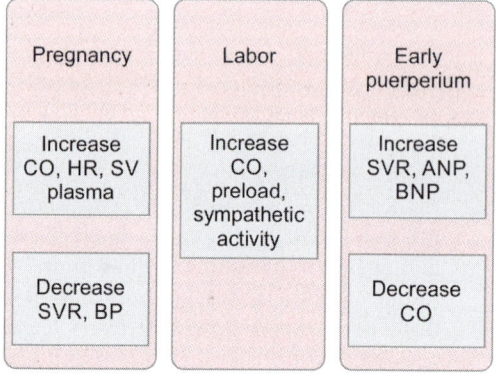

Fig. 1: Changes in maternal cardiovascular physiology during pregnancy. (ANP: atrial natriuretic peptide; BNP: brain natriuretic peptide; BP: blood pressure; CO: cardiac output; HR: heart rate; SV: stroke volume; SVR: systemic vascular resistance)

Rheumatic heart disease is the leading cause of heart failure in India and other developing countries whereas cardiomyopathy and congenital heart disease remain the leading cause in developed countries. In the antenatal period, about 75% of the cases are diagnosed while the rest 25% of HF cases are diagnosed during gestation.[5] Heart failure mimics many normal symptoms in pregnancy such as breathlessness, palpitation, and swelling of legs, making the diagnosis challenging. However, any type of arrhythmia, tachypnea, cyanosis, hypoxia, clubbing, diastolic murmur, marked peripheral edema, murmur with a thrill, or an evidence of pulmonary edema warrant further evaluation. The commonly observed symptoms in the pregnant women with HF are bilateral pitting pedal edema, dyspnea, elevated jugular venous pressure, cough, tender hepatomegaly, and third heart sound.[6]

THERAPEUTICS AND PRINCIPLES OF MANAGEMENT

The nature of the initial evaluation and management in pregnant patients with or at risk of initial evaluation varies according to the setting. However, stable as well as decompensated patients require joint cardiac and obstetric care; including baseline and follow-up echocardiogram, serial B-Natriuretic peptide (BNP) level as well as fetal ultrasound examinations.[7]

In stable HF patients, the management is similar to the management of a non-pregnant patient with the exception of teratogenic agents such as angiotensin-converting enzyme inhibitors, mineralocorticoid receptor antagonists, angiotensin II receptor blockers (ARB), atenolol, angiotensin receptor neprilysin inhibitors (ARNI), direct factor Xa inhibitors, SGLT-2 Inhibitors **(Table 1)**. So, the treatment's mainstay is beta-blockers (except atenolol), diuretics, hydralazine, and nitrates. In patients with signs and symptoms of heart failure diuretics should be used with caution as they have potential to cause electrolyte imbalance and reduce placental perfusion in the fetus.[8] Although there is less beneficial evidence available, nitrates and hydralazine appear to be safer in pregnancy than angiotensin-converting enzyme (ACE) inhibitors, and hence should be used only in the presence of severe LV dysfunction, hypertension, and/or indication of congestion in decompensated heart failure. The drugs that block beta receptors (beta-blockers) should be initiated at low doses, however the dose escalation is done gradually with caution. Once the woman is postpartum stage i.e., when there are less concerns regarding fetal maturity or teratogenicity, the patient is to be shifted to more standard therapy for heart failure.

In patients with acute heart failure with hemodynamic instability or cardiogenic shock, the initial goal is stabilizing the patient, confirming the diagnosis, assessing the severity of HF, assessing the fetal status and its viability. The precipitating factors such as infection, lower respiratory infection or pneumonia, pulmonary embolism, eclampsia-preeclampsia, or comorbidity usually anemia should be addressed and treated. Mechanical circulatory support should be considered in patients with cardiogenic shock despite vasopressor or inotropic therapy.[9,10] The severity of heart failure is determined by the following factors—hypotension (SBP <90 mm Hg), tachycardia or bradycardia (HR >130 or <45 beats/minute), respiratory rate <25 breaths/minute, systemic arterial saturation i.e., SpO_2 <90%, acidosis (lactate levels >20 mmol/L) or central venous oxygen saturation <60%, cold skin, and oliguria. The aim to treat these patients should be to optimize preload using diuretics and oxygenation. Intravenous vasodilator therapy with nitroglycerine can be considered (if SBP >110 mm Hg), and inotropes/vasopressors in

TABLE 1: Doses and potential side effects of commonly used drugs.

Drug	Dose	Potential side effects
• Furosemide • Torsemide	• 20–40 mg once or twice (intravenous preferred in symptomatic patients • 10–20 mg once	Safe, however caution should be taken regarding maternal hypovolemia and placental hypoperfusion
• Metoprolol succinate CR • Carvedilol	• 12.5–25 mg OD (target dose 200 mg) • 3.125 mg BD (maximum 25 mg BD)	Considered safe, however atenolol is to be avoided as it may be associated with low birth weight
Hydralazine	25–50 mg TDS	Safe, no major side effects maternal lupus like syndrome reported
Digoxin	0.125 mg/day	Usually safe
Nitroglycerin	20 µg/minute to maximum 400 µg/minute	
Levosimendan	12–24 µg/kg bolus over 10 minutes followed by infusion	Hypotension, tachycardia, and arrhythmias
• Dopamine • Dobutamine	• 2–20 µg/kg/minute • 2–20 µg/kg/minute	Tachycardia and arrhythmia
• Norepinephrine • Epinephrine	• 0.2–1.0 µg/kg/minute • 0.05–0.5 µg/kg/minute	Tachycardia, arrhythmia, and end-organ hypoperfusion

case of shock.[8] Peripartum cardiomyopathy patients are quite sensitive to the lethal effects of beta-blockers and hence it should be avoided (whenever possible) and the preferred inotropic agent is levosimendan.[11,12]

Delay in decision-making may lead to further deterioration of maternal health, therefore prespecified algorithm for management, rapid diagnosis, and decision-making is important **(Flowcharts 1 and 2)**.

■ DRUGS

Diuretics

Diuretics are given for symptomatic relief of heart failure. Treatment is preferred with loop diuretics, most commonly furosemide is used. Diuretics have shown association with maternal pancreatitis, neonatal jaundice, thrombocytopenia, and hyponatremia. Rather than initiated, hydrochlorothiazide (HCTZ) is mostly continued during gestation. HCTZ is found to have an association with lower child weights at birth, thrombocytopenia, bleeding diathesis, and neonatal jaundice however, till date no teratogenic effects of HCTZ have been reported.[13]

When ventricular dysfunction is the primary cause of pulmonary edema, diuretic therapy may be useful, whereas in other situations the use of diuretic agents may be less beneficial. Preeclampsia presenting as acute severe disease, is usually associated with increased vascular resistance and, in many cases, some degree of LV diastolic dysfunction.[14] Treatment with diuretics may further deteriorate the already constricted intravascular volume without reducing systemic vascular resistance. In such situation, reducing afterload with parenterally administered vasodilator decreases vascular resistance and increases LV stroke volume

Flowchart 1: Management of acute heart failure (AHF) in pregnancy.

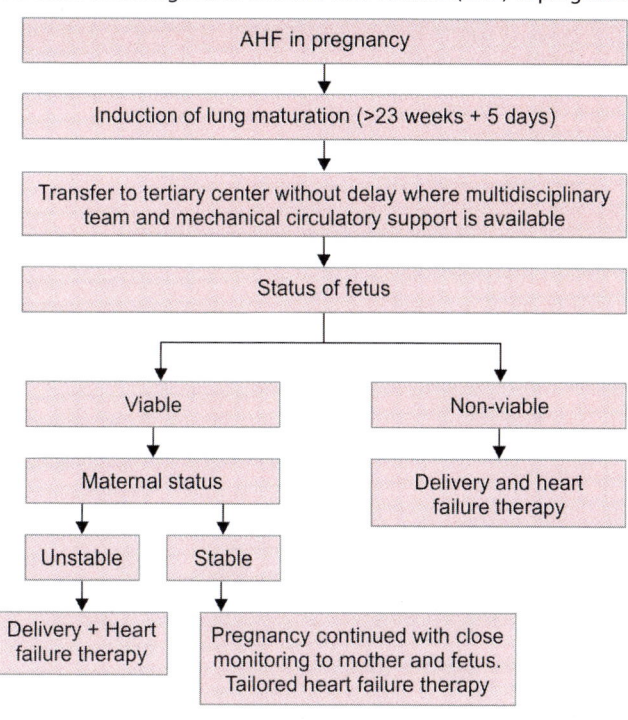

Source: Adapted from Regitz-Zagrosek V, Roos-Hesselink JW, Bauersachs J, Blomström-Lundqvist C, Cífková R, De Bonis M, et al. ESC Scientific Document Group. 2018 ESC Guidelines for the management of cardiovascular diseases during pregnancy. Eur Heart J. 2018;39(34):3165-3241.[8]

and cardiac output along with a secondary reduction in left-side filling pressures.[15]

Vasodilators

Hydralazine Plus Nitrates

An arterial vasodilator, that is used to treat heart failure as well as acute-onset and severe hypertension in pregnant patients is hydralazine which can be administered through oral or intravenous route. No effect on placental perfusion has been observed in patients with preeclampsia who administer oral hydralazine. Although the evidence for hydralazine plus nitrate therapy for heart failure with reduced ejection fraction (HFrEF) is not as strong as the evidence for ACE inhibitors. It should be used in pregnant patients with heart failure who are hypertensive and have severe LV dysfunction.[16]

Intravenous Nitroglycerine or Nitroprusside

Nitroglycerine which is a combined venous and arterial vasodilator, is usually used in pregnant patients who are acutely ill, and is hypertensive due to preeclampsia which is complicated by both left ventricular systolic failure especially if systolic blood pressure is >110 mm Hg.[8]

Nitroprusside may be considered when only when other interventions have failed and when maternal well-being is paramount. However minimal dose should be used due to the metabolism of the agent thiocyanate and cyanide, which has resulted in fetal cyanide toxicity in animal models.[17]

Flowchart 2: Management of acute heart failure (AHF) in pregnancy.

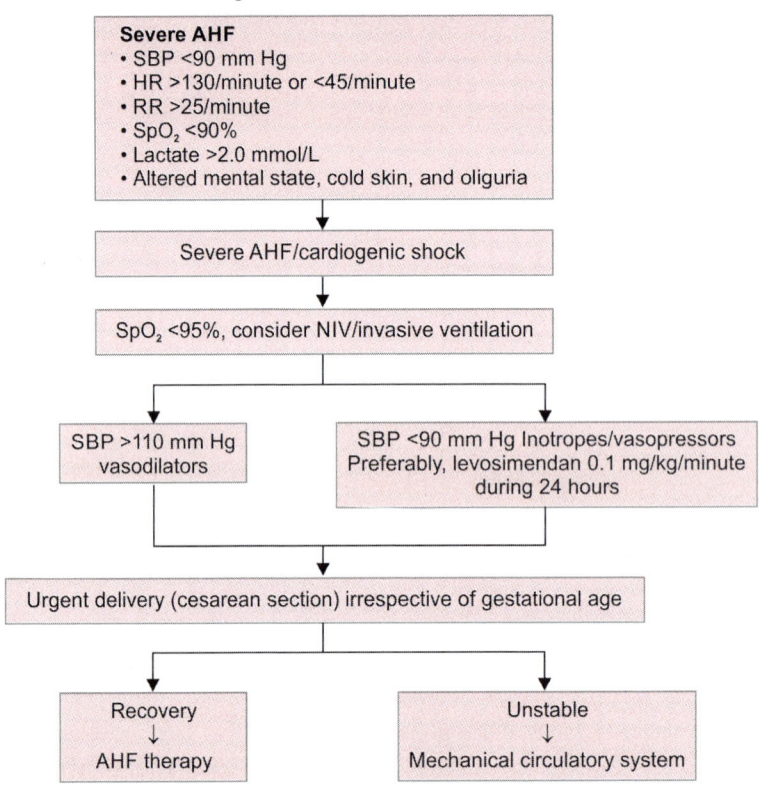

(HR: heart rate; NIV: noninvasive ventilation; SBP: systolic blood pressure)
Source: Adapted from Regitz-Zagrosek V, Roos-Hesselink JW, Bauersachs J, Blomström-Lundqvist C, Cífková R, De Bonis M, et al. ESC Scientific Document Group. 2018 ESC Guidelines for the management of cardiovascular diseases during pregnancy. Eur Heart J. 2018;39(34):3165-3241.[8]

Beta-blockers

The commonly used cardiovascular medications in pregnancy is beta-blockers and is because of its role in the treatment of valvular disease, atrial and ventricular arrhythmias hypertension and heart failure. In general, beta-1 selective agents are preferred, since these agents are less likely to interfere with beta 2-mediated peripheral vasodilation and uterine relaxation. Commonly used are labetalol and metoprolol. On comparison with controls, neonates who are exposed to beta-blockers had significantly more hypoglycemia and bradycardia. However, labetalol compared to metoprolol or atenolol, was widely associated with such observed effects. Hence the neonate should be observed for a few days for the beta-blockade effect (bradycardia and hypoglycemia).[18] Atenolol should not be used as it has been shown to be associated with fetal growth restriction.

Beta-blockers are not initiated in acute decompensated heart failure, and similarly, for patients who are already on beta-blockers, the dose is either reduced or withheld. Once the patient is stabilized beta-blockers are reintroduced in low doses with gradual escalation.

Metoprolol is usually considered safe in pregnancy and is used in most cases. A small study was conducted in 12 pregnant women as a result intrauterine growth retardation was observed in a one-half of the neonates however propranolol is usually considered safe in pregnancies.[19] Atenolol should not be used in pregnancy as it is known to cause fetal growth restriction. No growth restriction was associated on use of carvedilol.[20]

Inotropes and Vasopressor

There is limited data and no established guideline for the use of inotropic or vasopressor agents in critically ill pregnant patients. Dobutamine and dopamine which is used as inotrope support are found to be safe in pregnancy.[21] As dobutamine can lead to heart failure progression in patients with bromocriptine and peripartum cardiomyopathy (PPCM), levosimendan, a calcium sensitizer is suggested for management.[9] Vasopressors convey the risk of decreasing uterine blood stream although norepinephrine, which is ordinarily utilized as the first-line vasoactive agent, has not been shown to affect the fetus.[22]

Digitalis

Digitalis can be used as management in patients with overt HF with AF.

Anticoagulation

Thromboprophylaxis with low molecular weight heparin (LMWH), enoxaparin 40 mg OD is advised in patients with severe left ventricular dysfunction and heart failure.[8]

Patients with atrial fibrillation (AF) and RHD or prosthetic valve require anticoagulation with LMWH throughout the first trimester and after 36 weeks of pregnancy. Acenocoumarol or warfarin may be used. Acenocoumarol (3 mg) or warfarin (5 mg) is used when low dose is required during second and third trimesters. If dose required is high, LMWH should be continued and factor X level should be monitored once a week.[8]

Angiotensin receptor blockers (ARBS), ACE inhibitors, direct renin inhibitors, aldosterone antagonists, ARNI, and sodium-glucose transport protein-2 (SGLT-2) inhibitors

As soon as pregnancy is suspected or in the preconception period some medication such as ACE inhibitors, ARBs, direct renin inhibitors should be stopped as they can induce renal dysgenesis which often leads to fetal death. Antiandrogen effects were observed in first trimester on male fetus due to medication such as spironolactone, aldosterone antagonist, and eplerenone, also teratogenesis was observed in the rat model. During lactation ARNI and ARB should not be used as there are no data available, but ACE inhibitors such as captopril, enalapril, and benazepril must be used safely. Due to a lack of safety data, SGLT-2 inhibitors are not recommended in pregnancy or postpartum.

Bromocriptine and Peripartum Cardiomyopathy

When bromocriptine is added to standard HF therapy that could improve recovery and clinical outcomes in women with acute severe PPCM. In uncomplicated cases, bromocriptine (2.5 mg once daily) for at least 1 week may be used, whereas a prolonged treatment (2.5 mg twice daily for 2 weeks, then 2.5 mg once daily for 6 weeks) may be administered in patients with cardiogenic shock and/or EF <25%. Anticoagulation with heparin (UFH or LMWH) must be added in prophylactic dosages along with bromocriptine.[23,24] High resting heart rate indicates unfavorable results in patients with PPCM, and treatment with ivabradine may be beneficial if the patient is not pregnant or breastfeeding.[25,26] After improving of left ventricular function, treatment should be continued for at least 6 months followed by gradual tapering as relapse of PPCM has been reported after rapid tapering of HF therapies.[27]

DELIVERY CONSIDERATION

Irrespective of gestational duration, urgent delivery by cesarean section should be planned in women with persistent hemodynamic instability on severe HF even after treatment. Vaginal delivery with epidural anesthesia is better in women with stable HF. In vaginal delivery, instrumentation is mostly used to shorten the second stage of labor.[8]

PROGNOSIS

The diagnosis in pregnancy with HF varies from full recuperation in many patients with PPCM to lethal results. Prior to discharge, the following ought to be conveyed with the patients—evaluation of blood pressure and volume status; start of goal-directed restorative therapy; optimization of chronic oral HF therapy; assessment of renal function and electrolytes; discussion about treatment of the comorbid condition; contraception plans and lactation and about her health status. In patients with heart disease lactation should be allowed whenever possible but should be ceased in case of HF with reduced ejection fraction.[8]

KEY POINTS

- Heart failure in pregnancy requires joint obstetric and cardiac care.
- Modification of conventional HF therapy to exclude teratogenic drugs is paramount.
- Vaginal delivery should be promoted in uncomplicated cases, and in case of complication because of obstetric reasons cesarean section should be performed in patients with decompensated HF.
- The postpartum period should be used to improve the care of these vulnerable patients by optimizing heart failure treatment, risk stratification for a subsequent pregnancy, and contraceptive counseling.

REFERENCES

1. Ruys TP, Roos-Hesselink JW, Hall R, Subirana-Domènech MT, Grando-Ting J, Estensen M, et al. Heart failure in pregnant women with cardiac disease: data from the ROPAC. Heart. 2014;100(3):231-8.
2. Lima FV, Parikh PB, Zhu J, Yang J, Stergiopoulos K. Association of cardiomyopathy with adverse cardiac events in pregnant women at the time of delivery. JACC Heart Fail. 2015;3(3):257-66.
3. Watkins DA, Johnson CO, Colquhoun SM, Karthikeyan G, Beaton A, Bukhman G, et al. Global, regional, and national burden of rheumatic heart disease, 1990-2015. N Engl J Med. 2017;377(8):713-22.
4. Mogos MF, Piano MR, McFarlin BL, Salemi JL, Liese KL, Briller JE. Heart failure in pregnant women: a concern across the pregnancy continuum. Circ Heart Fail. 2018;11(1):e004005.
5. French KA, Poppas A. Rheumatic heart disease in pregnancy: global challenges and clear opportunities. Circulation. 2018;137(8):817-9.
6. Akinwusi PO, Adeniji AO, Atanda OO, Adekunle AD. Hospital-based incidence of maternal heart failure during pregnancy in Nigeria. Int J Gen Med. 2013;6:201-7.
7. Tanous D, Siu SC, Mason J, Greutmann M, Wald RM, Parker JD, et al. B-type natriuretic peptide in pregnant women with heart disease. J Am Coll Cardiol. 2010;56(15):1247-53.
8. Regitz-Zagrosek V, Roos-Hesselink JW, Bauersachs J, Blomström-Lundqvist C, Cífková R, De Bonis M, et al. ESC Scientific Document Group. 2018 ESC Guidelines for the management of cardiovascular diseases during pregnancy. Eur Heart J. 2018;39(34):3165-3241.
9. Bauersachs J, Arrigo M, Hilfiker-Kleiner D, Veltmann C, Coats AJ, Crespo-Leiro MG, et al. Current management of patients with severe acute peripartum cardiomyopathy: practical guidance from the Heart Failure Association of the European Society of Cardiology Study Group on peripartum cardiomyopathy. Eur J Heart Fail. 2016;18(9):1096-105.

10. Mebazaa A, Yilmaz MB, Levy P, Ponikowski P, Peacock WF, Laribi S, et al. Recommendations on pre-hospital & early hospital management of acute heart failure: a consensus paper from the Heart Failure Association of the European Society of Cardiology, the European Society of Emergency Medicine and the Society of Academic Emergency Medicine. Eur J Heart Fail. 2015;17(6):544-58.
11. Stapel B, Kohlhaas M, Ricke-Hoch M, Haghikia A, Erschow S, Knuuti J, et al. Low STAT3 expression sensitizes to toxic effects of β-adrenergic receptor stimulation in peripartum cardiomyopathy. Eur Heart J. 2017;38(5):349-61.
12. Labbene I, Arrigo M, Tavares M, Hajjej Z, Brandão JL, Tolppanen H, et al. Decongestive effects of levosimendan in cardiogenic shock induced by postpartum cardiomyopathy. Anaesth Crit Care Pain Med. 2017;36(1):39-42.
13. Hypertension in pregnancy. Report of the American College of Obstetricians and Gynecologists' Task Force on Hypertension in Pregnancy. Obstet Gynecol. 2013;122(5):1122-31.
14. Belfort MA, Anthony J, Kirshon B. Respiratory function in severe gestational proteinuric hypertension: the effects of rapid volume expansion and subsequent vasodilatation with verapamil. Br J Obstet Gynaecol. 1991;98(10):964-72.
15. Belfort M, Akovic K, Anthony J, Saade G, Kirshon B, Moise K Jr. The effect of acute volume expansion and vasodilatation with verapamil on uterine and umbilical artery Doppler indices in severe preeclampsia. J Clin Ultrasound. 1994;22(5):317-25.
16. Gudmundsson S, Gennser G, Marsal K. Effects of hydralazine on placental and renal circulation in pre-eclampsia. Acta Obstet Gynecol Scand. 1995;74(6):415-8.
17. Palmer RF, Lasseter KC. Drug therapy. Sodium nitroprusside. N Engl J Med. 1975;292(6):294-7.
18. Bateman BT, Patorno E, Desai RJ, Seely EW, Mogun H, Maeda A, et al. Late pregnancy β blocker exposure and risks of neonatal hypoglycemia and bradycardia. Pediatrics. 2016;138(3):e20160731.
19. Pruyn SC, Phelan JP, Buchanan GC. Long-term propranolol therapy in pregnancy: maternal and fetal outcome. Am J Obstet Gynecol. 1979;135(4):485-9.
20. Tanaka K, Tanaka H, Kamiya C, Katsuragi S, Sawada M, Tsuritani M, et al. Beta-blockers and fetal growth restriction in pregnant women with cardiovascular disease. Circ J. 2016;80(10):2221-6.
21. Canobbio MM, Warnes CA, Aboulhosn J, Connolly HM, Khanna A, Koos BJ, et al. Management of Pregnancy in Patients With Complex Congenital Heart Disease: A Scientific Statement for Healthcare Professionals From the American Heart Association. Circulation. 2017;135(8):e50-87.
22. Van Nimwegen D, Dyer DC. The action of vasopressors on isolated uterine arteries. Am J Obstet Gynecol. 1974;118(8):1099-103.
23. Haghikia A, Podewski E, Berliner D, Sonnenschein K, Fischer D, Angermann CE, et al. Rationale and design of a randomized, controlled multicentre clinical trial to evaluate the effect of bromocriptine on left ventricular function in women with peripartum cardiomyopathy. Clin Res Cardiol. 2015;104(11):911-7.
24. Hilfiker-Kleiner D, Haghikia A, Berliner D, Vogel-Claussen J, Schwab J, Franke A, et al. Bromocriptine for the treatment of peripartum cardiomyopathy: a multicentre randomized study. Eur Heart J. 2017;38(35):2671-9.
25. Libhaber E, Sliwa K, Bachelier K, Lamont K, Böhm M. Low systolic blood pressure and high resting heart rate as predictors of outcome in patients with peripartum cardiomyopathy. Int J Cardiol. 2015;190:376-82.
26. Haghikia A, Tongers J, Berliner D, König T, Schäfer A, Brehm M, et al. Early ivabradine treatment in patients with acute peripartum cardiomyopathy: subanalysis of the German PPCM registry. Int J Cardiol. 2016;216:165-7.
27. Hilfiker-Kleiner D, Haghikia A, Nonhoff J, Bauersachs J. Peripartum cardiomyopathy: current management and future perspectives. Eur Heart J. 2015;36(18):1090-7.

Section 4

Medical Management of Liver Disorders in Pregnancy

◢ **Intrahepatic Cholestasis**
   Neha Pruthi Tandon, Archana Chaurasia

◢ **Hepatitis and Hepatic Encephalopathy**
   Durgesh

Chapter 9

Intrahepatic Cholestasis

Neha Pruthi Tandon, Archana Chaurasia

■ DEFINITION

Intrahepatic cholestasis of pregnancy (IHCP), also known as obstetric cholestasis, is one of the most common liver diseases specific to pregnancy.[1] It usually manifests in the third trimester of pregnancy as skin itching and as elevation of serum levels of bile acids and liver enzymes. This condition worsens as pregnancy proceeds and resolves completely after delivery. The incidence ranges from <1 to 27.6% worldwide.[2] In Asian Indian population its incidence is around 1.2–1.5%.[3]

■ ETIOLOGY: MULTIFACTORIAL

The cause of IHCP is multifactorial and includes a combination of genetic susceptibility, environmental and hormonal factors **(Fig. 1)**.

■ RISK FACTORS

- Previous history of IHCP (recurrence)
- Preexisting hepatobiliary disease
- Chronic hepatitis C infection
- Multiple gestations
- Advance maternal age
- Family history

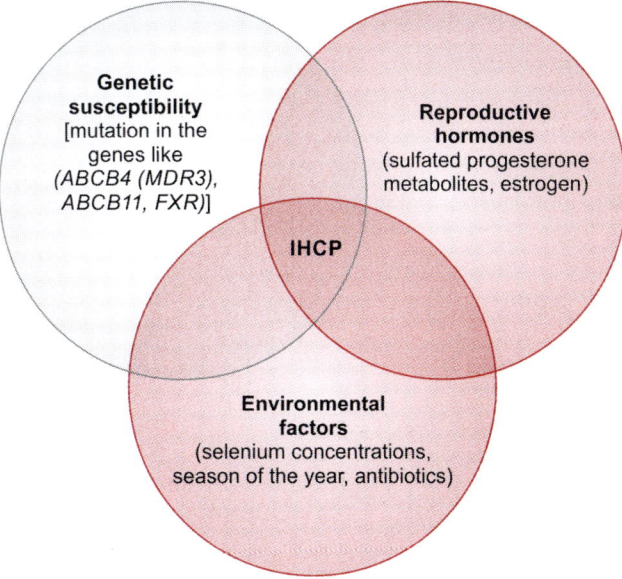

Fig. 1: Etiology of intrahepatic cholestasis of pregnancy (IHCP).

PATHOPHYSIOLOGY

Out of all known reproductive hormones, estrogen is found to be the main contributor in the development of IHCP. In a genetically susceptible female, estrogen decreases the expression of nuclear hepatic bile acid receptors and hepatic biliary canalicular transport proteins thereby leading to impairment in hepatic bile acid homeostasis, which in turn lead to increase in bile acids levels.

Pathophysiology of Adverse Pregnancy Outcome

The pathophysiology of pregnancy morbidity and fetal death in IHCP are poorly understood.

High level of bile acids can cause sudden vasospasm of placental chorionic surface vessels and development of fetal arrhythmias leading to sudden fetal death. Certain preexisting obstetric complications such as preeclampsia and gestational diabetes mellitus also play a very important role.

Rising bile acids are associated with increased expression of myometrial oxytocin receptors, which may lead to preterm labor and spontaneous preterm birth.

There is no established relationship between IHCP and weight of the baby at birth. In addition to this, oligohydramnios and fetal growth restriction is also not attributed to the disease process.

CLINICAL FEATURES

- Pruritus without primary skin condition
- Commonly on palms and soles
- More in night time
- Presents in second/third trimester
- Nausea, decreased appetite, right upper quadrant pain, sleep disturbances, and steatorrhea.

DIAGNOSIS

A pregnant female complaining of pruritus (especially in palms and soles) along with raised peak bile acid level of 19 µmol/L or more, the diagnosis of IHCP should be considered. Post-delivery, if the bile acid levels become normal and itching reduces, the diagnosis is more confirmatory. Diagnosis of IHCP as mild, moderate and severe can be made based on parameters listed in **Table 1**.

ADVERSE PERINATAL OUTCOMES

- Preterm birth (both spontaneous and iatrogenic)
- Meconium stained amniotic fluid
- Respiratory distress syndrome
- Still birth

MANAGEMENT/TREATMENT

- Role of drug treatment is to reduce maternal itching.
- No evidence of improvement in perinatal outcomes, reduction in bile acid levels.

Ursodeoxycholic Acid

Ursodeoxycholic acid (UDCA) is considered as treatment of choice for IHCP and recommended as the first-line agent for the treatment of maternal symptoms of

TABLE 1: Diagnosis of intrahepatic cholestasis of pregnancy (IHCP).

Diagnosis	Clinical features
Gestational pruritus	Pruritis and peak serum bile acid levels <19 µmol/L
Mild IHCP	Pruritis and raised peak serum bile acid levels 19–39 µmol/L
Moderate IHCP	Pruritis and raised peak serum bile acid levels 40–99 µmol/L
Severe IHCP	Pruritis and raised peak serum bile acid levels ≥100 µmol/L

IHCP (GRADE 1A) (SFMF)[3] **(Table 2)**. Ursodeoxycholic acid is the only treatment (proposed as disease modifying drug), which principally improves the biochemical test results along with maternal symptoms. Evidence from RCT has shown that treatment with UDCA does not reduce adverse perinatal outcome (still birth and preterm deliveries) in women with IHCP.[4] A systematic review and individual participant meta-analysis of ursodeoxycholic acid in IHCP which included four randomized controlled trials has shown that spontaneous preterm birth under 37 weeks' gestation was reduced in women taking ursodeoxycholic acid compared with placebo.

Mechanism of action (MOA): It is a naturally occurring bile acid (BA). It acts by displacing the more hydrophobic endogenous bile salts from BA pool. This action helps in protecting the hepatocyte membrane from the toxic effect of bile salts, thereby increasing the clearance of BA across the placenta from the fetus. It also increases biliary bile acid excretion through various mechanisms such as upregulation of hepatic metabolizing enzymes and bile acid transporters, stimulation of impaired hepatocellular secretion by post-transcriptional mechanisms, stabilization of the plasma membrane and protection of cholangiocytes of the biliary epithelium against cytotoxicity of bile acids. It also protects hepatocytes against bile acid-induced apoptosis.[5]

Dose: Starting dose for UDCA treatment is 10–15 mg/kg/day, which can be divided into 2 or 3 daily doses. If pruritus persist beyond 2 weeks, dose may be titrated to maximum of 21 mg/kg/day.[6] Typical regimens are 300–600 mg twice or three times daily. Maximum dose up to 2,000 mg/day.

Itching usually relieves/decreases in 1–2 weeks. However, biochemical changes take at least 3–4 weeks to show improvement.

Side effects: Nausea, diarrhea, stomach upset, constipation, headache, hair loss, stuffy nose.

Contraindication: In presence of any opaque stone or radiolucent bile pigment stone.

Drug interaction: With cholestyramine, estrogen, and antacid that contain aluminum.

Safety category: FDA category-B drug that has been found safe in first trimester also.

■ OTHER AGENTS (*see* TABLE 2)

The Royal College of Obstetricians and Gynaecologists (RCOG, 2022) recommends not offer other agents for treatment of IHCP outside of a research study or individualized specialist treatment.[7]

Rifampicin

It is a semisynthetic antibiotic which has a wide range of antimicrobial activity. Rifampicin is used as a first-line agent for treatment of tuberculosis, including pregnancy. It is also used in the management of cholestasis due to its action on decreasing the level of serum bile acid. A study was conducted on 30 patients where use of rifampicin (in divided doses of 300–1,200 mg) was combined with UDCA for treatment of refractory IHCP.[8,9] Itching was improved in 11/16 patients and many of them had decreased serum bile acid/aminotransferase levels. A good perinatal outcome was observed in all infants who delivered between 32 and 37 weeks.

Mechanism of action: Rifampicin is a pregnane X-receptor (PXR) agonist. It acts as a potent inducer of enzymes such as CYP3A4, CYP2D, UGT1A1, SULT2A1 which plays a

TABLE 2: Summary of drugs used in intrahepatic cholestasis of pregnancy (IHCP).

Drug	Dosage	MOA	Side effects	FDA pregnancy category
UDCA	10–15 mg/kg/day	Displaces more hydrophobic endogenous bile salts from bile acid pool	Nausea, diarrhea, stomach upset, constipation, headache, hair loss, and stuffy nose	Category B
Rifampicin	300–1,200 mg in divided doses	A potent inducer of enzymes such as CYP3A4, CYP2D, UGT1A1, SULT2A1 which plays a key role in liver and intestinal detoxification system	Red orange discoloration of body fluids, including urine, stools, saliva, sputum, sweat, and tears. Others include headache, bone and muscle pain, nausea, vomiting and abdominal cramps, diarrhea, urticaria	Category C
S-adenosyl-L-methionine	800 mg qd IV or 1,600 mg qd orally	It acts as a methyl group donor and plays an important role in the biosynthesis of phospholipids, which are helpful in maintaining the fluidity of hepatic cell membranes and excretion of estrogen metabolites	Dry mouth, nausea, gas, diarrhea, headache, anxiety, and palpitations insomnia	Category C
Cholestyramine	2–4 g/day	Inhibits the absorption of bile acids after it binds to the intestine. As a consequence, it may interfere with the absorption of fat-soluble vitamins, especially vitamin K	Constipation, abdominal pain and steatorrhea	
Phenobarbitone	100 mg qd	Increases the excretion of bile salts into the biliary tree and increases bile flow	Rare allergic reaction	Category D
Chlorpheniramine	4 mg orally every 4–6 hours	First-generation alkylamine antihistamine.	Sedation	Category B
Topical emollients (calamine lotion)	Local application	Antipruritic and antiseptic properties, suppresses histamine-induced itching	–	Calamine lotion is approved by FDA as over-the-counter medication

(FDA: Food and Drug Administration; MOA: mechanism of action; UDCA: ursodeoxycholic acid)

key role in liver and intestinal detoxification system.

Dose: 300 mg to be taken orally, two times a day.

Side effects: Commonly, body fluids, including urine, stools, saliva, sputum, sweat and tears, turn red-orange. Others include headache, bone and muscle pain, nausea, vomiting and abdominal cramps, diarrhea, and urticaria.

Drug interaction: With oral contraceptive pills.

S-Adenosyl-L-Methionine

S-adenosyl-L-methionine (SAMe) is produced in all mammalian cells and is a derivative of methionine and adenosine triphosphate (ATP). It is principally produced and metabolized in the liver. It acts as a methyl group donor and plays an important role in the biosynthesis of phospholipids, which are helpful in maintaining the fluidity of hepatic cell membranes and excretion of estrogen metabolites.

Mechanism of action: It acts as a precursor of glutathione and affects the composition and fluidity of hepatocyte plasma membranes thereby increases the methylation and biliary excretion of hormone metabolites.[10] Usually administered as intravenous therapy. However oral SAMe (1,600 mg/day) is preferred for treatment of cholestasis in nonpregnant patient.

Dose: Usually effective in a dose of 800 mg qd IV or 1,600 mg qd orally.

Cholestyramine

Cholestyramine is a resin that acts by inhibiting the absorption of bile salts from ileum, thereby enhancing their excretion in the feces.

Dose: Orally effective, with a starting dose of 2–4 g/day and it can be gradually increased up to a maximum dose of 16 g/day, depending on the need so as to control the symptoms.[11]

Side effects: Constipation, abdominal pain, and steatorrhea leading to deficiency of fat-soluble vitamins (e.g., vitamin K), especially when given in high doses (e.g., >4 g/day). Cholestyramine may interfere with the absorption of fat-soluble vitamins, especially vitamin K, which plays an important role in blood coagulation. This in turn increases the risk of postpartum hemorrhage in the pregnant women and intracranial hemorrhage in the fetus.

■ TOPICAL EMOLLIENT

They will not modifying the disease process, but may provide relief some of the discomfort associated with itching.
- Calamine lotion is a topical emollient and its role is yet to be established in clinical trials. It may provide temporary relief from itching in some women and is considered safe in pregnancy. It is a mixture of zinc oxide (ZnO) and 0.5% iron oxide (Fe_2O_3) and has both antipruritic and antiseptic properties.
- About 1–2% menthol in the form of aqueous cream is found to affect a delta type sensory nerve fibers and suppress histamine-induced pruritus.

Chlorpheniramine

It is a first-generation alkylamine antihistamine. The effectiveness of this treatment is uncertain in women with IHCP. Its use along with that of other H1—antagonist antihistamine has not been tested for use in IHCP, but it seems to provide a significant relief from the symptom of pruritis in certain women. Usually administered at night for its sedative effect.

Dose: Chlorpheniramine is given 4 mg per oral every 4–6 hours, maximum 24 mg/day. Hydroxyzine given in the dose of 25–50 mg every 4–6 hourly is also effective.

Side effects: Mild sedation but is otherwise considered safe in pregnancy.

Phenobarbitone

In 1968, Cunningham was first to establish the role of phenobarbitone in cholestasis. Studies done in some animal models suggest that it increases the excretion of bile salts into the biliary tree and thereby increases the bile flow. This drug crosses the placental barrier and distributes in fetal tissues, including the placenta, liver, and brain. Use during the first and third trimesters may be associated with an increased risk of teratogenicity and withdrawal symptoms in the newborn, respectively.

Dexamethasone

It is recommended only for lung maturity. In a randomized trial of about 130 patients of IHCP, it was concluded that this drug is not very effective in improving itching or reducing the level of serum aminotransferase and was also found to be less effective than UDCA 1,000 mg/day in decreasing bilirubin and bile acids levels.[12]

Others

It includes charcoal, ultraviolet light, certain herbal remedies. Their efficacy is uncertain, as only few patients were treated. There is insufficient evidence to indicate that SAMe, dexamethasone, cholestyramine, Yinchenhao decoction (YCHD), Danxioling pill (DXLP), Salvia, and Yiganling alone or in combination are effective in treating women with cholestasis of pregnancy.[13]

■ ROLE OF VITAMIN K

Routine use of vitamin K treatment in women with IHCP is not indicated. Maternal vitamin K treatment is considered only if there appears to be reduced absorption of dietary fats (e.g., presence of steatorrhea) and/or evidence of abnormal prothrombin time if coagulation studies are performed.

Vitamin K is a fat-soluble vitamin that affects coagulation pathways within the body.

Dose: Menadione IM injection 1 mL (10 mg).

Contraindications: Hereditary hypoprothrombinemia, renal impairment, and hypersensitivity to vitamin K.

Side effects: No known toxicity is associated with high doses of vitamin K_1 or vitamin K_2. Side effects are rare. A few have reported allergic reactions, bronchospasm and cardiac arrest reported with fast IV administration. The oral form of vitamin K does not seem to cause severe reactions.

■ KEY POINTS

- The diagnosis of intrahepatic cholestasis of pregnancy is based upon pruritus associated with elevated total serum bile acid levels, elevated aminotransferases, or both, and the absence of diseases that may produce similar laboratory findings and symptoms.
- Most preferred drug for the treatment is ursodeoxycholic acid (ursodiol or UDCA, a synthetic bile acid).
- The RCOG (2022) recommends not to offer other agents for treatment of IHCP outside of a research study or individualized specialist treatment.
- Routine use of vitamin K treatment in women with IHCP is not indicated. It is recommended on women with evidence of abnormal prothrombin time.
- Topical emollients and chlorpheniramine will not modifying the disease process, but may provide relief from discomfort associated with itching.

REFERENCES

1. Clinical Updates in Women's Health Care Summary: Liver Disease: Reproductive Considerations. Obstet Gynecol. 2017;129(1): 236.
2. Geenes V, Williamson C. Intrahepatic cholestasis of pregnancy. World J Gastroenterol. 2009;15:2049-66.
3. Society for Maternal-Fetal Medicine (SMFM). Electronic address: pubs@smfm.org, Lee RH, Mara Greenberg, Metz TD, Pettker CM. Society for Maternal-Fetal Medicine Consult Series #53: Intrahepatic cholestasis of pregnancy: Replaces Consult #13, April 2011. Am J Obstet Gynecol. 2021;224(2):B2-9.
4. Chappell LC, Bell JL, Smith A, Linsell L, Juszczak E, Dixon PH, et al. Ursodeoxycholic acid versus placebo in women with intrahepatic cholestasis of pregnancy (PITCHES): a randomised controlled trial. The Lancet. 2019;394:849-60.
5. Ovadia C, Sajous J, Seed PT, Patel K, Williamson NJ, Attilakos G, et al. Ursodeoxycholic acid in intrahepatic cholestasis of pregnancy: a systematic review and individual participant data meta-analysis. Lancet Gastroenterol Hepatol. 2021; 6(7):547-58.
6. Williamson C, Geenes V. Intrahepatic cholestasis of pregnancy. Obstet Gynecol. 2014;124(1):120-33.
7. Girling J, Knight CL, Chappell L. Intrahepatic cholestasis of pregnancy Green-top Guideline No. 43. BJOG. 2022;129:e95-114.
8. Liu J, Murray AM, Mankus EB, Ireland KE, Acosta OM, Ramsey PS. Adjuvant use of rifampin for refractory intrahepatic cholestasis of pregnancy. Obstet Gynecol. 2018;132(3):678-81.
9. Geenes V, Chambers J, Khurana R, Shemer EW, Sia W, Mandair D, et al. Rifampicin in the treatment of severe intrahepatic cholestasis of pregnancy. Eur J Obstet Gynecol Reprod Biol. 2015;189:59-63.
10. Ozkan S, Ceylan Y, Ozkan OV, Yildirim S. Review of a challenging clinical issue: Intrahepatic cholestasis of pregnancy. World J Gastroenterol. 2015;21(23):7134-41.
11. Mela M, Mancuso A, Burroughs AK. Review article: pruritus in cholestatic and other liver diseases. Aliment Pharmacol Ther. 2003;17(7):857-70.
12. Kong X, Kong Y, Zhang F, Wang T, Yan J. Evaluating the effectiveness and safety of ursodeoxycholic acid in treatment of intrahepatic cholestasis of pregnancy: A meta-analysis (a prisma-compliant study). Medicine (Baltimore). 2016;95(40):e4949.
13. Walker KF, Chappell LC, Hague WM, Middleton P, Thornton JG. Pharmacological interventions for treating intrahepatic cholestasis of pregnancy. Cochrane Database Syst Rev. 2020;7:CD000493.

Chapter 10

Hepatitis and Hepatic Encephalopathy

Durgesh

Hepatitis is an inflammation of the liver that is caused by a variety of infectious agents like viruses and noninfectious agents like drugs, etc.

There are five main strains of the hepatitis virus—type A, B, C, D, and E. Other viruses causing hepatitis are herpes simplex and cytomegalovirus (CMV).[1]

The modes of transmission, severity of the illness, geographical distribution, and prevention methods are different for all these strains. Types B and C lead to chronic disease and together are the most common cause of liver cirrhosis, liver cancer, and viral hepatitis-related deaths.[1,2]

Most of these viral infections are self-limiting but during pregnancy, there is a high chance of worsening of liver disease as well as mother-to-child transmission due to hepatitis.[3-5] Hence, judicious screening with preventive strategies, treatment of infection using antivirals and supportive treatment and immunoprophylaxis,[4] encouragement of safe breastfeeding practices and hygiene, along with active multidisciplinary involvement is warranted.[6]

■ HEPATITIS A

A pre-exposure and postexposure prophylaxis offers best treatment as no specific therapy is available for hepatitis A **(Table 1)**.

The prophylaxis is recommended for pregnant females:
- Who are working or traveling to countries with moderate-to-high hepatitis A virus (HAV) endemicity
- Who are at risk of infection or adverse outcome due to hepatitis A infection (e.g., in patients with pre-existing liver diseases)
- Who have high risk of exposure to HAV-infected persons.

HAV Vaccine Prophylaxis

Hepatitis A virus vaccine is prepared from the inactivated virus. The protective levels of antibodies develop after 2 weeks of first shot of HAV vaccine in majority of the individuals.

After receiving the second dose of HAV vaccine, antibodies are likely persist for at least 10–30 years or may be lifelong.[7]

Havrix (GlaxoSmithKline) and Vaqta (Merk) are single antigen inactivated vaccines. They are given as 1 mL, intramuscular injection on a two-dose schedule 0, 6–12 months apart. Another vaccine, which is combined hepatitis A and B, is also available in the market, but it is not recommended for postexposure prophylaxis.

Side effects—the vaccine is considered safe in pregnancy. It does not carry risks to the developing fetus.

TABLE 1: Hepatitis virus in pregnancy.

Key features	Hepatitis A	Hepatitis B	Hepatitis C	Hepatitis D	Hepatitis E
Virus characteristics[1]	Picornavirus family, single strand RNA virus	Hepadnavirus family, small DNA virus	Small, single-stranded, enveloped RNA virus in the Flavivirus family	Defective single strand, spherical, RNA virus	Hepeviridae family, single strand RNA virus
Mode of spread[1]	Fecal–oral route	Sexual contact, direct contact with body secretions	Direct percutaneous exposure to blood mainly, other secretions like saliva, semen, body fluids may rarely transmit the infection	Generally occurs as a co-infection with hepatitis B. Route of transmission is same as hepatitis B	Fecal–oral route
Effects on pregnancy	• Minimal impact on pregnancy • As such the virus is not teratogenic • It is generally self-limiting, but may occasionally lead to fulminant hepatitis[5]	Usually mild and is not associated with deleterious effects on mother and fetus, chances of chronic carrier, hepatocellular carcinoma, cirrhosis in later life[5]	Rarely causes fulminant liver disease in pregnancy, high risk of chronic liver disease in later life[5]	Usually mild but may cause serious co-infection with hepatitis B	High risk for fulminant hepatitis and acute liver failure (ALF) especially in late trimester[5]
Diagnosis	Serum anti-HAV immunoglobulin M (IgM) antibody	HBsAg, IgM antibodies to HBcAg	Anti-HCV antibody	Anti-HDV IgM	Anti-HEV IgM in serum or HEV RNA by PCR in serum or stool
Preventive measures	• Safe hygienic practices HAV vaccine and passive immunization can be considered in mothers at risk • Postexposure immunoglobulin should be given within 2 weeks of exposure of HAV and is safe to use in pregnancy	• Hygienic and safe sex practices and avoiding sharing of personal items • MTCT is reduced by avoiding use of fetal scalp electrodes, fetal blood sampling, assisted delivery, and vigorous airway suctioning of infant at birth	Safe sex practices and avoiding sharing of personal items and needles	Hygienic and safe sex practices	Hygienic practices, use of safe drinking water (boiling and chlorination may inactivate HEV), and avoiding uncooked or poorly cooked meat

Contd...

Contd...

Key features	Hepatitis A	Hepatitis B	Hepatitis C	Hepatitis D	Hepatitis E
Screening	No routine screening is recommended	• Standard routine test with HBsAg in all pregnant women (<12–14 weeks) is recommended • If HBsAg$^+$, then HBeAg, HBV DNA, ALT, and ultrasonography for liver	• Routine universal testing with anti-HCV antibody at first antenatal visit • If screening is positive, then HCV RNA level and testing for STDs (HIV, syphilis, HBV) are undertaken	IgM anti-hepatitis D Ag	No routine screening recommended
MTCT	Rare	The risk is otherwise up to 90% if mother has chronic HBV, HBeAg$^+$, HBV DNA >200,000 IU/m. Treatment reduces the risk for MTCT from 10 to 1–2%	Increased risk with maternal viral load, HIV co-infection, prolonged rupture of membranes, and fetal scalp monitoring. In the absence of these factors, risk is approximately 5%, and chronic HCV develops in 3% of infants	Rare	Increased risk in acute viremia especially in third trimester (range, 30–100%)
Immunization in mother	HAV vaccine is recommended in patients with specific risk factors	HBV vaccine is recommended in women with risk factors. If exposed, HBIG (within 72 hours of exposure) and HBV vaccine (within 7 days, at 1 and 6 months) are administered	No approved vaccine or immunoglobulin is available	No specific vaccine against hepatitis D available, but immunization against hepatitis B is helpful	No FDA-approved vaccine is available yet
Breastfeeding	No contraindication	No contraindication	To be avoided in high viral loads, HIV/HCV co-infection, and if nipples are cracked, or damaged	No contraindication	Generally considered safe with low risk for transmission

(ALT: alanine transaminase; FDA: Food and Drug Administration; HBIG: hepatitis B immunoglobulin; HBV: hepatitis B vaccine; HIV: human immunodeficiency virus; MTCT: mother-to-child transmission; PCR: polymerase chain reaction)

HEPATITIS B

There is a high risk of transmission of virus to fetus from 10% in first trimester to 90% in the third trimester, to as high as 90% especially in those mothers who are seropositive to HepBsAg and e antigen HbeAg (*see* **Table 1**).

Treatment of Hepatitis B in Pregnancy

Figure 1 describes the treatment of hepatitis B in pregnancy.

Prenatal management includes immunization both active and passive.

Hepatitis B Vaccines

Recombinant DNA vaccines are available which are given in a series of two or three IM injections, 0.5 mL, in deltoid preferably over 6-months interval (*see* **Table 1**). These vaccines are safe to use in pregnancy as well as in newborns.[8-10]

A combination (HAV and HBV) is also available for adults.

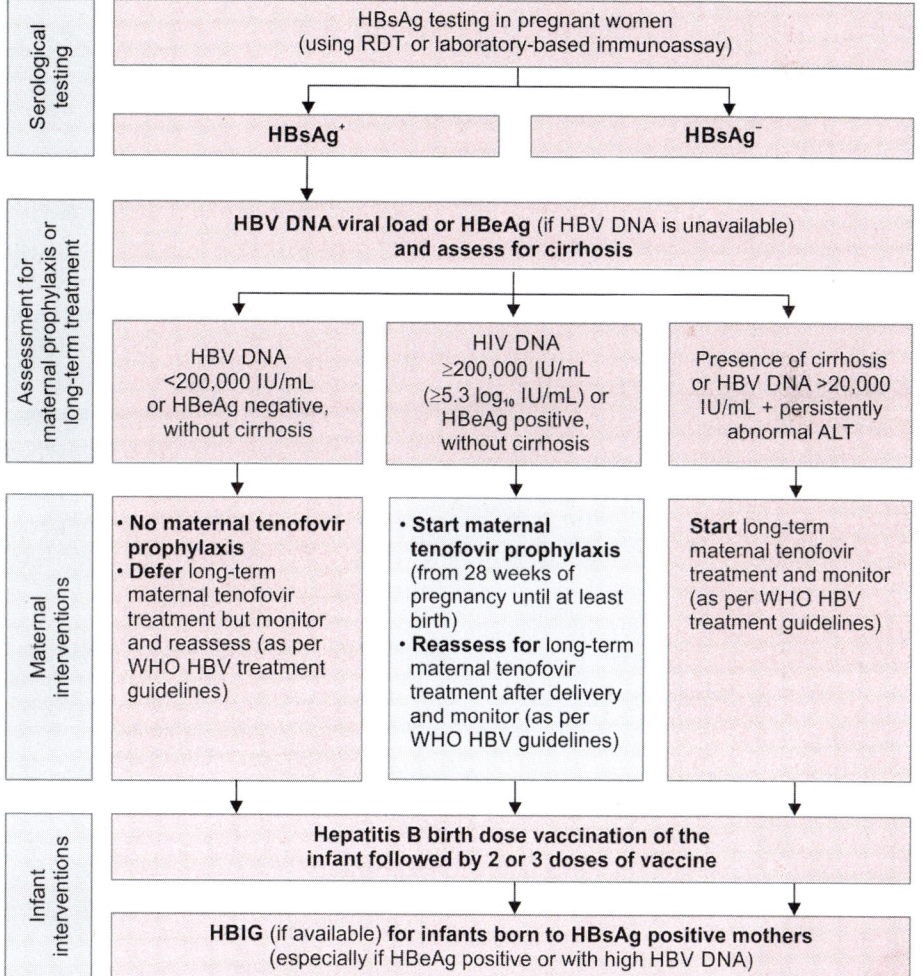

Fig. 1: Treatment of hepatitis B in pregnancy.[8-11] (ALT: alanine transaminase; HBIG: hepatitis B immunoglobulin; HBV: hepatitis B vaccine; HIV: human immunodeficiency virus; WHO: World Health Organization)

Drugs

Nucleoside/nucleotide analogs: Use of these analogs reduces the viral load; hence, they are helpful in reducing vertical transmission, and long-term sequelae related to hepatitis B virus in mother such as cirrhosis **(Table 2)**.

As per the recommendations of American Association for the study of Liver Diseases (AASLD), NICE guidelines, and the European Association for the Study of Liver (EASL), all the pregnant women in third trimester with viral load >10^6–10^8 copies/mL or 200,000 IU/mL should be given—tenofovir disoproxil fumarate as the first-line antiviral therapy. This should also be considered for the pregnant women with chronic HBV and cirrhosis.[10]

Drugs timelines for hepatitis B:

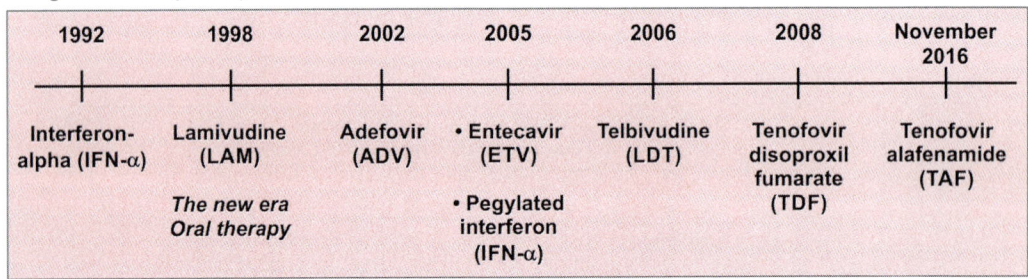

Clinical trials are still undergoing to establish safety profile of tenofovir alafenamide which is newer drug in pregnancy, hence it is still not recommended to be used in pregnancy.[12]

World Health Organization recommends that pregnant women testing positive for HBV infection (HBsAg positive) with an HBV DNA ≥5.3 $\log_{10}$ IU/mL (≥200,000 IU/mL^2) receive tenofovir prophylaxis from the 28th week of pregnancy till delivery, to prevent mother-to-child transmission of HBV.[12]

Various studies have shown that risk of mother-to-child transmission (MTCT) reduces to as low as 80% with the use of tenofovir.

Newborns of mothers known to have hepatitis B must receive both:
- Monovalent hepatitis B vaccine
- Hepatitis B immunoglobulin (HBIG)

These should both be given at birth, at the same time in separate thighs.

The dose of HBIG is 100 IU given by IM injection. Infants should receive HBIG immediately after birth—within 12 hours of birth and certainly within 48 hours.

Monovalent hepatitis B vaccine is given preferably within 24 hours of birth, and within 7 days. This regimen results in seroconversion rates of >90% in neonates, even with concurrent administration of HBIG.

Vaccination must not be delayed beyond 7 days after birth.

Immunoprophylaxis by HBV vaccine and HBIG, given at birth with scheduled doses, reduces MTCT from 60–90% to 5–10%.[13]

WHO aims to reduce maternal to child transmission to 0.1% by 2030.[14]

■ HEPATITIS D IN PREGNANCY

It generally occurs as a co-infection or superinfection and the risk increases with high hepatitis B viral load especially in the third trimester of pregnancy. There is no specific antiviral against hepatitis D, hence supportive treatment plays a key role (*see* **Table 1**).

■ HEPATITIS C IN PREGNANCY

None of the antiviral therapies recommended for HCV infection are currently approved for use in antenatal women (*see* **Table 1**).

TABLE 2: Drugs in hepatitis B.

Name	Mechanism of action	Excretion	Side effects	Treatment	FDA category
Pegylated interferon alpha (IFN-α)	The exact mechanism is unknown. It is thought to act on various parts of the HBV lifecycle as well as augmenting cell-mediated immunity. It inhibits HBV replication by decreasing RNA transcription	• Pegylated IFN-α is distributed to both the liver and kidney, whereas standard IFN-α localizes principally in the kidney. Pegylated IFN-α requires hepatic metabolism by nonspecific proteases • Active renal excretion is <5%. Thus, pegylated IFN-α has significantly lower renal clearance than standard IFN-α and this prolongs antiviral activity	Flu-like symptoms, hematological toxicity, raised transaminases, nausea, fatigue, psychiatric sequelae	180 μg per week	C
Lamivudine	It is a nucleoside reverse transcriptase inhibitor (NRTI) with activity against hepatitis B (HBV) to disrupt viral DNA synthesis. When phosphorylated, lamivudine forms active metabolites which compete for incorporation into viral DNA	Approximately 5% is recovered in the urine as a trans-sulfoxide metabolite and 70% is excreted unchanged in the urine	• Headache • Diarrhea • Heartburn • Difficulty Falling asleep or staying asleep • Depression • Cough • Joint pain	100 mg orally once daily	C
Adefovir	It inhibits HBV DNA polymerase (reverse transcriptase) by competing with the natural substrate deoxyadenosine triphosphate and by causing DNA chain termination after its	It has renal excretion by a combination of glomerular filtration and active tubular secretion	Weakness, headache, fever, cough, nausea, vomiting, diarrhea	10 mg once a day	C

Contd...

Contd...

Name	Mechanism of action	Excretion	Side effects	Treatment	FDA category
Entecavir	It is a nucleoside analog (deoxyguanosine analog) that belongs to a class of carbocyclic nucleosides and inhibits reverse transcription, DNA replication, and transcription in the process of viral replication	Renal excretion (through glomerular filtration and tubular secretion)	• Abdominal or stomach discomfort • Decreased appetite • Difficulty with swallowing • Tachycardia • Tachypnea • General feeling of discomfort • Hives, itching, or rash • Muscle pain or cramping	0.5–1 mg or 10 to 20 mL OD	C
Telbivudine	It is activated by phosphorylation and is efficiently metabolized to 5-triphosphate derivative. 5-triphosphate metabolite of β-L-2-deoxynucleosides interacts with the viral polymerase and cause inhibition of viral replication resulting in obligate chain termination of DNA synthesis	Eliminated primarily by renal excretion of unchanged drug	Rash, hives, swollen, red blistered, or peeling skin with or without fever, itching, wheezing, tightness in the chest or throat; trouble breathing, swallowing, or talking, hoarseness	600 mg or 30 mL OD	B
Tenofovir	It is a nucleotide analog that inhibits viral replication by competing with natural nucleotides for binding to the active site of HBV polymerase	It is mainly excreted via the kidneys, both by glomerular filtration and by tubular secretion	• Weakness or tiredness • Unusual muscle pain • Shortness of breath or fast breathing • Stomach pain with nausea or vomiting • Cold or blue hands or feet • Dizziness • Tachycardia	300-mg per oral daily	B

(FDA: Food and Drug Administration)

Ribavirin, which is a nucleoside analog, is contraindicated in pregnancy due to its association with embryocidal and/or teratogenic effects in all animal species studied. Ribavirin use has been found to be associated with malformations of the gastrointestinal tract, skull, palate, jaw, limbs, skeleton, and eye in animal models.[15] Additionally, since Ribavirin can persist in non-plasma compartments for a period up to 6 months, the US Food and Drug Administration (FDA) advises that pregnancy should be avoided in women taking Ribavirin as well as in female partners of male patients taking Ribavirin until 6 months after completing therapy.

There are limited studies on the effects of second-generation DAA (direct acting antiviral agents) therapy in pregnancy.

The FDA has not categorized most of these drugs in terms of pregnancy safety, since many of them were introduced after the FDA began eliminating A-B-C-D-X pregnancy drug categories in 2014.[16]

Limited animal studies have shown *Sofosbuvir* and Ombitasvir/Paritaprevir/Ritonavir do not confer a risk to the fetus.[16,17]

Drugs such as velpatasvir, daclatasvir, ombitasvir/paritaprevir/ritonavir/dasabuvir, ledipasvir, and elbasvir/grazoprevir have not been included in approved FDA drug category.[16]

However, the limited animal data that exists has not shown a risk to the fetus due to the lack of human studies, no DAA therapy has yet been approved to treat HCV infection in pregnancy. A recent clinical trial on the pharmacokinetics of ledipasvir/sofosbuvir during pregnancy in women has shown some promising results after a 12-week treatment course.[17]

If a woman becomes pregnant while taking one of the DAA therapies, animal data do not suggest teratogenic risk, but women should be counseled that human data are lacking.[18]

HEPATITIS E IN PREGNANCY

The symptoms of hepatitis E range from mild to severe—fulminant course in pregnancy. Hepatitis E infection in pregnancy carries a very high risk of liver failure with high risk of mortality. There is no available treatment option for hepatitis E in pregnancy as of now. Although for nonpregnant patients, available options include ribavirin and interferons alpha.[18-20]

Since this infection is primarily water and foodborne, hence preventive measures are always emphasized (*see* **Table 1**).

In case of HEV-induced acute liver failure (ALF), liver transplantation may offer some help.

Further trials are still undergoing to establish the efficacy and safety of hepatitis E vaccines in pregnancy.[18,20]

HEPATIC ENCEPHALOPATHY IN PREGNANCY

The wide spectrum of neurological or psychiatric manifestations ranging from subclinical alterations to coma caused due to deteriorating liver condition is defined as hepatic encephalopathy. As hepatic encephalopathy is a manifestation of serious liver impairment, its outcome depends upon the severity of underlying liver disease, its clinical course, and its treatment.[18,21]

During pregnancy, most common causes of liver failure include acute fatty liver of pregnancy and HELLP syndrome, viral infections—HBV, HAV, HEV, and herpes simplex. Other nonpregnant causes include drug-induced liver diseases, toxins, mushroom poisoning, shock, trauma, and decompensation of pre-existing liver diseases.

There is a high incidence of maternal mortality in these cases due to hepatic encephalopathy, renal failure, coagulopathy, metabolic acidosis, and sepsis.[21,22]

Early diagnosis can be made based on proper history and examination, epidemiological, clinical, and laboratory findings. Prompt management can save both mother and baby.

The principles of management include supportive care to mother and prompt delivery of the fetus with following keys points:[22]

- Multidisciplinary team approach with senior obstetricians, obstetric anesthetists, gastroenterologists, neurologists, and intensivists.
- Treatment is usually similar to that of hepatic encephalopathy in the absence of pregnancy.
- Hemodynamic stabilization including maintaining patency of airways, careful monitoring of oxygen saturation, and other parameters.
- Fluid correction has to be done carefully as these patients have low systemic vascular resistance and volume depletion. The possibility of pulmonary edema and volume overload due to hypoalbuminemia and concomitant development of renal insufficiency has to be kept in mind.
- Correction of metabolic and electrolyte disturbances and coagulation profile with fresh frozen plasma (FFP) and platelet transfusion
- *Lowering of ammonia*: As ammonia is produced by glutamine, by enterocytes, as well as generated by colonic bacteria through catabolism of nitrogenous sources. Due to liver failure, serum ammonia gets elevated, concomitant renal failure can worsen it. This is further aggravated by hypokalemia, which increases renal ammonia production. So, lactulose enema, restriction of dietary protein, antibiotics should be given.
- Nephrotoxic drugs should be avoided due to high risk of renal failure.[8] After stabilization of patient, termination of pregnancy to be considered.
- High-risk labor management protocols to be followed under expert team guidance and care with proper precautions to control postpartum hemorrhage (PPH).

Viral infection, acute hepatitis related to hepatitis E virus and herpes simplex virus, is known to have an increased risk of acute liver failure in pregnant patient although the course of acute viral hepatitis is unaffected by pregnancy.

Acute fatty liver of pregnancy: Swansea diagnostic criteria[23] is helpful in diagnosis—six or more of the following features in the absence of another explanation:

- Vomiting
- Abdominal pain
- Polydipsia/polyuria
- Encephalopathy, high bilirubin (>14 µmol/L)
- Hypoglycemia (<4 mmol/L)
- High uric acid (>340 µmol/L)
- Leukocytosis (>11 × 106/L)
- Ascites or bright liver on ultrasound
- High aspartate transaminase (AST)/alanine transaminase (ALT) (>42 IU/L)
- High ammonia (>47 µmol/L)
- Renal impairment (creatinine >150 µmol/L)
- Coagulopathy [PT >14 seconds or activated partial thromboplastin time (aPTT) >34 seconds]
- Microvesicular steatosis on liver biopsy

The definitive treatment of acute fatty liver in pregnancy (AFLP) and HELLP is delivery. If possible, vaginal delivery is induced, but if the maternal or fetal condition does not permit this, operative delivery must be achieved as soon as safely possible. After delivery, the mother must be observed carefully for deterioration in the hemodynamic status because of the risk of clotting failure.

Liver transplants have been a last and rare resort in AFLP when women show irreparable liver failure even after delivery and despite intensive medical support, or hepatic encephalopathy, severe metabolic acidosis, or worsening coagulopathy.[22,23]

■ KEY POINTS

- Hepatitis in pregnancy can be caused by various viruses and other agents. It may have variable presentation from asymptomatic, mild to fulminant course. There are chances of vertical transmission also.
- Hepatitis A is spread by feco-oral route and generally has a benign course in pregnancy. Pre- and postexposure vaccine prophylaxis is recommended for individuals including pregnant ladies as no specific treatment is available.
- HBV infection is transmitted through parenteral as well sexual contact. There are high chances of vertical transmission in pregnancy from 10 to 90%, especially high during third trimester and delivery. Early pregnancy screening is recommended for all antenatal ladies multidisciplinary team approach while treating hepatitis B in pregnancy is advisable for better patient outcome.
- Preconception counseling and immunization of ladies, judicious use of antiviral therapy (Tenofovir) shows promising results against hepatitis B. Active and passive immunization of infants is recommended to avoid lifelong complications and morbidity associated with hepatitis B virus.
- Hepatitis C is caused by RNA virus and may coexist with hepatitis B virus during pregnancy. It is managed symptomatically during pregnancy as no specific antiviral therapy/vaccine is approved. Early screening in pregnancy is recommended.
- Hepatitis E virus is the most important non-A and non-B hepatitis virus worldwide. It has variable presentation from asymptomatic to fulminant hepatitis with high chance of mortality during pregnancy. Safe hygiene practices are recommended since no antiviral therapy or vaccine is available.

■ REFERENCES

1. Lemon SM, Ott JJ, Van Damme P, Shouval D. Type a viral hepatitis: a summary and update on the molecular virology, epidemiology, pathogenesis and prevention. J Hepatol. 2018;68:167-84.
2. Lanini S, Ustianowski A, Pisapia R, Zumla A, Ippolito G. Viral Hepatitis: etiology, epidemiology, transmission, diagnostics, treatment, and Prevention. Infect Dis Clin North Am. 2019;33:1045-62.
3. Elinav E, Ben-Dov IZ, Shapira Y, Daudi N, Adler R, Shouval D, et al. Acute hepatitis a infection in pregnancy is associated with high rates of gestational complications and preterm labor. Gastroenterology. 2006;130:1129-34.
4. WHO. Position paper on hepatitis a vaccines. Wkly Epidemiol Rec. 2012;28:261-75.
5. Dahiya M, Kumar A, Kar P, Gupta RK, Kumar A. Acute viral hepatitis in third trimester of pregnancy. Indian J Gastroenterol. 2005;24:128-9.
6. World Health Organization. Global Hepatitis Report, 2017. Geneva: WHO; 2017.
7. Groom HC, Smith N, Irving SA, Koppolu P, Vazquez-Benitez G, Kharbanda EO, et al. Uptake and safety of hepatitis A vaccination during pregnancy: a vaccine safety datalink study. Vaccine. 2019;37:6648-55.
8. US Department of Health and Human Services. (2019). Hepatitis B basic information. [online] Available from: https://www.hhs.gov/hepatitis/learn-about-viral-hepatitis/hepatitis-b-basics/index.html. [Last accessed December, 2023].
9. Su WJ, Chen SF, Yang CH, Chuang PH, Chang HF, Chang MH. The impact of universal infant hepatitis B immunization on reducing the hepatitis B carrier rate in pregnant women. J Infect Dis. 2019;220;1118-26.
10. European Association for the Study of the Liver (EASL). EASL 2017 Clinical practice Guidelines on the management of hepatitis B virus infection. J Hepatol. 2017;67(2):370-98.
11. NHS Infectious Diseases in Pregnancy Screening Programme. Laboratory handbook 2016-2017. [online] Available from:

https://www.gov.uk/government/publications/infectious-diseases-in-pregnancy-screening-programme-laboratory-handbook/infectious-diseases-in-pregnancy-screening-programme-laboratory-handbook. [Last accessed December, 2023].
12. Razavi-shearer D, Gamkrelidze I, Nguyen MH, Chen DS, Van Damme P, Abbas Z, et al. Global prevalence, treatment, and prevention of hepatitis B virus infection in 2016; a modelling study. Lancet Gastroenterol Hepatol. 2018;(6):383-403.
13. World Health Organization. Hepatitis B. (2023). https://www.who.int/news-room/fact-sheets/detail/hepatitis-b. [Last accessed December, 2023].
14. May S, Mandal S, Keel P, Haywood B, Ngui SL, Ramsay M, et al. Hepatitis B virus immunization and neonatal acquisition of persistent infection in England and Wales. J Infect Dis. 2018:218(5):726-33.
15. US National Library of Medicine. Drug label information: ribavirin tablet. US National Library of Medicine Daily Med. [online] Available from: https://dailymed.nlm.nih.gov/dailymed/drugInfo.cfm?setid=eee304d0-c2ea-44f4-97d9-92a414d31b6c. [Last accessed December, 2023].
16. US National Library of Medicine. Drug label information: Sovaldie sofosbuvir tablet, film coated. US National Library of Medicine Daily Med. [online] Available from: https://dailymed.nlm.nih.gov/dailymed/drugInfo.cfm?setid=80beab2c-396e-4a37-a4dc-40fdb62859cf. [Last accessed December, 2023].
17. Chappell CA, Scarsi KK, Kirby BJ, Suri V, Gaggar A, Bogen DL, et al. Ledipasvir plus sofosbuvir in pregnant women with hepatitis C virus infection: a phase 1 pharmocokinetic study. The Lancet Microbe. 2020;1(5):e200-8.
18. Berglov A, Hallager S, Weis N. Hepatitis E during pregnancy: maternal and fetal case—fatality rates and adverse outcomes—a systematic review. J Viral Hepat. 2019;26(11): 1240-8.
19. WHO. (2023) Hepatitis E fact sheet. [online] Available from: https://www.who.int/news-room/fact-sheets/detail/hepatitis-e. [Last accessed December, 2023].
20. Perez-Gracia MT, Suay-Garcia B, Mateos-Lindermann ML. Hepatitis E and pregnancy: current state. Rev Med Virol. 2017; 27(3):e1929.
21. Westbrook RH, Dusheiko G, Williamson C. Pregnancy and liver disease. J Hepatol. 2016;64(4):933-45.
22. Pandey CK, Karna ST, Pandey VK, Tandon M. Acute liver failure in pregnancy: challenges and management. Indian J Anaesth. 2015:59(3):144-9.
23. Nelson DB, Byrne JJ, Cunningham FG. Acte fatty liver of pregnan. Obstet Gynecol. 2021:137:535-46.

Section 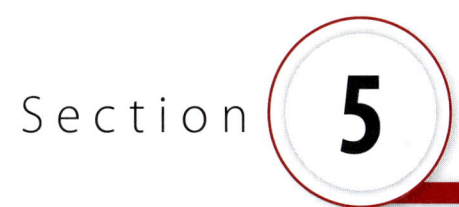 5

Medical Management of Respiratory Disorders in Pregnancy

- **Bronchial Asthma**
  Ajay Chauhan

- **Respiratory Infections**
  Rekha Bharti, Vitusha Suri

Chapter 11

Bronchial Asthma

Ajay Chauhan

Bronchial asthma is one of the most common respiratory illnesses, encountered during pregnancy.

Asthma is a heterogeneous disease, characterized by chronic airway inflammation. It is defined by the history of respiratory symptoms, such as wheezing, shortness of breath, chest tightness, and cough, that vary over time and in intensity, together with variable expiratory airflow limitation.[1]

■ DIAGNOSIS

Bronchial asthma is a clinical diagnosis, characterized by variable respiratory symptoms, such as wheezing, chest tightness, cough, and shortness of breath.

- Symptoms are varying in intensity and timing.
- Symptoms are worsened at night or upon waking up.
- Symptoms are exacerbated by exercise, laughter, allergens, and cold air.
- Symptoms appear or are exacerbated by viral infections.

Diagnosis is confirmed by:
- Documented expiratory flow limitation [forced expiratory volume in 1 second/forced vital capacity (FEV_1/FVC): <0.75–0.80]
- *Documented variability in expiratory flow limitation:*
  - *Bronchodilator responsiveness:* FEV_1 increases by >12%
  - Excessive variability in twice daily peak expiratory flow (PEF) (>10%)
  - Significant increase in respiratory functions over 4 weeks of inflammatory therapy (FEV_1 increases by 12%)
  - Positive exercise challenge test (fall in FEV_1 by >10%)
  - Positive methacholine challenge test (fall in FEV_1 by ≥20%).

The course of the disease during pregnancy is highly heterogenous and varies from patient to patient.[2] Over one-third of the bronchial asthma cases report worsening of symptoms during pregnancy, one-third have a stable course over pregnancy, and over one-third have reported an improvement of symptoms during pregnancy.[3] Various physiological changes occur due to pregnancy, and they affect the disease process of asthma, and the manifestations and exacerbations of asthma also have an effect on the outcome of the pregnancy.[4]

Figure 1 shows the management of bronchial asthma in pregnancy.

The advantages of actively treating bronchial asthma during pregnancy markedly outweighs the potential risks of the usual controller and reliever medications.

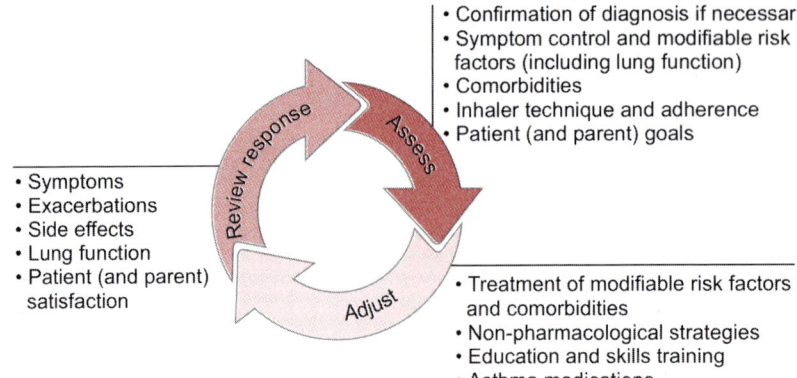

Fig. 1: Management of bronchial asthma in pregnancy.

TABLE 1: Drug therapy of bronchial asthma.	
Symptoms	**Therapy**
Step 1: Infrequent asthma symptoms <2 times a week	• Low-dose ICS plus rapid-onset LABA (e.g., budesonide–formoterol combination MDI 160 μg/4.5 μg per inhalation, or DPI 200 μg/6 μg per inhalation) one inhalation as and when needed Or • Low-dose ICS plus SABA whenever needed
Step 2: Asthma symptoms and inhaler need >2 times a week	• Low-dose ICS–formoterol as needed Or • Low-dose ICS daily and SABA when needed
Step 3: Troublesome asthma most days of the week, nocturnal awakening due to asthma at least once per month or risk factor exacerbations present	• *Preferred:* Low-dose ICS–formoterol as maintenance and reliever therapy Or • Low-dose ICS–LABA daily with SABA as and when needed
Steps 4–5: Severely uncontrolled asthma with ≥3 of the following: • Daytime symptoms >2 times a week • Nocturnal awakening due to asthma >2 times a week • Reliever needed >2 times a week • Activity limitation due to asthma Or • Acute exacerbation (Step 5)	*Step 4:* • Medium-dose ICS–formoterol as reliever and maintenance therapy Or • Medium-dose ICS–LABA daily plus SABA as and when needed *Step 5:* • Medium-dose ICS–LABA as reliever and maintenance therapy, plus LAMA daily Or • Medium-dose ICS–LABA plus LAMA daily, plus SABA as and when needed

(DPI: dry powdered inhaler; ICS: inhaled corticosteroids; LABA: long-acting beta agonists; LAMA: long-acting muscarinic agonists; MDI: metered dose inhaler; SABA: short-acting beta agonists)

TABLE 2: Drugs used in bronchial asthma.

Drug class	Form	Dosage	Side effects	Safety in pregnancy
Short-acting beta agonists—rescuer drugs: Salbutamol	• HFA: 90 µg/puff • DPI: 90 µg/puff • Nebulized solution: 5 mg/mL and 0.63, 1.25, and 2.5 mg/3 mL	• Two puffs every 4–6 hours as needed and two puffs 15–30 minutes before exercise • Two puffs every 4–6 hours as needed and two puffs 15–30 minutes before exercise • 1.25–5 mg in 3 mL saline every 4–6 hours as needed	Increase in heart rate, tremors	Safe in pregnancy
Long-acting beta-agonists—used in combination therapy: • Arformoterol • Formoterol • Salmeterol	• Nebulized solution: 15 µg/2 mL • Nebulized solution: 20 µg/2 mL • HFA: 21 µg/puff • DPI: 50 µg/puff	• 15–25 µg every 12 hours • 20 µg every 12 hours • Two puffs every 12 hours • One puff every 12 hours	Increase in heart rate, tremors	Safe in pregnancy
Ultra-long-acting beta-agonists—used in combination therapy: • Indacaterol • Olodaterol	• DPI: 75 µg/puff • SMI: 2.5 µg/puff	• One puff once a day • Two puffs once a day	• Runny nose and sneezing • High blood pressure • Cough • Headache	Safe in pregnancy
Anticholinergics—used in combination therapy, but not as first line: • Ipratropium • Tiotropium	• HFA: 17 µg/puff • Nebulized solution: 500 µg (0.02%, 2 mL) • SMI: 1.25 µg/puff • DPI: 18 µg/capsule	• Two puffs every 6 hours as needed • 500 µg every 6–8 hours as needed • Two puffs once a day (maximum 2 puffs/day) • 18 µg (1 capsule) once a day	• Dry mouth • Rapid heart rate	Generally safe for intermittent usage in pregnancy

Contd...

Contd...

Drug class	Form	Dosage	Side effects	Safety in pregnancy
Inhaled corticosteroids—first-line therapy: • Beclomethasone • Budesonide • Fluticasone propionate	• HFA: 40–80 µg/puff • DPI: 90 or 180 µg/puff • HFA: 44, 110, or 220 µg/puffs • DPI: 50, 100, or 250 µg/puff	• One to two puffs every 12 hours • 360–720 µg twice a day • If previously taking bronchodilators alone, initial dose of 88 µg twice a day (maximum 440 µg twice a day) • If previously taking inhaled corticosteroids, initial dose of 88–220 µg twice a day (maximum 440 µg twice a day) • If previously taking oral corticosteroids, initial dose of 440–880 µg twice a day (maximum 880 µg twice a day) • If previously taking bronchodilators alone, initial dose of 100 µg twice a day (maximum 500 µg twice a day) • If previously taking inhaled corticosteroids, initial dose of 100–250 µg twice a day (maximum 500 µg twice a day) • If previously taking oral corticosteroids, initial dose of 500–1,000 µg twice a day (maximum 1,000 µg twice a day)	Fungal infection of the mouth (thrush)	Safe in pregnancy
Systemic corticosteroids (oral)—acute severe asthma, status asthmaticus: • Prednisone • Methylprednisolone	• Tablets: 1, 2.5, 5, 10, 20, or 50 mg • Tablets: 2, 4, 8, 16, or 32 mg	• 7.5–60 mg once a day in the morning or every other day in the morning • Short-course burst: 40–60 mg once a day for 3–10 days	• Weight gain • Elevated blood sugar levels • Rarely, psychosis • Osteoporosis • Cataracts • Skin thinning and easy bruising • Insomnia	Adverse effects were recorded, but when indicated in acute exacerbations, they potentially outweigh the risk of asthma exacerbation

Contd...

Contd...

Drug class	Form	Dosage	Side effects	Safety in pregnancy
Mast cell stabilizers: Cromolyn	Nebulized solution: 20 mg/ampule	One ampule three or four times a day	Coughing or wheezing	Limited studies available
Leukotriene modifiers: • Montelukast • Zafirlukast	Tablets, chewable tablets, and granules: 4, 5, or 10 mg	• 10 mg orally once a day in the evening • 20 mg orally in the evening	Eosinophilic granulomatosis with polyangiitis	Safe in pregnancy, but studies are limited
Methylxanthines: Theophylline	• Tablet: 10 or 20 mg • Tablet, extended-release: 100, 200, 400, 450, or 600 mg	Initial dose of 10 mg/kg/day up to 600 mg/day, then adjusted to achieve a serum concentration of 5–15 μg/mL at steady state	• Increased heart rate • Shakiness • Stomach upset • Seizures (if the blood level is high) • Arrhythmias	Limited usage, but safety recorded on clinical experience
Immunomodulators				Limited studies to comment upon

(DPI: dry powder inhaler; HFA: hydrofluoroalkane; MDI: metered-dose inhaler; PEF: peak expiratory flow; SMI: soft mist inhaler)

Goals of treatment:
- Achieve and maintain remission
- Prevent acute exacerbations

Effective communication with the patient regarding the hesitation of taking the essential drugs during pregnancy forms an important aspect of management.[5]

NON-PHARMACOLOGICAL MANAGEMENT

- Educating the patient regarding the nature and course of the disease during pregnancy, drugs, and their potential adverse effects, and how the benefits of taking the essential drugs far outweigh the risk of potential adverse effects.
- Monthly follow-up (as opposed 2 or 3 months once in nonpregnant patients)
- Routine evaluation with fractional exhaled nitric oxide (FENO) and Asthma Control Questionnaire (ACQ)
- To avoid potential triggers of exacerbation, such as pollen, cigarette-smoking, animal dander, dust, change in weather, and emotions
- To ensure proper technique of inhaler use.

PHARMACOLOGICAL MANAGEMENT

Drug therapy of bronchial asthma during pregnancy remains largely unaltered, as various studies have proven that the drugs used for long-term management of bronchial asthma can be safely used during pregnancy as well **(Tables 1 and 2)**.[6]

Biologics like omalizumab even though not to be started on a pregnant patient can be continued if the patient is already on it.[7]

Approximately 10% of the patients have acute exacerbations during labor, mainly due to hyperventilation causing bronchoconstriction. Short-acting beta agonists (SABAs) are used during acute exacerbations, but they may cause neonatal hypoglycemia. Blood glucose monitoring to be done for at least 24 hours post delivery. In uncontrolled exacerbations, systemic corticosteroids can also be used. Intravenous (IV) magnesium sulfate can be used as an adjunct to corticosteroids, for acute exacerbation of asthma.

KEY POINTS

- Bronchial asthma is one of the most common respiratory illnesses, encountered during pregnancy.
- An early diagnosis by peak flow meter followed thereafter with titration of treatment can go a long way in avoiding acute worsening.
- Patient education is necessary to avoid potential triggers of exacerbation, such as pollen, cigarette-smoking, animal dander, dust, change in weather, and emotion. It is mandatory to teach proper technique of inhaler use.
- Benefits of instituting pharmacologic therapy at right time far outweighs its risks.

REFERENCES

1. Global Initiative for Asthma (GINA) (2022). Global Strategy for Asthma Management and Prevention. [online] Available from: https://ginasthma.org/gina-reports/ [Last accessed December, 2023].
2. Gluck JC, Gluck PA. The effect of pregnancy on the course of asthma. Immunol Allergy Clin North Am. 2006;1:63-80.
3. Schatz M, Harden K, Forsythe A, Chilingar L, Hoffman C, Sperling W, et al. The course of asthma during pregnancy, post partum, and with successive pregnancies: a prospective analysis. J Allergy Clin Immunol. 1988; 3:509-17.
4. Grindheim G, Toska K, Estensen ME, Rosseland LA. Changes in pulmonary function during pregnancy: a longitudinal cohort study. BJOG. 2012;1:94-101.

5. Popa M, Peltecu G, Gica N, Ciobanu AM, Botezatu R, Gica C, et al. Asthma in Pregnancy. Review of Current Literature and Recommendations. Maedica (Bucur). 2021;16(1):80-7.
6. Scottish Intercollegiate Guidelines Network; British Thoracic Society. (2019). SIGN158 British guideline on the management of asthma. [online] Available from: https://www.sign.ac.uk/media/1773/sign158-updated.pdf [Last accessed December, 2023].
7. National Asthma Council. (2022). Australian Asthma Handbook. [online] Available from: https://www.nationalasthma.org.au/health-professionals/australian-asthma-handbook [Last accessed December, 2023].

Chapter 12

Respiratory Infections

Rekha Bharti, Vitusha Suri

Respiratory tract infections (RTIs) include infections of upper and lower respiratory tract. Most of the outpatient visits of adults and children are due to RTIs, involving mainly upper respiratory tract.[1] Although, the main etiological factor is viral infection, it is also the most important cause of antibiotic misuse.[2] Other causes include bacterial and fungal infections.

Various types of upper respiratory tract infections (URTIs), their common presentations, causes and management are described in **Tables 1 and 2**.

COMMUNITY-ACQUIRED PNEUMONIA

Clinical Presentation

In women with RTI, findings suggestive of bacterial pneumonia include fever, productive cough with purulent sputum, shortness of breath, and pleuritic chest pain. Patient looks ill and has dyspnea, tachypnea, tachycardia, and abnormal breath sound including crackles, rales, and signs of parenchymal consolidation. In viral community-acquired pneumonia (CAP) onset of illness is gradual with low-grade temperature, nonproductive cough, and wheezing. The disease shows seasonal trend and is more often seen in the fall or winter.[11,15-17]

Causes

Common causative bacteria include *Streptococcus pneumoniae*, *Mycoplasma pneumoniae*, *Haemophilus influenzae*, and *Staphylococcus aureus*, and most of viral infections are due to influenza A and B, COVID-19 (coronavirus disease 2019), and varicella zoster virus. Fungal causes include histoplasmosis, blastomycosis, coccidioidomycosis, and aspergillosis.

Diagnostic Tests

The diagnostic tests include chest radiograph, sputum gram stain and culture, blood counts, and blood cultures.

Management

Line of management depends on the severity of illness and epidemiologic evidence of causative pathogens that may progress rapidly to severe disease, e.g., COVID-19, influenza, postviral bacterial pneumonias, severe acute respiratory syndrome, and Middle East respiratory syndrome. With presence of organisms that can rapidly progress to severe disease, a close clinical follow-up of women is needed who may initially present with mild disease. Pregnant women in particular are at increased risk of rapidly progressing disease and may need close observation.

CHAPTER 12: Respiratory Infections

TABLE 1: Upper respiratory tract infections (URTIs)—presentations, causes, and management.

URTI	Presentation	Causes	Diagnosis	Treatment	Pregnancy and lactation

Common cold	• *Most common symptom:* Nasal congestion
	• *Common symptoms:* Sore throat, cough, malaise
	• *Less common:* Fever, conjunctivitis
		Rhinoviruses	Clinical	*Self-limiting:* Generally resolves in 10 days
				• *Nasal congestion:* Heated humidified air, saline nasal sprays
				• *Pharmacotherapy:* Ipratropium bromide nasal spray: 0.06%, two 42 µg sprays per nostril three to four times a day. Intranasal cromolyn sodium (aqueous): 5.2 mg/dose, one spray per nostril up to six times per day, may cause transient bronchospasm; use with caution in asthmatics
				• *Sore throat/pharyngitis, headache, fever:* Tab acetaminophen 500 mg PO SOS. Maximum dose <3 g/day
				• *Cough:* Honey or honey-containing preparations guaifenesin—100–400 mg PO q4h; not to exceed 2.4 g/day; dextromethorphan syrup—10–20 mg PO q4 hr OR 30 mg q6–8h
					• *Ipratropium bromide nasal spray:* Animal studies have not shown adverse effects. Negligibly absorbed systemically. Studies have not identified a drug-associated risk of major birth defects, miscarriage, or adverse maternal or fetal outcomes
					  – *Lactation:* Distribution in breastmilk not known
					• *Intranasal cromolyn sodium:* There are no controlled data in human pregnancy
					  – *Lactation:* Considered compatible with breastfeeding as per WHO
					• *Acetaminophen:* Normal doses not associated with miscarriage or still birth; it is associated with a decrease of some congenital anomalies related to maternal hyperthermia[3]
					• *Guaifenesin:* Most studies suggest that guaifenesin is not associated with an increased risk of birth defects over background risk
					  – *Lactation:* Distribution in breast not known
					• *Dextromethorphan:* Available data has not demonstrated major teratogenic risk
					  – *Lactation:* Distribution in breast not known

Contd...

Contd...

URTI	Presentation	Causes	Diagnosis	Treatment	Pregnancy and lactation
Acute bronchitis D/D: Common cold and pneumonia	• Acute-onset persistent cough without clinical findings of pneumonia, sputum production Initially symptoms resemble common cold, but cough persists for 1–3 weeks • Fever is more common with influenza or pneumonia • Purulent sputum is reported in 50% cases,[4] and does not signify bacterial infection	• Virus in 90% cases, include influenza A and B, parainfluenza virus 3, coronavirus, adenovirus, metapneumovirus, rhinovirus, and respiratory syncytial virus • *Occasional:* *Mycoplasma pneumoniae,* *Chlamydia pneumoniae,* or *Bordetella pertussis*	Chest radiograph can be done safely in pregnancy and abnormalities on chest radiography distinguishes acute bronchitis from pneumonia	• *Viral:* Symptomatic treatment same as common cold, antibiotics are not beneficial • *Nonviral:* Treat *pertussis* during the first 1–2 weeks before coughing paroxysms occurs. Treatment is ineffective if started late in the course of illness. Antibiotic therapy (Tab azithromycin 500 mg PO on day 1 followed by 250 mg OD from day 2–5) for pregnant patients • Women near term with clinical or microbiologic diagnosis of *pertussis* should receive antibiotics within 6 weeks after cough onset to prevent transmission to neonates[5] • *Mycoplasma pneumoniae* or *Chlamydia pneumoniae:* Antibiotics are not required in absence of pneumonia	• No drug-associated risks for major birth defects, miscarriage, or adverse maternal or fetal outcomes are reported • *Lactation:* No serious adverse reactions or effect on lactation is reported • S/E: Nausea, vomiting, diarrhea, hepatitis, cholestatic jaundice, hepatic failure, hepatic necrosis, QT interval prolongation

Contd...

Contd...

URTI	Presentation	Causes	Diagnosis	Treatment	Pregnancy and lactation

Acute sinusitis	• Classic findings: Nasal congestion, purulent nasal discharge, maxillary tooth discomfort, hyposmia, and facial pain or pressure that is worse when bending forward. Pregnant women with common cold are at increased risk of developing rhinosinusitis and Eustachian tube dysfunction due to nasal congestion from hormonal effects[6]
	• Uncomplicated cases resolve in 7–10 days
		• Most common viruses
		• Secondary bacterial: In small fraction
			• Criteria to diagnose acute bacterial rhinosinusitis: In pregnant patients:[2,7-9]
			  – Persistent symptoms or signs for ≥10 days without improvement
			  – Temperature >39°C, purulent nasal discharge, or facial pain for at least 3–4 consecutive days at the beginning of the URTI
			  – Worsening of symptoms or signs (such as doubling in severity or the new onset of fever, headache, nasal discharge, following a typical viral URTI that lasted 5–6 days and was initially improving)
			• Sinus radiographs: In resistant cases
				• Symptomatic management for 7 days in suspected acute bacterial rhinosinusitis. Antibiotic therapy
				  – Cap amoxicillin 500 mg PO TDS or amoxicillin–clavulanate 625 mg TDS or third-generation cephalosporin with or without clindamycin in case of penicillin allergy. Fluoroquinolones and doxycycline should be avoided
				  – *S/E*: Amoxicillin diarrhea, antibiotic-associated diarrhea due to *Clostridium difficile* candidal diaper rash, skin rash, urticaria, nausea, vomiting
				• *Clindamycin*: Diarrhea, antibiotic-associated diarrhea due to *C. difficile*, nausea, vomiting, flatulence, metallic taste, anorexia, esophagitis, Maculopapular skin rash
				• *Adjunctive treatments*: Saline nasal spray, acetaminophen, and steroid nasal sprays (beclomethasone or budesonide) to relieve nasal congestion and pain
				• No role of antihistamines,[6] decongestants or guaifenesin
					• *Amoxicillin*: No drug-associated risks for major birth defects, miscarriage, or adverse maternal or fetal outcomes reported
					  – *Lactation*: Secreted in breast milk and diarrhea in breastfed infant; no effect on lactation
					• *Amoxicillin–clavulanate*:
					  – *Pregnancy*: No teratogenic effects; may be associated with an increased risk of necrotizing enterocolitis in neonates
					  – *Lactation*: Except for risk of sensitization no known adverse effects for the breastfed infant
					• Cephalosporins and clindamycin are generally considered safe during pregnancy

(OD: once a day; PO: per oral; q4h: every 4 hours; S/E: side effect; SOS: as needed; TDS: three times a day)

TABLE 2: Antimicrobials used for treatment of pneumonia.

Type of infection	Antimicrobials	Doses	Pregnancy and lactation	Side effects (S/E) and contraindications (C/I)
Bacterial	No comorbidities and no antibiotic use in previous 3 months—azithromycin	Azithromycin:[10] 500 mg once a day on day 1, followed by 250 mg once a day on days 2–5	No drug-associated risks for major birth defects, miscarriage, or adverse maternal or fetal outcomes • Lactation: No serious adverse reactions or effect on lactation is reported	Azithromycin common S/E: Diarrhea, nausea, abdominal pain, hypersensitivity, prolonged QT interval leading to cardiac arrhythmia and torsades de pointes, exacerbations of symptoms of myasthenia gravis
	Presence of comorbidities or use of antibiotics in previous 3 months or inpatient, non-ICU treatment—Beta-lactam plus azithromycin	Cefotaxime:[10] 1–2 g IV or IM 8 hourly	Although cefotaxime has been reported to cross the placental barrier and appear in cord blood, the effect on the human fetus is not known • Lactation: Drug enters breast milk; use with caution	Cefotaxime: Rapid bolus through central line can lead to potentially life-threatening arrhythmia, use for >10 days can cause granulocytopenia, use with caution in patients with penicillin allergy and history of colitis, may potentiate effects of nephrotoxic drugs, including aminoglycosides, NSAIDs, and furosemide
	Inpatient, ICU treatment: Beta-lactam (cefotaxime, ceftriaxone or ampicillin–sulbactam) plus either azithromycin	Ceftriaxone:[10] 1–2 g IV 12–24 hourly	No drug-associated risks for major birth defects, miscarriage, or adverse maternal or fetal outcomes reported • Lactation: No serious adverse reactions or effect on lactation is reported	• S/E ceftriaxone: Induration after IM injection, eosinophilia, thrombocytosis, diarrhea, elevated hepatic transaminases, leukopenia, rash, increased blood urea nitrogen (BUN), induration at IV site • Contraindications include documented hypersensitivity; hyperbilirubinemia in neonates; neonates <28 days if they receive calcium-containing IV products • C/I: Hypersensitivity, previous history of cholestatic jaundice/hepatic dysfunction associated with ampicillin sulbactam • In renal failure dose adjustment is required
		Ampicillin–sulbactam:[10] 1.5 g (1 g ampicillin + 0.5 g sulbactam) to 3 g (2 g ampicillin + 1 g sulbactam) IV 6 hourly	Ampicillin–sulbactam: Both ampicillin and sulbactam cross the placenta. Based on available data, penicillin antibiotics are generally considered compatible for use during pregnancy • Lactation: Excreted in milk, caution is advised but no major fetal effect reported	S/E Ampicillin–sulbactam: Diarrhea, IV injection site pain, thrombophlebitis, rash, hepatitis, cholestasis, hyperbilirubinemia, jaundice, abnormal hepatic function, melena, gastritis, stomatitis, dyspepsia, and *Clostridium difficile*-associated diarrhea

Contd...

Contd...

Type of infection	Antimicrobials	Doses	Pregnancy and lactation	Side effects (S/E) and contraindications (C/I)
Suspected Pseudomonas infection	Antipneumococcal, antipseudomonal beta-lactam (piperacillin–tazobactam, cefepime, imipenem, or meropenem) plus an aminoglycoside and azithromycin (for penicillin-sensitive patients, replace beta-lactam with aztreonam)	Piperacillin–tazobactam:[10] 4.5 g IV 6 hourly	Crosses placenta but insufficient data available for fetal effects Lactation: Piperacillin is excreted in human milk; tazobactam is not studied. No information available regarding effect on breastfed baby	Piperacillin–tazobactam: Diarrhea is major side effect • C/I: Allergy to penicillins, cephalosporins, imipenem, beta-lactamase inhibitors • Caution: Hypernatrenia due to high Na$^+$ content and in hypokalemia • Renal dose adjustment is required
		Cefepime:[10] 1–2 g IV 8–12 hourly	No drug exposure during pregnancy has been reported Lactation: Excreted in breast milk, no information on effect on baby	Cefepime—S/E: Positive Coombs test without hemolysis • C/I: Hypersensitivity to cefepime, penicillins, or other beta-lactam antibiotics
		Imipenem:[10] 500–750 mg IV 12 hourly to 500 mg 6 hourly	Imipenem: Insufficient data available on use in pregnancy and lactation	Imipenem: Phlebitis, seizures, transient increase in BUN and creatinine, false positive Coombs test
		Meropenem:[10] 1 g IV 8 hourly	• Meropenem: Few cases of exposure in pregnancy—no effect on fetus reported • Lactation: No data on effects on breastfed baby	Meropenem: Constipation, diarrhea, nausea, vomiting, irritation at site of injection
		Aztreonam:[10] 2 g IV/IM 6–8 hourly, maximum 8 g/day	• Aztreonam: Animal studies have not shown teratogenicity. However there is no controlled data from human pregnancy studies • Lactation: Excreted in milk in low concentrations; according to American Academy of Pediatrics committee drug is compatible with nursing	Aztreonam: Pain at injection site, increase in serum transaminases, neutropenia • C/I: Hypersensitivity • Dose adjustment in renal failure is required

Contd...

Contd...

Type of infection	Antimicrobials	Doses	Pregnancy and lactation	Side effects (S/E) and contraindications (C/I)
CA-MRSA	Beta-lactam (cefotaxime, ceftriaxone or ampicillin–sulbactam) plus azithromycin either vancomycin or linezolid	• Vancomycin:[10] 2 g/day either as 500 mg 6 hourly or 1 g 12 hourly • Initial daily dose ≥15 mg/kg Linezolid:[10] 600 mg orally or IV 12 hourly for 10–14 days	• Potential ototoxicity and nephrotoxicity • Lactation: secreted in breast milk, stop lactation or the drug • No reported risk of major birth defects, miscarriage, or adverse maternal or fetal outcomes • Lactation: Secreted in breast milk, diarrhea, and vomiting are common. Not much data available on adverse effects on breastfed baby	• S/E: Nausea, abdominal pain, hypokalemia, ototoxicity, nephrotoxicity • C/I: Hypersensitivity • Vancomycin infusion reaction due to rapid administration can cause pruritus and erythema of upper body neck, and upper torso Linezolid: • S/E: Common—headache, diarrhea, nausea, vomiting • C/I: Hypersensitivity, within 14 days of taking MAO inhibitor
Varicella zoster virus	Acyclovir	10–15 mg/kg IV 8 hourly for 7–10 days, renal dose adjustment required	• Use of acyclovir is not associated with an increase in birth defects. • Lactation: compatible with breastfeeding	S/E: Rashes, sweating, emesis, hypotension, tremors, disorientation
Influenza A and B virus	Oseltamivir Zanamivir Peramivir	Start within 48 hours of symptom onset. Most commonly used is oseltamivir:[11] 75 mg PO BD for 5 days • Zanamivir:[11] 10 mg (two 5 mg inhalations) twice daily for 5 days • Peramivir:[11] 600 mg IV as a single dose, renal dose adjustment required	Oseltamivir: • Pregnancy: Not associated with adverse fetal effects (based on epidemiological data) • Lactation: No reported adverse effects in breastfed babies Zanamivir: • Pregnancy: No risk of birth defects or adverse maternal or fetal outcomes • Pregnancy and lactation: Safety not proven	Oseltamivir: • S/E: Abdominal pain, insomnia, nausea, vomiting, vertigo • C/I: Hypersensitivity Zanamivir: • S/E: Headache, throat, cough • C/I: Hypersensitivity, can lead to bronchospasm in patients with asthma/COPD • Not effective for severe infection Peramivir: • S/E: Diarrhea, increased serum glucose (>160 mg/dL), creatine phosphokinase (≥6 × ULN), constipation, insomnia, AST and ALT increased, hypertension • C/I: Hypersensitivity

Contd...

Type of infection	Antimicrobials	Doses	Pregnancy and lactation	Side effects (S/E) and contraindications (C/I)
COVID-19	Antiviral	• *Remdesivir* for severe COVID-19 who are not on mechanical ventilation • *Dose:* 200 mg IV on day 1 followed by 100 mg IV daily for 5 days total (with extension to 10 days if there is no clinical improvement)	Insufficient data available on use in pregnancy and lactation	S/E: Nausea, vomiting, transaminase elevations, bradycardia[12,13]

Fungal pneumonia	*Blastomycosis and histoplasmosis:*[14] Most common fungal pneumonia, mild and self-limiting; other rare causes include coccidioidomycosis and aspergillosis	• Liposomal amphotericin B (AmB): 3 mg/kg/day IV or AmB lipid complex 5 mg/kg/day IV or AmB deoxycholate 0.7–1 mg/kg/day IV for 1–2 weeks followed by itraconazole 200 mg PO every 8 hours for the first 3 days, then 200 mg PO twice daily for a total of 12 weeks
		• Methylprednisolone: 0.5–1 mg/kg/day IV for 1–2 weeks for respiratory complications (e.g., hypoxemia or respiratory distress)
			• AmB: No adequate and well-controlled studies in pregnant women
			  – *Lactation:* It has potential for serious adverse reactions in breastfed infants, and decision should be made whether to discontinue nursing or discontinue drug
			• Itraconazole:
			  – *Pregnancy:* No reported major birth defects, inconclusive findings on risk of miscarriage
			  – *Lactation:* Insufficient data on secretion in human milk and effects on breastfed child or effects on milk production
				• AmB S/E: Nausea, vomiting, fever, chills, headache, nephrotoxicity, hypokalemia, hypomagnesemia, hyperchloremic acidosis
				• Itraconazole: Rash, vomiting, edema, headache, abnormal liver function test results, diarrhea, fever, fatigue, hypertension, pruritus, abdominal pain, dizziness, hypokalemia, hypertriglyceridemia

(ALT: alanine transaminase; AST: aspartate transaminase; BD: twice a day; COPD: chronic obstructive pulmonary disease; COVID-19: coronavirus disease 2019; CR-MRSA: community-acquired methicillin-resistant *Staphylococcus aureus*; ICU: intensive care unit; IM: intramuscular; IV: intravenous; MAO: monoamine oxidase; NSAIDs: nonsteroidal anti-inflammatory drugs; PO: per oral; ULN: upper limit of normal)

Outpatient Management

Women with milder illness can be treated on outpatient basis, but they should be closely followed due to increased risk of progressing to severe disease. Various scoring systems are used for prognostication of patients with CAP, the two most commonly used systems are Pneumonia Severity Index (PSI) and CURB-65.

Supportive Management

Maintain oxygen saturation ≥95%, treat with oxygen supplementation, and if required provide assisted ventilation to maintain maternal partial pressure of oxygen (pO_2) >70 mm Hg. Normal partial pressure of carbon dioxide (pCO_2) in pregnancy is 25–33 mm Hg and a value of 35 mm Hg indicates CO_2 retention and patient may be heading toward respiratory failure. Treat fever with acetaminophen and maintain hydration. Maintain left lateral position to relieve aortocaval pressure. Pregnant women confined to bed should also receive prophylaxis for venous thromboembolism. If indicated, bronchoscopy can be performed safely in pregnant patients. Due to increased renal clearance, higher and frequent antibiotic doses are required to treat pneumonia in pregnancy. Tetracyclines, clarithromycin, and fluoroquinolones are avoided in pregnancy.

Management of COVID-19

Steroid for patients on oxygen support or ventilator, Tab dexamethasone 6 mg per oral (PO)/intravenous (IV) per day for 10 days or until discharge (whichever is earlier). Tab prednisolone 40 mg once daily (OD) or Tab methylprednisolone 32 mg OD for systemic disease.[18-22] Side effects include hyperglycemia, increased risk of infections, and weight gain. *Thromboprophylaxis* is recommended in hospitalized pregnant women with either low-molecular-weight heparin (LMWH) or unfractionated heparin (UFH). LMWH does not cross placenta, and not excreted in breast milk. UFH does not increase adverse maternal or fetal outcomes and there is no information regarding effects on breastfed infant. *Interleukin 6 (IL-6) inhibitor* (tocilizumab) is recommended for women on respiratory support with glucocorticoid coverage, increased C-reactive protein (CRP) >75 mg/dL, and increased IL-6 levels. Side effects include *secondary infections*.[23,24]

Respiratory tract infections are the most common infections that affect pregnant women. Most of these infections are caused by viruses and respond to supportive management. Antibiotics are not required for URTIs unless complicated by secondary bacterial infection. Pregnant women are at an increased risk of developing lower respiratory infections and need close monitoring with aggressive treatment. Various scoring systems are available for deciding type of care and prognostication of disease. Influenza, varicella zoster, and many viral infections usually have self-limiting course but can lead to life-threatening complications in pregnancy. Antiviral drugs should be started within 48 hours of start of symptoms. If indicated radiological investigations and bronchoscopy can be safely done during pregnancy. Appropriate antimicrobials should be started considering safety during pregnancy and lactation but drugs with compatibility not proven may be given if documented adverse maternal and fetal effects are not available. Adjuvant therapy like respiratory support, steroids, thromboprophylaxis, and IL-6 inhibitor should be given when indicated.

KEY POINTS

- Viral respiratory infections are self-limiting and do not require antibiotics unless complicated by superimposed bacterial infection.
- Pregnant women in are at increased risk of rapid deterioration and need close observation.
- In pregnancy, maintain oxygen saturation ≥95%.
- Normal pCO_2 in pregnancy is 25–33 mm Hg and pCO_2 ≥35 mm Hg indicates CO_2 retention.
- In pregnancy, left lateral position relieves aortocaval pressure.
- If not ambulatory, venous thromboembolism prophylaxis should be initiated.
- The diagnostic procedures like radiological investigations and bronchoscopy can be performed safely in pregnant women.
- If indicated, antiviral drugs should be started within 48 hours of onset of symptoms.
- Appropriate antibiotics with minimal maternal and fetal effects should be administered.
- Higher and frequent antibiotic doses are required to treat pneumonia in pregnancy.

REFERENCES

1. Mahashur A. Management of lower respiratory tract infection in outpatient settings: Focus on Clarithromycin. Lung India. 2018;35(2):143-9.
2. Harris AM, Hicks LA, Qaseem A. High Value Care Task Force of the American College of Physicians and for the Centers for Disease Control and Prevention. Appropriate Antibiotic Use for Acute Respiratory Tract Infection in Adults: Advice for High-Value Care From the American College of Physicians and the Centers for Disease Control and Prevention. Ann Intern Med. 2016;164:425-34.
3. Feldkamp ML, Meyer RE, Krikov S, Botto LD. Acetaminophen use in pregnancy and risk of birth defects: findings from the National Birth Defects Prevention Study. Obstet Gynecol. 2010;115:109-15.
4. Wenzel RP, Fowler AA 3rd. Clinical practice. Acute bronchitis. N Engl J Med. 2006;355:2125-30.
5. Centers for Disease Control and Prevention. (2022). Pertussis (Whooping Cough). Treatment. [online] Available from: https://www.cdc.gov/pertussis/clinical/treatment.html [Last accessed December, 2023].
6. Incaudo GA. Diagnosis and treatment of allergic rhinitis and sinusitis during pregnancy and lactation. Clin Rev Allergy Immunol. 2004;27:159-77.
7. Rosenfeld RM, Piccirillo JF, Chandrasekhar SS, Brook I, Ashok Kumar K, Kramper M, et al. Clinical practice guideline (update): adult sinusitis. Otolaryngol Head Neck Surg. 2015;152:S1-S39.
8. Chow AW, Benninger MS, Brook I, Brozek JL, Goldstein EJ, Hicks LA, et al; Infectious Diseases Society of America. IDSA clinical practice guideline for acute bacterial rhinosinusitis in children and adults. Clin Infect Dis. 2012;54:e72-e112.
9. American Academy of Family Physicians. Twenty Things Physicians and Patients Should Question. Choosing Wisely. [online] Available from: https://www.choosingwisely.org/societies/american-academy-of-family-physicians/ [Last accessed December, 2023].
10. Metlay JP, Waterer GW, Long AC, Anzueto A, Brozek J, Crothers K, et al. Diagnosis and Treatment of Adults with Community-acquired Pneumonia. An Official Clinical Practice Guideline of the American Thoracic Society and Infectious Diseases Society of America. Am J Respir Crit Care Med. 2019;200(7):e45-e67.
11. ACOG Committee Opinion No. 753: Assessment and Treatment of Pregnant Women With Suspected or Confirmed Influenza. Obstet Gynecol. 2018;132:e169-e173. Reaffirmed 2021.
12. Barkas F, Styla CP, Bechlioulis A, Milionis H, Liberopoulos E. Sinus Bradycardia Associated with Remdesivir Treatment in COVID-19: A Case Report and Literature Review. J Cardiovasc Dev Dis. 2021;8:18.
13. Touafchia A, Bagheri H, Carrié D, Durrieu G, Sommet A, Chouchana L, et al. Serious bradycardia and remdesivir for coronavirus 2019 (COVID-19): a new safety concerns.

14. Wheat LJ, Freifeld AG, Kleiman MB, Baddley JW, McKinsey DS, Loyd JE, et al. Clinical practice guidelines for the management of patients with histoplasmosis: 2007 update by the Infectious Diseases Society of America. Clin Infect Dis. 2007;45:807-25.
15. Grohskopf LA, Blanton LH, Ferdinands JM, Chung JR, Broder KR, Talbot HK, et al. Prevention and Control of Seasonal Influenza with Vaccines: Recommendations of the Advisory Committee on Immunization Practices - United States, 2022-23 Influenza Season. MMWR Recomm Rep. 2022;71:1-28.
16. Uyeki TM. Influenza. Ann Intern Med. 2021;174:ITC161-ITC176.
17. Uyeki TM, Bernstein HH, Bradley JS, Englund JA, File TM, Fry AM, et al. Clinical Practice Guidelines by the Infectious Diseases Society of America: 2018 Update on Diagnosis, Treatment, Chemoprophylaxis, and Institutional Outbreak Management of Seasonal Influenza. Clin Infect Dis. 2019;68:e1-e47.
18. National Institutes of Health. (2023). Coronavirus Disease 2019 (COVID-19) Treatment Guidelines. [online] Available from: https://covid19treatmentguidelines.nih.gov/ [Last accessed December, 2023].
19. Department of Health and Social Care. (2020). World first coronavirus treatment approved for NHS use by government. [online] Available from: https://www.gov.uk/government/news/world-first-coronavirus-treatment-approved-for-nhs-use-by-government [Last accessed December, 2023].
20. Infectious Diseases Society of America. (2023). IDSA Guidelines on the Treatment and Management of Patients with COVID-19. [online] Available from: https://www.idsociety.org/practice-guideline/covid-19-guideline-treatment-and-management/ [Last accessed December, 2023].
21. World Health Organization. (2020). Corticosteroids for COVID-19: Living guidance. [online] Available from: https://www.who.int/publications/i/item/WHO-2019-nCoV-Corticosteroids-2020.1 [Last accessed December, 2023].
22. Agarwal A, Hunt B, Stegemann M, Rochwerg B, Lamontagne F, Siemieniuk RA, et al. A living WHO guideline on drugs for COVID-19. BMJ. 2020;370:m3379.
23. Mariette X, Hermine O, Tharaux PL, Resche-Rigon M, Steg PG, Porcher R, et al. Effectiveness of Tocilizumab in Patients Hospitalized With COVID-19: A Follow-up of the CORIMUNO-TOCI-1 Randomized Clinical Trial. JAMA Intern Med. 2021;181:1241-3.
24. Guaraldi G, Meschiari M, Cozzi-Lepri A, Milic J, Tonelli R, Menozzi M, et al. Tocilizumab in patients with severe COVID-19: a retrospective cohort study. Lancet Rheumatol. 2020;2:e474.

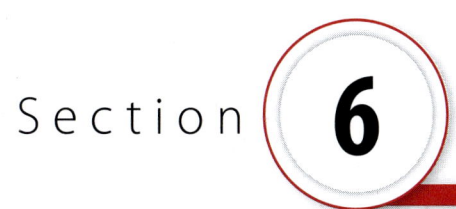

Section 6

Medical Management of Labor and Puerperium

▲ **Preterm Labor**
Anjum Ara

▲ **Induction and Augmentation of Labor**
Kanika Kumari

▲ **Cesarean and Vaginal Delivery: Antibiotic Therapy**
Madhavi M Gupta, Vaishnavi Jayaram

▲ **Postpartum Sepsis**
Jyotsna Suri, Ankita Jain

▲ **Postpartum Hemorrhage**
Renuka Malik, Meghna Reddy

Chapter 13

Preterm Labor

Anjum Ara

Regular uterine contractions resulting in the dilatation of cervix after week 24 and before 37th week of pregnancy is known as preterm labor.[1] It may result in premature birth which is a significant cause of perinatal mortality and morbidity. The earlier the premature birth occurs, the greater are the risks for neonate.[1,2]

Complications associated with a premature birth include immature lungs, difficulty regulating body temperature, poor feeding, and slow weight gain.

Premature babies may need longer or more intense nursery care, medication, and sometimes surgery.

Drugs used in preterm labor can be divided as per usage into therapeutic and prophylactic.

■ THERAPEUTICS

Drug used in preterm labor can be divided into:
- *Prophylactic:* Progesterone
- *Therapeutics* **(Table 1)**

TABLE 1: Therapeutic drugs.

Maternal	• Progesterone • Tocolysis
Fetal	• Steroid coverage • Magnesium sulfate ($MgSO_4$) for fetal neuroprotection

Progesterone

Progesterone by maintaining the uterine quiescence helps in both treatment and prevention of preterm birth. The exact mechanism of the onset of both term and preterm labor in humans is a complex interaction of many different hormonal pathways, culminating in coordinated uterine contractile activity, mediated by the production of prostaglandins.[3]

Progesterone achieves uterine quiescence through suppression of the calcium–calmodulin–myosin light chain kinase system, reducing calcium flux and altering the resting potential of smooth muscle.

In humans, the progesterone receptor (PR) has two major subtypes: PR-A and PR-B. An increase in the myometrial PR-A to PR-B expression ratio occurs at the onset of labor at term, resulting in an increase in myometrial PR-A and leading to functional withdrawal of progesterone and increased sensitivity to contractile stimuli. Prostaglandins produced prior to the onset of labor, also act to increase the PR-A/PR-B expression ratio.[4]

In labor, there occurs increase in inflammatory markers like tumor necrosis factor alpha (TNF-α), interleukin-1 (IL-1) and IL-6, and decrease in levels of anti-inflammatory markers like IL-10. Inflammatory cytokines alter enzyme expression and increase prostaglandin production prior to the onset of labor.[5] These inflammatory mediators may then interact at the fetoplacental level and precipitate preterm birth. In particular, inflammatory cytokines interleukin-1 and TNF-α act to increase prostaglandin production and IL-10 and progesterone have a negative effect on prostaglandin production and thus help in stopping the preterm labor.

Indications:
- Previous history of preterm labor
- Short cervical length on ultrasonography (USG)

Contraindications:
- History of venous thromboembolism
- Liver dysfunction
- Carcinoma breast

Dosage and preparations:
- Micronized progesterone 200 mg or 300 mg can be given orally/vaginally
- 17-hydroxyprogesterone caproate injections
- These preparations are given till 36 weeks

Tocolysis

Tocolysis is delaying the preterm labor by medicines to stop uterine contraction in order to provide a time for steroid cover or in utero transfer of fetus to centers with neonatal intensive care unit (NICU) facility.

Common tocolytics drugs:
- Calcium channel blockers
- Magnesium sulfate
- Oxytocin antagonist
- Beta blockers
- Nitric oxide
- *Prostaglandin antagonists:* Indomethacin, sulindac, ketorolac

Contraindications:
- A gestational age above 34 weeks
- Chorioamnionitis
- Maternal bleeding with hemodynamic instability
- Intrauterine fetal demise
- Lethal fetal anomaly
- Nonreassuring fetal status
- Severe preeclampsia or eclampsia
- Specific contraindications to tocolytic agents

Calcium Channel Blockers

Calcium channel blockers are the first-line agent used for tocolysis. These agents act to inhibit calcium influx across cell membranes, thereby decreasing tone in the smooth muscle of the vasculature. The voltage dependent L-type calcium channels have been identified in uterine myometrium by electrophysiological, pharmacological, and molecular studies. The Ca^{2+} channels are complex proteins composed of five distinct subunits (α1, α2, β, δ, and γ) encoded by multiple genes.[6] Dihydropyridines (DHPs) such as nifedipine bind to the DHP-binding side of the voltage-gated (VG) L-type channels, which is located on the α1 subunit.

The half-life of nifedipine is 8 hours.

Side effects: These include headache, hypotension, tachycardia, and sometimes pulmonary edema in patients with comorbidities.

Pulse rate monitoring is required. Avoid giving with magnesium as it can enhance the neuromuscular blocking effects.

Contraindications: These are tachycardia, hypotension, cardiac, or renal disease.

Preparation: This includes oral tablets as Depin and Depin Retard.

Magnesium Sulfate

Magnesium sulphate is a calcium competitor in the sarcoplasmic reticulum. It diminishes the interaction of calcium with the actin–myosin complex and interferes with myometrium repolarization. It also acts competitively in blocking the entry of calcium into synaptic endings, thereby altering neuromuscular transmission.

It has a dual advantage of neuroprotection and prevents of cerebral palsy in severe premature infants.[1,7] The mechanism for the neuroprotection in preterm infants is still not well understood but the following mechanisms have been proposed:
- Stabilization of cerebral circulation by regulating blood pressure and cerebral blood flow
- Prevention of excitatory injury by stabilization of neuronal membranes and blocking excitatory neurotransmitters, such as glutamate

Magnesium sulfate ($MgSO_4$) given in antenatal period to the mother crosses placenta within 30 minutes and neonatal magnesium sulfate concentrations remained elevated up to 24 hours.

It should be administered when early preterm birth <30 weeks is planned or expected and should be considered for patient between 30 and 33^{+6} weeks. When birth is planned, $MgSO_4$ should commence as close as possible to 4 hours before birth. If delivery is planned or expected to occur sooner than 4 hours $MgSO_4$ should be administered, as there is still likely to have advantage with the administration.[1,2]

Contraindications: These include myasthenia gravis, renal damage, and cardiac dysfunction.

Preparation: Intravenous (IV) injection given 4 mg bolus followed by 1 g IV maintenance.

Monitoring is done by knee jerks, renal output, and respiratory rate as magnesium toxicity can occur.

TABLE 2: Magnesium sulfate ($MgSO_4$) levels and toxicity.

$MgSO_4$ levels	Toxicity
5–10 mEq/L	Electrocardiogram (ECG) changes
>7 mEq/L	Loss of tendon reflex
15 mEq/L	Respiratory depression
20 mEq/L	Cardiac arrest

Side effects: The side effects are flushing, nausea, headache, blurring of vision, pulmonary edema, and respiratory distress.

Toxicity: Patient on $MgSO_4$ needs to be monitored for magnesium toxicity as levels >7 mmol/L are associated with toxicity **(Table 2)**.

Oxytocin Antagonist

Atosiban is a synthetic peptide oxytocin antagonist. It resembles oxytocin with modifications at the 1, 2, 4, and 8 positions. The N-terminus of the cysteine residue is deaminated to form 3-mercaptopropanic acid at position 1, at position 2 L-tyrosine is modified to D-tyrosine with an ethoxy group replacing the phenol, threonine replaces glutamine at position 4, and ornithine replaces leucine at position 8.

It binds to membrane-bound oxytocin receptors on the myometrium and prevents oxytocin-stimulated increases in inositol triphosphate production. This ultimately prevents release of stored calcium from the sarcoplasmic reticulum and subsequent opening of VG calcium channels. This shutdown of cytosolic calcium increase prevents contractions of the uterine muscle, reducing the frequency of contractions and inducing uterine quiescence.[8]

Dosage: This includes 6.5 mg IV stat over 1 minute followed by 18 mg/h for 3 hours, and then 6 mg/h for 45 hours with half-life 3 hours.

Side effects: The side effects are tachycardia, palpitation, hypotension, chest pain, nausea, vomiting, and headache.

Contraindications: These are hepatic and renal disorders.

Nitric Oxide Donors

Nitric oxide donors, such as nitroglycerin, have been used to relax the uterus. Nitroglycerine works by inducing myometrial guanylyl cyclase to produce cyclic GMP (cGMP). Increases in cGMP inhibit the ability of intracellular calcium levels to rise. Furthermore, cGMP is also used to dephosphorylate myosin heads which halts the ability for contractions to proceed.[9]

The two routes for nitroglycerine administration are IV and transdermal. The half-life is 3 minutes and it undergoes hepatic metabolism.

Side effect profile is better when compared to beta-adrenergic receptor agonists. Common ones are headache, palpitation, tremors, and restlessness.

Contraindications: Raised intracranial temperature (ICT), severe anemia, myocardial infarction, or hypersensitivity are the contraindications.

Dosage: 100 µg IV bolus followed by 1 µg/min, 50 µg transdermal patch for 24 hours

Preparation: It includes Nitrostat, Nitroquick, and Nitro-bid

Beta Agonist

Beta-adrenergic receptor agonists specifically work on the beta-2 receptor. Activation of the beta-2 receptors causes an increase in cyclic AMP (cAMP) which leads to increased smooth muscle relaxation.[10]

The most common medication in this class is terbutaline. Hexoprenaline is used in many countries still needs approval by the US Food and Drug Administration. Ritodrine is also used internationally for tocolysis, but is not approved in the United States. There has been a black box warning by the US Food and Drug Administration against the use of injectable terbutaline in prolonged preterm labor management (over 72 hours) due to maternal cardiac complications. These complications result from terbutaline's activity at beta-1 receptors located in cardiac muscle.[10]

Side effects are headache, tachycardia, hypotension, nausea, vomiting, hyperglycemia in diabetics, and cardiac arrhythmias. It may also lead to fetal tachycardia **(Table 3)**.

Prostaglandins Antagonists (Cyclooxygenase-2 Inhibitors)

Prostaglandins contract uterine muscles by causing an increase in free intracellular calcium levels and amplifying activation of myosin light chain kinas. Prostaglandins have an important role in the onset and maintenance of labor. Cyclooxygenase (COX) enzymes convert arachidonic acid into prostaglandins and inhibition of COX activity results in decreased production of prostaglandins, thus reducing uterine contractions.

The COX-2 inhibitors like indomethacin, sulidac, ketorolac, and celecoxib have been reported in literature for use in preterm. COX inhibitors appear to have few maternal side effects, however, adverse effects reported in the fetus, like constriction of the fetal ductus arteriosus (DA), bronchopulmonary dysplasia, and oligohydramnios, are a major concern **(Tables 4 and 5)**.[11]

■ CORTICOSTEROIDS

Corticosteroids have proven role in accelerating fetal lung maturity and

TABLE 3: Beta-2 agonist in preterm labor.

Drugs	Routes	Dosage	Side effects	Contraindications
Ritodrine (FDA-approved)	Oral IV	40 mg TDS or BD 50 µg/min increase half hourly to maximum of 350 µg/min	Tachycardia, palpitation, hyperglycemia, hallucination, pulmonary edema	Heart disease, dysrhythmias, PIH, uncontrolled diabetes
Terbutaline	Oral SC IV	2.5 mg TDS × 1–2 weeks 250–500 µg QID 90–300 µg/h for 8–10 hours	Headache, palpitation, tremors, hyperglycemia	Dysrhythmias, uncontrolled diabetes, uncontrolled thyroid disorders
Isoxsuprine	Oral IV/IM	10–20 mg every 6 hours for 48 hours 200–500 µg/min IV infusion till controlled then 10 mg injection every 8 hourly for 1 week	Headache, palpitation, tremors, hyperglycemia	Dysrhythmias, uncontrolled diabetes, uncontrolled thyroid disorders

(BD: twice a day; IM: intramuscular; IV: intravenous; PIH: pregnancy-induced hypertension; QID: four times a day; SC: subcutaneous; TDS: thrice a day)

TABLE 4: Prostaglandins antagonists.

Drug	Route	Dosage	Indication	Side effects	Contraindications
Indomethacin	Oral	50–100 mg followed by 25–50 mg IM every 4–6 hours for 48 hours	Preterm labor associated with polyhydramnios	• Premature closure of DA • Oligohydramnios	• Peptic ulcer • Drug-induced asthma • Coagulation disorder
Sulindac	Oral	200 mg OD/BD for 24–48 hours			
Ketorolac	IM	60 mg IM followed by 30 mg IM every 6 hours for 24–48 hours			

(BD: twice a day; DA: ductus arteriosus; IM: intramuscular; OD: once a day)

decreasing the incidence and severity of respiratory distress syndrome and thereby decreasing neonatal morbidity and mortality.[12]

Drugs: Betamethasone and dexamethasone

Dose:
- Inj. Betamethasone 12 mg intramuscularly two doses 24 hours apart are given.
- Inj. Dexamethasone 6 mg intramuscularly 4 doses given 12 hours apart

Single course is recommended for women between 24 and 34 weeks' gestation who are at risk for delivery in 7 days.[1,2]

In women between 34 and 35[+6] weeks' antenatal steroids can be considered.[1]

- American College of Obstetricians and Gynecologists (ACOG) recommends

TABLE 5: Drugs.

Name	Progesterone	Calcium channel blockers	MgSO₄	Corticosteroids	Oxytocin agonist	Nitric oxide
Dosage	200–300 mg	10–20 mg	4 mg IV followed by 1 mg/h	12 mg two dose	6.5 mg IV followed by 6–18 mg/h	100 µg IV bolus followed by 1 µg/min 50 µg transdermal
Route	Oral/vaginal/IM	Oral	IM/IV	IM	IV	IV/transdermal
Side effects	Headache, breast tenderness, gastric discomfort	Headache, hypotension, tachycardia and sometimes pulmonary edema	Flushing, nausea, headache, blurring of vision, pulmonary edema and respiratory distress	Hyperglycemia in mother	Tachycardia, palpitation, hypotension, chest pain, nausea, vomiting and headache	Headache, palpitation, tremors, and restlessness
Contraindications	• History of venous thromboembolism • Liver dysfunction • Carcinoma breast	Tachycardia, hypotension, cardiac, or renal disease	Myasthenia gravis, renal damage, and cardiac dysfunction	Chorioamnionitis and uncontrolled diabetes	Hepatic and renal disorders	Raised ICT, severe anemia, myocardial infarction
Pharmacokinetics	Suppression of the calcium–calmodulin–myosin light chain	Inhibit calcium influx across cell membranes	Act as calcium competitor and prevent its interaction with the actin–myosin complex	Induces enzymes for synthesis of pulmonary surfactant	Oxytocic antagonist	Induces myometrial guanylyl cyclase to produce cyclic GMP

(GMP: guanosine monophosphate; ICT: intracranial temperature; IM: intramuscular; IV: intravenous)

single course can also be given in females between 34 and 36^{+6} weeks.[13]
- In a meta-analysis, Crowther and colleagues concluded that a single-rescue course of corticosteroids should be considered in women whose prior course was administered at least 7 days previously and who were <34 weeks' gestation. ACOG also recommends rescue dose in such cases.[14]

Optimal benefit: Begins 24 hours after therapy and lasts for 7 days

Advantages: Reduces incidence of the following in first week of life:
- Respiratory distress syndrome
- Necrotizing enterocolitis
- Intraventricular hemorrhage
- Bronchopulmonary dysplasia
- Patent ductus arteriosus
- Systemic infections

Fetal lung maturation decreases the need for mechanical ventilation and hence, reducing the neonatal morbidity and mortality.

Mechanism of action: Corticosteroids induce enzymes for synthesis of pulmonary surfactant. They release surfactant stored in type 2 pneumocytes and increase lung compliance. Corticosteroids even potentiate the response of postnatal administration of surfactant.

Contraindications:
- Chorioamnionitis (may flare up infection)
- Uncontrolled diabetes (increases blood sugar levels).

Side effects:
- Neonatal hypoglycemia
- Cerebral palsy (especially on repeated doses)
- Reduced birthweight (on repeated doses)
- Increase risk for fetal growth restriction (on repeated doses).

■ KEY POINTS

- Preterm labor remains a significant cause of preterm morbidity and mortality. Management is aimed to prevent labor at least for steroid coverage or in utero transfers.
- Progesterone prophylaxis can be considered in patient those at risk of preterm labor.
- Tocolytics like calcium channel blockers and beta agonists are effective in gaining time for steroid coverage.
- Corticosteroids and $MgSO_4$ are clinically proven to improve adverse fetal outcomes because of prematurity.

■ REFERENCES

1. Thomson AJ; Royal College of Obstetricians and Gynaecologists. Care of Women Presenting with Suspected Preterm Prelabour Rupture of Membranes from 24+0 Weeks of Gestation: Green-top Guideline No. 73. BJOG. 2019;126:e152-e166.
2. National Institute for Health and Care Excellence. (2019). Preterm labour and birth. Quality Standard (QS135). [online] Available from: https://www.nice.org.uk/guidance/qs135 [Last accessed December, 2023.
3. Care A, Nevitt S J, Medley N, Donegan S, Good L, Hampson L et al. Interventions to prevent spontaneous preterm birth in women with singleton pregnancy who are at high risk: systematic review and network meta-analysis BMJ. 2022;376:e064547.
4. Dodd JM, Crowther CA. The role of progesterone in prevention of preterm birth. Int J Womens Health. 2009;1:73-84.
5. Cao XL, Zhou XY, Xu NX, Chen SC, Xu CM. Association of IL-4 and IL-10 Polymorphisms With Preterm Birth Susceptibility: A Systematic Review and Meta-Analysis. Front Immunol. 2022;13:917383.
6. Flenady V, Wojcieszek AM, Papatsonis DN, Stock OM, Murray L, Jardine LA, Carbonne B. Calcium channel blockers for inhibiting preterm labour and birth. Cochrane Database Syst Rev. 2014;2014(6):CD002255.
7. Shennan A, Suff N, Jacobsson B; FIGO Working Group for Preterm Birth. FIGO good practice recommendations on magnesium

sulfate administration for preterm fetal neuroprotection. Int J Gynaecol Obstet. 2021;155:31-3.
8. Flenady V, Reinebrant HE, Liley HG, Tambimuttu EG, Papatsonis DNM. Oxytocin receptor antagonists for inhibiting preterm labour. Cochrane Database Syst Rev. 2014;6:CD004452.
9. Duckitt K, Thornton S, O'Donovan OP, Dowswell T. Nitric oxide donors for treating preterm labour. Cochrane Database Syst Rev. 2014;2014(5):CD002860.
10. Chung JE, Choi SA, Hwang HS, Park JY, Lee KE, Yee J, et al. Association between ß2-adrenergic receptor gene polymorphisms and adverse events of ritodrine in the treatment of preterm labor: a prospective observational study. BMC Genet. 2017; 18(1):96.
11. Reinebrant HE, Pileggi-Castro C, Romero CL, Dos Santos RA, Kumar S, Souza JP, et al. Cyclo-oxygenase (COX) inhibitors for treating preterm labour. Cochrane Database Syst Rev. 2015;2015(6):CD001992.
12. McGoldrick E, Stewart F, Parker R, Dalziel SR. Antenatal corticosteroids for accelerating fetal lung maturation for women at risk of preterm birth. Cochrane Database Syst Rev. 2020;12:CD004454.
13. Committee on Obstetric Practice. Committee Opinion No. 713: Antenatal Corticosteroid Therapy for Fetal Maturation. Committee Opinion No. 713 Obstet Gynecol. 2017; 130:e102-e109.
14. Crowther CA, Middleton PF, Voysey M, Askie L, Zhang S, Martlow TK, et al. PRECISE Group. Effects of repeat prenatal corticosteroids given to women at risk of preterm birth: An individual participant data meta-analysis. PLoS Med. 2019; 16(4):e1002771.

Chapter 14

Induction and Augmentation of Labor

Kanika Kumari

Induction of labor is defined as intervention designed to artificially initiate uterine contractions leading to progressive dilatation and effacement of cervix and birth of baby in the women with intact membrane or absent membrane but who are not in labor. It is indicated only when it is agreed that the mother or the fetus will benefit from higher probability of a healthy outcome than if birth is delayed and it should be done only when vaginal delivery is the appropriate route of delivery.[1-3]

Augmentation of labor defined as active interventions during labor to promote the frequency, duration, and amplitude of uterine contractions.

After confirmation of indication of induction of labor and rule out contraindication of induction of labor following counseling should be done **(Table 1)**.

■ COUNSELING BEFORE INDUCTION

- The reason for induction of labor.
- Induced labor is more painful than spontaneous labor.
- More likely to have additional interventions such as assisted or operative birth including cesarean birth.
- Options available should be discussed.
- The efficacy and possible adverse effects for the women and her baby associated with each method should be discussed.
- Cesarean birth might be needed if induction is not successful.
- Increased likelihood of neonatal intensive care unit (NICU) admission of baby.

TABLE 1: Name of pharmacological agents for induction and augmentation of labor.

S. no.	Name	FDA approved	Bishop's score	Clinical setting
1.	Dinoprostone PGE2	Yes	<6	Without scarred uterus
2.	Misoprostol PGE1	No	<6	Without scarred uterus
3.	Oxytocin	Yes	>6	Can be used with scarred uterus
4.	Mifepristone	No	<6	• In research settings • Can be used with scarred uterus
5.	Isosorbide mononitrate	No	<6	In research setting
6.	Relaxin	No	<6	In research setting
7.	Dexamethasone	No	<6	In research setting

(FDA: Food and Drug Administration; PGE1: prostaglandin E1; PGE2: prostaglandin E2)

- Continuous fetal and uterine monitoring will be done.[4]

DINOPROSTONE PROSTAGLANDIN E2

It is a naturally occurring prostaglandins. It is the Food and Drug Administration (FDA) approved drug for labor induction **(Table 2)**.

Mechanism of Action

Exact mechanism is unknown. It releases PGF2α that increases the sensitivity of myometrium to oxytocin. It also stimulates contractions in the myometrium via direct stimulation. It binds to EP receptors in the myometrium and act via cell membrane calcium channels and intracellular cyclic 3′5′-adenosine monophosphate.[5] It also promotes cervical dilatation, effacement, and softening. By increase in collagenase secretion which activates the digestion of some of the structural collagen network of the cervix so by increase the glycosaminoglycan, hyaluronic acid, and decrease the dermatan sulfate in the cervix.[6] And thus causes softening of cervix which is dilatable.

Pharmacokinetics

It is absorbed at the rate of 0.3 mg/h in case of vaginal insert or vaginal delivery system and much faster in case of intracervical gel. Its half-life is 2.5–5 minutes. Peak plasma level time is 0.5–0.75 hour. It is a locally acting substance and is rapidly inactivated locally so it does not causes systemic toxicity.

Rapid metabolism of dinoprostone occurs primarily in the local tissues; any systemic absorption of the medication is cleared mainly in the maternal lungs and, secondarily, at sites such as liver and kidneys.

Its metabolites are mainly excreted in urine and small amount in feces.

Contraindications

- Previous history of hypersensitivity to drug
- Previous history of uterine surgery
- Asthma
- Glaucoma
- Active pulmonary disease, heart disease, hepatic and renal disease, and active pulmonary disease in case of vaginal tablet or suppository
- Surgery on cervix.

Side Effects

- Gastrointestinal symptoms such as nausea, vomiting, and diarrhea
- Uterine hyperstimulation with or without non reassuring fetal heart rate pattern
- Fever
- Dizziness
- Flushing of skin
- Fever and headache
- Rarely anaphylactic reactions.

TABLE 2: Different formulations of dinoprostone.

S. no.	Form	Route of administration	Strength	Storage
1.	Intracervical	Endocervical	0.5 mg/3.0 g gel	2–8°C
2.	Insert/vaginal delivery system	Vaginally in posterior fornix	10 mg	–10 to –25°C
3.	Vaginal suppository	High in the vagina	20 mg	–20 to –40°C
4.	Vaginal tablet	High in the vagina	3 mg	–10 to –20°C
5.	Intravaginal gel	In posterior fornix	1 mg or 2 mg	2–8°C

TABLE 3: Comparison of success rate of dinoprostone intravaginal pessary and intracervical gel.[7]

S. no.	Characteristics	Pessary	Gel
1.	Vaginal delivery	85%	83.3%
2.	LSCS	15%	16.7%
3.	Time of insertion of the agent to onset of active labor • Primigravida • Multigravida	• 6 hours • 4 hours	• 13 hours • 6 hours
4.	Time of insertion of the agent to vaginal delivery • Primigravida • Multigravida	• 12.7 hours • 8.5 hours	• 23.4 hours • 17.3 hours
5.	Apgar score at 5 minutes	7	8
6.	No NICU admission	95%	93.3%
7.	Patient satisfaction	83.3%	78.3%

(LSCS: lower segment cesarean section; NICU: neonatal intensive care unit)

Drug Interactions

- It should not be administered along with oxytocin and misoprostol.
- The interval between last dose of dinoprostone gel is 6–12 hours.

Intracervical Gel

- It comes in the prefilled syringe.
- After removing from refrigerator it should be administered immediately.
- After passing urine, patient should be lied down in lithotomy position and under vision it should be instilled endocervically. Patient should be kept in recumbent position for 30 minutes. Then fetal heart rate monitoring and maternal uterine activity should be monitored regularly.
- *Administration*: It should be administered as 0.5 mg 6–12 hourly maximum three doses or 1.5 mg **(Table 3)**.[2,3]

VAGINAL DELIVERY SYSTEM/INSERT

It is used for induction of labor at term. It is a thin, flat, and polymeric slab which contains 10 mg dinoprostone in a hydrogel within the pouch of polyester retrieval system as a long tape designed to aid retrieval at end of dosing interval or earlier, if required. It is so designed to release drug at the rate of 0.3 mg per hour. It is placed in the posterior fornix in moist environment. It absorbs water, swell, and release dinoprostone. It must be kept frozen before insertion. It is kept in the posterior fornix transversely. A minimal amount of water-miscible lubricant may be used to assist insertion. After insertion patient must be kept in recumbent position for 2 hours thereafter may be ambulatory.

Only one dose over 24 hours is recommended.[4] It is to be removed after 24 hours whether labor induced or not or to be removed earlier if adequate uterine contractions established, uterine hyperstimulation encountered, nonreassuring fetal heart rate pattern noticed, rupture of membranes occurred, or hypersensitive reactions occur. Oxytocin administration should be delayed at least 30 minutes after removal of insert.

Advantages

Less vaginal examination required so minimizes discomfort to the female as it can be put for 24 hours, its ability to reverse uterine hyperstimulation/tachysystole by quick removal of insert and its allowance of quick retrieval in case of abnormal fetal heart rate tracing.

Disadvantages

Risk of cesarean section is elevated in nulliparous women as the time from labor induction to active labor is more and rate of uterine tachysystole with or without fetal distress is more.

■ VAGINAL SUPPOSITORY

This formulation is not available in India. It is available in 20 mg dosage. It is used for termination of pregnancy from 12 to 20 weeks or evacuation of uterus in case of Intrauterine demise (IUD) at or >28 week and management of nonmetastatic gestational trophoblastic disease. It is to be administered in posterior fornix as 20 mg next dose to be repeated after 3–5 hours till the expulsion of fetus occurs but not to be given for >48 hours. Within the earlier mentioned recommended intervals administration time should be determined by abortifacient progress, uterine contractility response, and by patient tolerance.

PROSTIN E2 Vaginal Suppositories are available in foil strips of five individually sealed suppositories. Each suppository contains 20 mg of dinoprostone in a mixture of glycerides of fatty acids.

■ DINOPROSTONE TABLETS

It is available in a strength of 1 mg and 2 mg. It is used for labor induction at term. In primigravida, the initial dose is 2 mg then second dose after 6 hours is 1 mg or 2 mg maximum two doses/4 mg. In multigravida, first dose is 1 mg or 2 mg then second dose is also 1 mg or 2 mg maximum two doses up to 3 mg.[8]

■ DINOPROSTONE VAGINAL GEL

This form is not available in India. 1 mg vaginal gel is to be administered in the posterior fornix high up. If labor does not induce then second dose of 1 mg or 2 mg to be administered after 6 hours. Only two doses are recommended. The national institute for health and care excellence (NICE) prefers vaginal gel or vaginal tablets for labor induction at term.[7]

■ MISOPROSTOL PROSTAGLANDIN E1

Misoprostol is a synthetic analog of prostaglandin E1. It is not the FDA approved drug for labor induction **(Table 4)**.

Pharmacology

Mechanism of Action

Misoprostol is deesterified to active metabolite to misoprostol acid. This active metabolite causes degradation of collagen in the connective tissue of the stroma of cervix and reduces the cervical tone which induces

TABLE 4: Pharmacokinetics of misoprostol.[10]

S. no.	Route of administration	Onset of action	Duration of action
1.	Oral	8 minutes	2 hours
2.	Sublingual	11 minutes	3 hours
3.	Vaginal	20 minutes	4 hours
4.	Rectal	100 minutes	4 hours

softening, effacement, and dilatation of cervix. It causes contraction of muscle fibers of myometrium which facilitates cervical opening.[9]

It is mainly secreted in urine. It is heat stable drug and is kept/stored at room temperature.

Side Effects

- Hyperthermia with chills and rigors secondary to the effect on the hypothalamus
- Nausea and vomiting
- Flatulence and dyspepsia
- Vertigo
- Hypotension
- Tachysystole
- Nonreassuring fetal heart rate and fetal hypoxemia
- Meconium staining of liquor
- Rarely hypersensitive and anaphylactic reactions.[10]

Contraindications

- Previous history of allergic reactions or hypersensitive reaction to prostaglandins
- Those at a risk of gastric ulcers secondary to nonsteroidal anti-inflammatory drug (NSAID) use
- Previous history of uterine surgery.

Drug Interactions

Should not be given with other uterotonics and oxytocin. Oxytocin should be started after 4–6 hours of last dose of misoprostol.

Dosage

- Vaginal misoprostol 25 µg 6-hourly maximum up to 24 hours
- Oral misoprostol 25 µg 2-hourly maximum up to 24 hours[11]
- Sublingual misoprostol 25 µg 3-hourly maximum up to 5 doses
- Buccal (dissolves between gum and cheek) misoprostol 25 µg 4-hourly.[12]

■ OXYTOCIN

It is the FDA approved and most commonly used pharmacological agent for induction and augmentation of labor **(Table 5)**.

Pharmacology

It is a recombinant hormone used to induce or strengthen uterine contractions. It is parenterally administered and fully bioavailable drug. It is colorless and generally available in ampoules containing 5 IU in 1 mL with intravenous (IV) use. Its half-life is approximately 3–12 minutes, depending

TABLE 5: Administration of oxytocin by infusion pump.

Preparation of oxytocin infusion	Low dose regime	High dose regime
• Mix 1 mL/5 IU oxytocin + 4 mL RL solution = 1 U/mL oxytocin • Take 2 mL premixed oxytocin + 48 mL RL solution = 50 mL diluted oxytocin • Put it in infusion pump and then administer	6 mL/h = 2 mU	12 mL/h = 4 mU
	12 mL/h = 4 mU	18 mL/h = 8 mU
	15 mL/h = 6 mU	21 mL/h = 12 mU
	18 mL/h = 8 mU	24 mL/h = 16 mU
	21 mL/h =12 mU	27 mL/h = 20 mU
	24 mL/h = 16 mU	30 mL/h = 24 mU
	27 mL/h = 20 mU	36 mL/h = 30 mU

on its dilution. On start of infusion, uterine contractions is elicited within 3–5 minutes, reaching a steady state within 20–40 minutes. Discontinuation or reduction of the infusion rate leads to rapid decline in contractile activity. At low infusion rates it causes rhythmic uterine contractions. In higher doses, it has a direct relaxing effect on vascular smooth muscles resulting in transient hypotension, reflex tachycardia, and flushing.

The uterus is more sensitive to oxytocin as pregnancy advances, in younger women, in parous women, in women with lower body mass index, in female with spontaneous labor, after prostaglandin administration, in late first stage, and in the second stage of labor. However, there is a large biological variability in the infusion dose required to achieve adequate uterine contractions that is why there is no absolute safe rate and there is a need of constant titration of oxytocin infusion rate according to the frequency, strength, and duration of uterine contractions. It is removed from the body by liver and kidney.

Toxicity

Its supratherapeutic dose can lead to:
- Myocardial ischemia
- Tachycardia
- Arrhythmias
- Hypotension
- Postpartum hemorrhage (PPH)
- Maternal and neonatal hyponatremia
- In uterus can cause hypertonicity and rupture and fetal hypoxia
- >200 MIU in 24 hours can lead to water intoxication and can lead to seizures, coma, and death.

Dosage of Oxytocin for Induction of Labor (Table 6)

Oxytocin to be given as IV infusion. The oxytocin infusion should be delayed at least 6–12 hours after administration of prostaglandins preparations as the effect of prostaglandins on uterine contractility is heightened with oxytocin. It can be given in two regimen as follows:

1. *Low dose oxytocin regimen:* Initial dose of 2 mU/minute increased by 2 mU/minute every 15–40 minutes up to a maximum of 20 mU/minute.
2. *High dose oxytocin regimen:* Initial dose of 4–6 mU/minute increased by 4 mU/minute every 15–40 minutes up to a maximum dose of 32 mU/minute.[1,3]

TABLE 6: Administration of oxytocin by infusion.[13]

Time	No uterine scar		Previous uterine scar	
	mIU/min	mL/hour	mIU/min	mL/hour
Start	2	12	1	6
0.5 hour	4	24	2	12
1 hour	6	36	3	18
1.5 hours	8	48	4	24
2 hours	10	60	5	30
2.5 hours	12	72	6	36
3 hours	14	84	7	42
3.5 hours	16	96	8	48
Medical review				
4 hours	18	108	9	54
4.5 hours	20	120	10	60
5 hours	22	132	Maximum dose	
5.5 hours	24	144		
6 hours	26	156		
6.5 hours	28	168		
7 hours	30	180		
Maximum dose				

■ MIFEPRISTONE

It is also called as Roussel-Uclaf (RU)-486. It is 19-norsteroid with antiprogesterone and antiglucocorticoid activity. It modifies the cervical consistency and increase the sensitivity to prostaglandins and convert the quiet pregnant uterus into organ of spontaneous activity. It is used for labor induction in research settings only.

It is used for cervical ripening and induction of labor in normal uterus and in patients with previous lower segment caesarean section.[14,15] In these studies, 200 mg of mifepristone was given and Bishop's score was assessed after 24 hours. 80.7% patients went into labor no case of uterine rupture even in previous lower segment cesarean section (LSCS) patient. Even the NICE recommends that in cases of intrauterine fetal death if labor induction is required then offer 200 mg mifepristone followed by vaginal dinoprostone or oral or vaginal misoprostol.[4]

ISOSORBIDE MONONITRATE

- It improves cervical ripening score on administration of 40 mg vaginally in two doses 24 hours apart.
- It seems to be safe and effective agent for preinduction cervical ripening as it does not causes much changes in maternal hemodynamics and does not cause uterine hyperstimulation.
- It improves cervical score both in primigravida and multigravida and reduces both duration of induction to the active phase of labor and induction to delivery time.[16]

RELAXIN

It is a protein hormone. The recombinant relaxin was used as cervical ripening agent. In the studies it was found that it does not cause uterine hyperstimulation with fetal heart rate changes. Although the rate of cesarean section was not different from noninduced females but there was a reduction in the risk of the cervix remaining unfavorable on induction with relaxin.

DEXAMETHASONE

It is used for induction of labor on the basis of the fact that during pregnancy the placenta and fetal membranes secrete large amount of corticotropin-releasing hormone (CRH). CRH levels in plasma increases during labor with peak levels at vaginal delivery. There is a considerable evidence for the effect of dexamethasone on the duration of labor stages.

Dexamethasone by any route of administration shortens the interval between induction and active phase of labor, the length of first, second, and third stages of labor. It does not imparts any adverse effects on maternal and neonatal outcomes.[17]

KEY POINTS

- Correct period of gestation, indication, and contraindications must be confirmed before starting induction of labor.
- Proper counseling must be done, informed consent must be taken and documented in the case file, and all the arrangements must be done before induction of labor.
- In leaking per vaginum vaginal route of administration of dinoprostone should be avoided due to unpredictable response.
- Mifepristone may be the good option in previously scarred uterus although further studies are required to prove its efficacy and safety profile.
- Oxytocin infusion is the FDA approved for induction and augmentation of labor even with scarred uterus but its efficacy is good with Bishop's score ≥6.
- After starting the process proper and continuous monitoring of mother for side effects of drug and fetal heart monitoring should be done.

REFERENCES

1. Royal College of Obstetrician and Gynaecologists. Induction of Labour. Evidence-based Clinical Guideline Number 9. London: RCOG Press; 2001.

2. World Health Organization. WHO Recommendations on Induction of Labour, At or Beyond Term. Geneva: World Health Organization; 2018.
3. ACOG Practice Bulletin No. 107: Induction of labor. Obstet Gynecol. 2009;114:386-97.
4. NICE. (2021). NICE Guideline [NG207]: Inducing Labour. [online] Available from: https://www.nice.org.uk/guidance/ng207. [Last accessed December, 2023].
5. Sugimoto Y, Narumiya S. Prostaglandin E receptors. J Biol Chem. 2007;282(16):11613-7.
6. MacLennan AH, Katz M, Creasey R. The morphologic characteristics of cervical ripening induced by the hormones relaxin and prostaglandin F2 alpha in a rabbit model. Am J Obstet Gynecol. 1985;152:691-6.
7. Nisiya KS, Devi U, Ahmed FM. A prospective study on comparison of effectiveness and safety of dinoprostone intracervical gel and dinoprostone vaginal insert on induction of labour. Int J Clin Obstet Gynaecol. 2022;6(1):152-60.
8. NICE. NICE Clinical Guidelines No. 70. Induction of labour. London: NICE; 2008.
9. Bakker R, Pierce S, Myers D. The role of prostaglandins E1 and E2, dinoprostone, and misoprostol in cervical ripening and the induction of labor: a mechanistic approach. Arch Gynecol Obstet. 2017;296(2):167-79.
10. Tang OS, Gemzell-Danielsson K, Ho PC. Misoprostol: pharmacokinetic profiles, effects on the uterus and side-effects. Int J Gynaecol Obstet. 2007;99 Suppl 2:S160-7.
11. World Health Organization. WHO Recommendations: Induction of Labour. Geneva: World Health Organization; 2011.
12. Weeks AD, Lightly K, Mol BW, Frohlich J, Pontefract S, Williams MJ; the Royal College of Obstetricians and Gynaecologists. Evaluating misoprostol and mechanical methods for induction of labour. Int J Obstet Gyanecol. 2022;129:e61-5.
13. Nunes I, Dupont C, Timonen S, de Campos DA, Cole V, Schwarz C. European guidelines on perinatal care—Oxytocin for induction and augmentation of labor. J Matern Fetal Neonatal Med. 2022;35(25):7166-72.
14. Lata G, Kaur SP, Sharma S. Mifepristone for cervical ripening and induction of labour in patients with lower segment caesarean section—a prospective case control study. Galore Int J Health Sci Res. 2019;4(3):165-9.
15. Priyanka, Shetty SS. The effect of mifepristone in induction of labour at term. MedPulse Int J Gynaecol. 2021;17(2):32-5.
16. Agrawal M, Acharya N, Joshi K, Shrivastava D. Effectiveness of isosorbide mononitrate in cervical ripening before induction of labor in full-term antenatal patients. J South Asian Feder Obst Gynae. 2019;11(2):96-9.
17. Mohaghegh Z, Siahkal SF, Bahmaei H, Sharifipour F, Leyli EK, Zahedian M. The effect of dexamethasone on labor induction: a systematic review. BMC Pregnancy Childbirth. 2021;21:563.

Chapter 15

Cesarean and Vaginal Delivery: Antibiotic Therapy

Madhavi M Gupta, Vaishnavi Jayaram

Direct maternal infections acquired during the process of delivery account for roughly 10% of maternal mortality. Peripartum infections are also associated with severe morbidity and long-term consequence such as pelvic inflammatory disease (PID), chronic pelvic pain, and secondary infertility. It also contributes to neonatal mortality.[1] Many factors have been found to increase risk of acquiring peripartum infections, which are given in **Table 1**.

Strategies to decrease risk of acquiring these infections are mainly directed at preventive measures in high-risk conditions. The most commonly used intervention globally for preventing peripartum infections and its associated morbidity and mortality has been prophylactic antibiotic therapy. However, inadvertent use of antibiotics during labor has been found to have implications on global efforts to restrict the emerging resistant strains of bacteria, and consequently, on global health.[2]

■ VAGINAL DELIVERY

- *Uncomplicated vaginal birth:*
  - Defined as vaginal birth in the absence of any of the specific risk factors or clinical signs of peripartum infection.[1]
  - Routine antibiotic prophylaxis is not recommended.
  - However, careful monitoring of all these women after birth is of utmost importance to promptly recognize any sign of infection and institute necessary antibiotic treatment.
- *Vaginal birth with episiotomy:*
  - Routine antibiotic prophylaxis for women with episiotomy is not recommended.
  - Antibiotics should be given when there are clinical signs of infection of the episiotomy wound.
  - Second-degree perineal tears are anatomically like episiotomies and do not require use of prophylactic antibiotics.
- *Third and fourth degree perineal tear:*
  - Third and fourth degree perineal tears are prone to infections in the postpartum period.

TABLE 1: Factors increasing risk of peripartum infections.

Preexisting maternal conditions:	Conditions during labor and delivery:
• Malnutrition • Severe anemia • Diabetes • Obesity • Bacterial vaginosis • Group B *Streptococcus* infections	• Prolonged rupture of membranes • Multiple vaginal examinations • Manual removal of placenta • Perineal tears • Cesarean section

- Wound infection might lead to aggravation of long-term consequences of these tears such as involuntary loss of flatus and fecal incontinence.
- Routine antibiotic prophylaxis is indicated in these cases.
- The Royal College of Obstetricians and Gynaecologists (RCOG) recommends use of broad-spectrum antibiotics in the postpartum period after obstetrical anal sphincter injuries (OASIS) repair.[3]
- The recommended antibiotic combinations include:[4]
    - Cefazolin + metronidazole
    - Clindamycin + gentamycin
- *Manual removal of placenta:*
  - Manual removal of placenta poses a high risk of infection during the postpartum period due to the invasive nature of uterine manipulation required.
  - Routine antibiotic prophylaxis is required in all such cases.[1]
  - *Recommended*: Single dose of ampicillin or first-generation cephalosporin.
- *Operative vaginal birth*:
  - Term used for delivery of the fetal head which is assisted by vacuum extractor or forceps.
  - Associated with increased risk of infection due to bladder catheterization, multiple vaginal examinations, and instrumentation during procedure and also risk of trauma to the perineum.
  - Routine antibiotic prophylaxis is recommended for all women undergoing operative vaginal birth.[5]
- *Recommended:* single dose IV amoxicillin (1 g) and clavulanic acid (200 mg). To be given as soon as possible after birth, within 6 hours.
- If this combination is unavailable, use of a class of antibiotics with a similar activity spectrum should be used based on local antibacterial resistance patterns, safety profile, availability, and cost.

■ CESAREAN SECTION

- Most important risk factor for infection in the early postpartum period. 5–20-fold increased risk compared to vaginal delivery.
- Cesarean section increases the risk of surgical site infection, endometritis, and urinary tract infections (UTIs). Rarer and more serious complications include bacteremia, pelvic abscess, septic shock, septic pelvic thrombophlebitis, and necrotizing fasciitis.
- These risks can be reduced by sound surgical techniques, using the right topical antiseptics and antibiotic prophylaxis.[2]
- *Recommended:* Single dose of first-generation cephalosporin or penicillin.
- If these are unavailable, other classes of antibiotics may be used based on local bacteriological patterns of post cesarean infectious morbidity, safety profile, clinician's experience, availability, and cost.
- Prophylactic antibiotics are to be given to women undergoing emergency as well as elective cesarean sections and need to be administered 30–60 minutes before the skin incision.

Summary of various antibiotics used during delivery is mentioned in **Table 2**.

TABLE 2: Summary of various antibiotics used during delivery.

Name of drug	Class	Mechanism of action	Target organisms	Route dosage	Pharmacokinetics	Mechanism of resistance	Postdelivery uses	Side effects/contraindications	Pregnancy safety
Penicillin	Beta lactams	Inhibition of cell wall synthesis; binding to penicillin-binding proteins	Gram-positive bacteria	*Oral dose:* 500 mg	60–73% bioavailability, crosses placenta, hepatic metabolism, eliminated through urine	Production of enzyme penicillinase	Cesarean section	• Nausea, vomiting, urticaria, anemia, oral candidiasis • *Contra-indications:* Allergy to penicillin	Safe
Ampicillin Amoxicillin	Beta lactams Aminopenicillin	Inhibition of cell wall synthesis; binding to penicillin-binding proteins	Gram-positive, Gram-negative bacteria	*Oral dose:* 500 mg tid or qid	74–92% bioavailability, hepatic metabolism, eliminated through urine	Production of enzyme penicillinase, modification of penicillin-binding proteins	Operative vaginal birth, manual removal of placenta	Headache, nausea, vomiting, diarrhea, AST/ALT elevation, anaphylaxis • *Contra-indications:* Known allergy	Safe
Cefazolin Cefalexin	First-generation cephalosporins	Inhibition of cell wall synthesis; binding to penicillin-binding proteins	Gram-positive bacteria	*Intravenous dose:* 1 g tid 250–1,000 mg 6–8 hourly PO	Peak plasma time—5 minutes, crosses placenta, minimally metabolized in liver, excreted in urine mostly as unchanged drug	Modification of penicillin-binding proteins	Third and fourth degree perineal tears, manual removal of placenta, cesarean section	Nausea, vomiting, leukopenia, eosinophilia, fever • *Contra-indications:* Documented hypersensitivity	Safe
Clindamycin	Lincosamides	Inhibits bacterial protein synthesis by binding at the level of 50 S ribosome	Aerobic gram-positive cocci, anaerobic gram-positive and negative bacteria	*Oral dose:* 150–300 mg qid 200–600 mg IV 8-hourly	90% bioavailability, crosses placenta, hepatic metabolism, excreted in urine and feces	Target site modification (mutation of ribosomal sites), efflux pumps	Third and fourth degree perineal tears	• Abdominal pain, agranulocytosis, hypotension, diarrhea • *Contra-indications:* Hypersensitivity	• Safe in second and third trimesters • Safety data in first trimester use is not available

Contd...

Contd...

Name of drug	Class	Mechanism of action	Target organisms	Route dosage	Pharmacokinetics	Mechanism of resistance	Postdelivery uses	Side effects/ contraindications	Pregnancy safety
Gentamicin	Aminoglycoside	Inhibits bacterial protein synthesis by binging at the level of 30 S ribosome	Aerobic organisms including gram-negative bacteria and mycobacteria	*Intravenous dose:* 80 mg IV/IM 3–5 mg/kg/day either as single or divided in three 8-hourly doses	<30% is protein bound, crosses placenta, half-life is 2–3 hours, excreted in urine, renal clearance is directly related to renal function	Reduced uptake or decreased cell permeability, alterations at the ribosomal binding sites, or production of aminoglycoside modifying enzymes	Third and fourth degree perineal tears	• Gait instability, ototoxicity, nephrotoxicity, neurotoxicity • *Contra-indications:* Hypersensitivity, renal failure, myasthenia gravis	Unsafe
Metronidazole	Nitroimidazoles	Inhibits bacterial nucleic acid synthesis by forming nitroso radicals, disrupting bacterial cells	Gram-positive and negative anaerobic bacteria, protozoa	*Oral dose:* 500 mg BD 400 mg tid	<20% is protein bound, metabolized through glucuronide conjugation, excreted in urine and feces	Inactivation or deletion of genes with nitroreductase activity, efflux pumps	Third and fourth degree perineal tears	• Disulfiram reaction, nausea, vomiting, headache, ataxia, appetite loss, dark urine • *Contra-indications:* Known allergy, use of disulfiram within past 2 weeks, consumption of alcohol within 3 days	Unsafe

(ALT: alanine transaminase; AST: aspartate transaminase; IM: intramuscular; IV: intravenous)

CHAPTER 15: Cesarean and Vaginal Delivery: Antibiotic Therapy

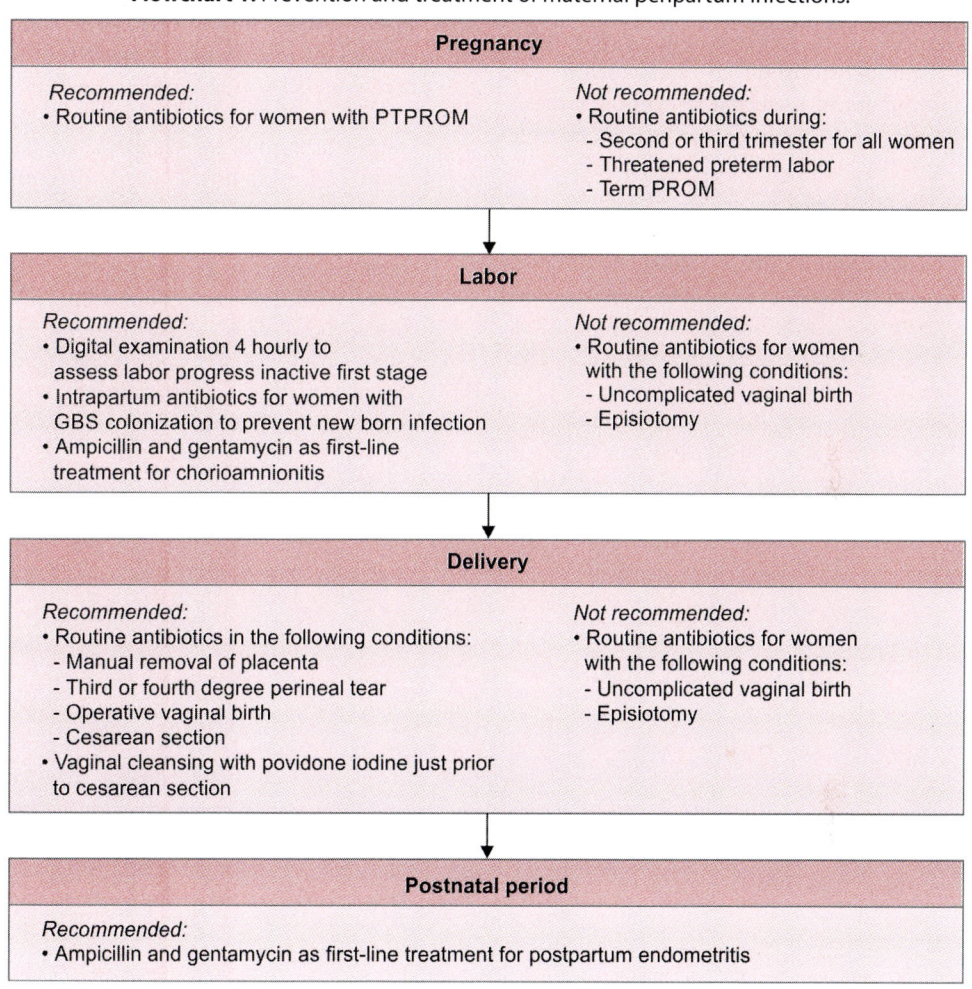

Flowchart 1: Prevention and treatment of maternal peripartum infections.

(GBS: group B *Streptococcus*; PTPROM: preterm premature rupture of membrane)

Summary of practices for prevention and treatment of maternal peripartum infections is given in **Flowchart 1**.

■ KEY POINTS

- 10% maternal morbidity due to direct infection acquired during delivery.
- Routine antibiotic prophylaxis is not recommended in uncomplicated vaginal birth including with episiotomy.
- Antibiotic prophylaxis recommended for (i) operatie vaginal delivery, third and fourth degree perineal tears, (ii) manual removal of placenta, (iii) single dose of 1st generation cephalosporin.
- Prophylactic antibiotic single dose to be given to women undergoing emergency and elective cesarean section.
- Factors increasing risk of peripartum infection include both maternal factors (anemia, malnutrition, etc.) and conditions during labors and delivery.

REFERENCES

1. World Health Organization. (2015). WHO recommendations for prevention and treatment of maternal infections. [online] Available from: https://apps.who.int/iris/handle/10665/186171. [Last accessed December, 2023].
2. World Health Organization. (2021). WHO recommendation on prophylactic antibiotics for women undergoing caesarean section. [online] Available from: https://apps.who.int/iris/handle/10665/341865. [Last accessed December, 2023].
3. Royal College of Obstetricians and Gynaecologists. (2015). The Management of Third- and Fourth-Degree Perineal Tears: Green-top Guideline No. 29. [online] Available from: https://www.rcog.org.uk/media/5jeb5hzu/gtg-29.pdf. [Last accessed December, 2023].
4. Duffy CR, Baptiste C, Huang Y, Wright D, Alton D, Friedman AM, et al. Trends in antibiotic use with third and fourth degree perineal lacerations. Am J Obstet Gynecol. 2019;220(1):s411-2.
5. World Health Organization. (2021). WHO recommendation on routine antibiotic prophylaxis for women undergoing operative vaginal birth. [online] Available from https://apps.who.int/iris/handle/10665/341862. [Last accessed December, 2023].

Chapter 16

Postpartum Sepsis

Jyotsna Suri, Ankita Jain

DEFINITIONS

Sepsis

Sepsis is defined as a life-threatening organ dysfunction caused by a dysregulated host response to infection. It is clinically characterized by a change in sequential organ failure assessment (SOFA) score ≥2 points, which denotes organ dysfunction.

Maternal Sepsis

The World Health Organization defines maternal sepsis as a life-threatening condition with organ dysfunction resulting from infection during pregnancy, childbirth, postabortion, or postpartum period.[1-3] *Postpartum sepsis* is a subset of maternal sepsis.

Puerperal Sepsis

Puerperal sepsis is a bacterial infection of the genital tract or its surrounding tissues occurring at any time between the onset of rupture of membranes or labor and the 42nd day postpartum in which two or more of the following are present: Pelvic pain, fever, abnormal vaginal discharge, abnormal smell/foul odor discharge, or delay in uterine involution.[1] Hence, all puerperal sepses are a part of postpartum sepsis whereas postpartum sepsis includes other conditions causing sepsis in the postpartum period such as pyelonephritis and pneumonia.

Septic Shock

It is a subset of sepsis in which circulatory, cellular, and metabolic abnormalities are associated with a greater risk of mortality than with sepsis alone (40% vs. 10%).[2] It is clinically identified by a serum lactate >2 mmol/L and a vasopressor requirement to maintain a mean arterial pressure ≥65 mm Hg that persists despite adequate fluid resuscitation.[2,4]

Systemic Inflammatory Response Syndrome

This is a terminology which is no longer used. It was characterized by ≥2 criteria exceeding thresholds for temperature, heart rate, respiratory rate, and white blood count. Formerly used in combination with infection to identify "sepsis" but now discarded as often represents an appropriate (i.e., nonpathological) host response to any inflammatory (i.e., nonspecific for infection) insult.[1,2]

SEPSIS SCREENING

Early identification of sepsis and prompt management is the key to improved outcomes in sepsis. Over the years various tools have been developed to pick sepsis early in obstetric patients. Some of these tools are quick sequential organ failure assessment (qSOFA) score, National Early Warning Score (NEWS), and Modified Early Warning Score (MEWS).[2] Modified Early Obstetric Warning Score (MEOWS), which is a modification of MEWS for use in obstetrics, or Carle's Obstetric Early Warning Score (OEWS) can be used for obstetric patients **(Fig. 1)**.[4] All these tools vary in diagnostic accuracy. Recently, it has been observed that qSOFA score **(Table 1)** is not a very effective screening tool but rather the NEWS and MEWS are more sensitive triaging tools for sepsis.

MANAGEMENT

Early institution of intravenous (IV) fluids, collecting and sending samples, and broad-spectrum antibiotics are the mainstay of management of sepsis and septic shock. Sepsis is one of the components of deadly triad of maternal mortality in India. Hence, it requires aggressive management. The Surviving Sepsis Campaign guidelines now emphasize on 1 hour bundle reinforcing the role of early management of sepsis to prevent its compliactions.[2] The UK Sepsis Trust in its Yellow Manual has protocolized "SEPSIS 6" as the key approach to a patient of sepsis.[1] **Table 2** depicts the SEPSIS 6 protocol

Clinical intensive care national audit and research center obstetric early warning score							
	3	2	1	Normal	1	2	3
Systolic blood pressure, mm Hg	<80	80–89		90–139	140–149	150–159	160
Diastolic blood pressure, mm Hg				<90	90–99	100–109	110
Respiratory rate/min	<10			10–17	18–24	25–29	30
Heart rate/min	<60			60–110		111–149	150
%O₂ required to maintain SpO₂ 96%				Room air	24–39%		40%
Temperature, °C	<34.0		34.0–35.0	35.1–37.9	38.0–38.9		39
Conscience level				Alert			Not alert

Fig. 1: Carle's Obstetric Early Warning Score (OEWS).[4] (SpO₂: oxygen saturation)

TABLE 1: Sepsis screening: qSOFA score.[2,3]

qSOFA score		
Altered mentation	Systolic BP <100 mm Hg	Respiratory rate >22 breaths/min
Any two criteria if present denote risk of sepsis and should undergo full SOFA score		
(BP: blood pressure; qSOFA: quick sequential organ failure assessment)		

TABLE 2: *SEPSIS 6 and severe sepsis bundle:* (Mnemonic: "SEPSIS").[1,2]

Senior obstetrician for help	
Ensure SpO$_2$ >95% and admit to ICU	• Oxygenation by mask at 8 L/min • Admit to ICU
Parenteral access and IV fluids	• IV access with wide bore cannula • IV crystalloids 30 mL/kg within first 3 hours • Monitored by dynamic tests to guide fluid resuscitation (echo, fluid bolus and change in pulse pressure, and passive leg raise test) • Start vasopressors early if MAP <65 mm Hg with fluid resuscitation • If on vasopressors, target MAP >65 mm Hg
Samples	*Before starting antibiotics:* CBC, ABG (serum lactate), coagulation profile, LFT, KFT, SE, relevant cultures, and infection/fever screen
Infection control	• IV broad-spectrum antibiotics within 1 hour of diagnosis • Beta lactams, MRSA cover, gram negative, and anaerobic cover • Consider patient weight and KFTs • Source control, e.g., doing D&E in case of presence of retained products of conception
See (monitor)	• Vitals, temperature, intake-output • Catheterize

(ABG: arterial blood gas; CBC: complete blood count; D&E: dilation and evacuation; ICU: intensive care unit; IV: intravenous; KFT: kidney function test; LFT: liver function test; MAP: mean arterial pressure; MRSA: methicillin-resistant *Staphylococcus aureus*; SpO$_2$: oxygen saturation)

TABLE 3: Common sources of infection in maternal sepsis.[5]

Source	Antepartum	Postpartum
Obstetric	• Septic abortion • Chorioamnionitis	• Endometritis • Wound infection
Nonobstetric	• Urinary tract infection • Pneumonia • Appendicitis	• Urinary tract infection • Pneumonia • Gastrointestinal

which comprises of six steps which can be remembered by the mnemonic SEPSIS.

Administration of appropriate antibiotics is an important step in managing sepsis. This necessitates the collection of samples from various sites for culture and antibiotic sensitivity, and starting empirical treatment till reports arrive. *However, if the facility for obtaining culture is not available, the antibiotics should not be withheld on this ground as every hour in delay in starting antibiotics increases the risk of mortality exponentially.*

The most frequently isolated organisms have been reported to be *Escherichia coli*, *Streptococcus* group A and B; followed by Staphylococci, gram negative, and anaerobic bacteria. The common sources of infection in maternal sepsis are listed in **Table 3**.[5]

The commonly used drug combinations in maternal sepsis in intensive care unit (ICU) are described in **Table 4**.[6-8] These drug therapies are based on the likely source of infection, the most frequently isolated organisms from these sites and the usual antibiotic therapies they respond to.

Table 5 discusses the IV fluids, commonly used antibiotics in the Indian setup and vasopressor drugs in detail.[6-8] It summarizes the drugs and their mechanism of action, dose, route, frequency, and side effects.

Most of the antibiotics have been seen to be safe in lactation. The Food and Drug Administration (FDA) categories for pregnancy and lactation (A, B, C, D, and X) have been withdrawn in 2015 and now it uses the Pregnancy and Lactation Labeling Rule (PLLR) instead. **Table 6** lists some commonly used antimicrobials and their risks in pregnancy and lactation.[8,9]

TABLE 4: Empirical antibiotics in sepsis.[6]

Source of infection	Proposed antibiotics
Endomyometritis	Ampicillin, gentamicin, and metronidazole (or clindamycin)
Chorioamnionitis	Ampicillin plus gentamicin. Add anaerobic cover (clindamycin or metronidazole) if cesarean delivery required
Urinary tract infections	Gentamicin with ampicillin or carbapenem or piperacillin-tazobactam
Community-acquired pneumonia	Cefotaxime, ceftriaxone, ertapenem, or ampicillin plus azithromycin/clarithromycin/erythromycin
Hospital-acquired pneumonia	• *Low-risk patients:* Piperacillin-tazobactam, meropenem, imipenem, or cefepime • *Patients with high risk of mortality:* Additionally; coverage for *Pseudomonas* (beta lactam plus aminoglycoside/quinolone) and methicillin-resistant *Staphylococcus aureus* (MRSA) coverage with vancomycin or linezolid
Abdominal infections	• Ceftriaxone/cefotaxime/ceftazidime/cefepime plus metronidazole • *Complicated cases:* Carbapenem or piperacillin-tazobactam
Skin and soft tissues (necrotizing)	Vancomycin plus piperacillin-tazobactam

TABLE 5: *Management of postpartum sepsis:* Drug dose, route, and frequency.[6-8]

Drug name	Information	Dose and route	Side effects	Remarks
IV fluids-crystalloids				
Ringer lactate (RL)	Contains 0.31 g/L sodium, 0.03 g/L potassium, osmolarity: 275 mosm/L, 130 mEq/L sodium and 4 mEq/L potassium	20–30 mL/kg; IV	Fluid overload, pulmonary edema, allergy, phlebitis, hyperkalemia	RL is the fluid of choice in septic shock for fluid resuscitation

Contd...

Contd...

Drug name	Information	Dose and route	Side effects	Remarks
Normal saline (NS)	0.9% NS contains 9 g/L sodium chloride (NaCl) osmolarity-308 mosm/L, 154 mEq/L sodium and 154 mEq/L chloride	20–30 mL/kg; IV	Fluid overload, pulmonary edema, allergy, phlebitis	
Antibiotics				
Injection ampicillin (penicillin derivative)	Binds to bacterial cell wall, broad spectrum, gram positive and negative coverage	2 g IV stat followed by 1 g 6 h	Nausea, vomiting, diarrhea, allergy	Take empty stomach
Injection ceftriaxone (third-generation cephalosporin)	Gram positive and negative coverage	2 g IV stat f/b 1 g 12 h	Nausea, vomiting, diarrhea, allergy, rash, CDAD, hemolytic anemia	Do not mix with calcium-containing diluents
Injection metronidazole	Anaerobic, antiprotozoal, produces free radicals	500 mg IV 8 h	Gastritis, vomiting, diarrhea, disulfiram reaction	
Injection gentamicin (aminoglycoside)	Inhibits bacterial protein synthesis	5 mg/kg in single or two divided doses	Nephrotoxic, neurotoxic, allergy, Fanconi-like syndrome	Avoid in renal impairment
Injection amoxicillin-clavulanic acid	Penicillin derivative and beta lactam inhibitor	1.2 g IV stat f/b 625 mg 8 h or 1.2 g 8 h	Gastritis, diarrhea, abdominal pain	
Injection piperacillin-tazobactam (extended spectrum penicillin)	Binds to bacterial cell wall and causes cell lysis	4.5 g IV 8 h	Constipation, gastritis, diarrhea, headache insomnia	Dose adjusted in renal impairment
Injection clindamycin (lincosamide)	Anaerobic cover, reserved for more serious infections, penicillin allergy	300–600 mg IV 8h	Nausea, vomiting, abdominal pain, diarrhea, skin rash	Dose adjusted in renal impairment
Injection meropenem (carbapenem)	Complicated and severe sepsis	2 g IV stat f/b 500 mg to 1 g 8 h	Nausea, vomiting, headache, diarrhea, skin rash	Dose adjusted in renal impairment
Vasopressors				
Injection noradrenaline (α1 and β1) receptors	First-line vasopressor: • ↑ venous and arterial tone • ↑ preload, ↑ contractility	8–12 μg/min and titrate as per MAP	Cardiac arrhythmia, peripheral ischemia, inadvertent immunomodulation	1 amp = 2 mg/2 mL. 2 amp in 46 mL 5% dextrose

Contd...

Contd...

Drug name	Information	Dose and route	Side effects	Remarks
Injection vasopressin (V1a, V2, and V1b) receptors	Second-line: • ↑ venous and arterial tone, platelet aggregation • ↑ water retention, release of coagulation factors • ↑ corticotropic axis stimulation, insulin secretion	Started at 2.4 mL/h	Peripheral ischemia, mesenteric ischemia, cardiac arrhythmia	1 amp = 20 units/mL, 46 mL NS
Injection adrenalin (α1, β1, and β2) receptors	• ↑ contractility, ↑ preload • ↑ venous and arterial tone • ↑ heart rate	Started at 0.2 mL/h	Tachycardia, tachyarrhythmia, splanchnic and peripheral ischemia, increased myocardial oxygen consumption, lactic acidosis, hyperglycemia	1 amp = 1 mg/mL, 48 mL

(amp: ampoule; CDAD: *Clostridium difficile*-associated diarrhea; ↑: increases; IV: intravenous)

TABLE 6: Fetal risks and safety during lactation for common antimicrobials.[8,9]

Drug name/class	Fetal risks	Maternal risks	Lactation
Antibacterials			
Penicillins			
Penicillin G, procaine penicillin G, and benzathine penicillin G	Nonexistent/very low		Compatible
Cloxacillin	Nonexistent/very low		Compatible
Ampicillin and sulbactam/ampicillin	Limited evidence T1-oral clefts		Compatible
Amoxicillin and amoxicillin/clavulanic acid	• Limited evidence T1-oral clefts • T3-necrotizing enterocolitis		Compatible
Piperacillin	Nonexistent/very low		Compatible
Cephalosporins			
First generation: Cefadroxil cefazolin cephalexin	Nonexistent/very low		Compatible
Second generation: Cefotetan, cefoxitin, cefuroxime	Nonexistent/very low		Compatible
Third generation: Cefixime, cefoperazone, cefotaxime, ceftriaxone	Nonexistent/very low		Compatible

Contd...

Contd…

Drug name/class	Fetal risks	Maternal risks	Lactation
Fourth generation	Nonexistent/very low		Compatible
Carbapenems			
Imipenem-cilastatin	Limited data available		Probably compatible
Meropenem	Limited data available		Probably compatible
Glycopeptides			
Vancomycin	Nonexistent/very low		Probably compatible
Teicoplanin	Limited data available		Probably compatible
Monobactams			
Aztreonam	Limited data available		Compatible
Fosfomycin	Nonexistent/very low		Probably compatible
Tetracyclines	Contraindicated after 15 week-interfere with bone mineralization	Hepatotoxic	Compatible
Macrolides			
Erythromycin	Nonexistent/very low	Estolate salt: Hepatotoxic	Compatible
Clarithromycin	Increased risk in animal studies		Compatible
Azithromycin	Nonexistent/very low		Compatible
Lincosamide			
Clindamycin	Nonexistent/very low		Compatible
Oxazolidinones			
Linezolid	Limited data, compatible-maternal benefit >> embryo-fetal risk		Probably compatible
Aminoglycosides			
Gentamycin	Low	Dose-related nephrotoxicity	Compatible
Amikacin	Low	Dose-related nephrotoxicity	Compatible
Sulfonamides	Contraindicated in T3, near term		Limited data: Potential toxicity
Trimethoprim/sulfamethoxazole	Trimethoprim is teratogenic-cardiovascular and neural tube defects; oral clefts		Limited data: Potential toxicity
Nitrofurantoin	Safe in T1, 2 T3: Risk of hemolytic anemia of newborn		Probably compatible

Contd…

Contd…

Drug name/class	Fetal risks	Maternal risks	Lactation
Quinolones			
Nalidixic acid–withdrawn from market	*T3:* Pyloric stenosis in the newborns		
• Norfloxacin • Ciprofloxacin • Ofloxacin • Levofloxacin	*Contraindicated:* *T3:* Fetal cartilage damage		*Limited data:* Potential toxicity
Chloramphenicol	*Avoid in T3:* Gray baby syndrome		*Limited data:* Potential toxicity
Antifungals			
Azoles			
Ketoconazole itraconazole	*Limited data:* Probably low risk, best avoided in T1		*Limited data:* Probably compatible
Fluconazole	Multiple doses. Teratogenic in T1		Compatible
Antiviral			
Acyclovir valacyclovir	Nonexistent/very low		Compatible
Anti-influenza			
Amantadine, rimantadine	Benefit outweighs risk. T1-teratogenic		*Limited data:* Potential toxicity
Oseltamivir, zanamivir	Benefit extremely outweighs risk		Compatible
Antimalarials			
Chloroquine	Benefit extremely outweighs risk		Compatible
Primaquine	*Contraindicated:* Hemolytic anemia	Hemolytic anemia in G6PD deficient mothers	*Limited data:* Potential toxicity
Hydroxychloroquine, mefloquine	Nonexistent/very low		Probably compatible
Antiprotozoals			
Metronidazole	Low risk		• Metallic taste of breast milk • Potential toxicity if prolonged use
Antihelmintic			
Albendazole, mebendazole, ivermectin	Nonexistent/very low		Probably compatible

T1, T2, T3: First, second, and third trimesters, respectively; FDA drug categories are now obsolete. Maternal risks during pregnancy and lactation as per PLLR.

(FDA: Food and Drug Administration; G6PD: glucose-6-phosphate dehydrogenase; PLLR: Pregnancy and Lactation Labeling Rule)

KEY POINTS

- The World Health Organization defines maternal sepsis as a life-threatening condition with organ dysfunction resulting from infection during pregnancy, childbirth, postabortion, or postpartum period.
- Postpartum sepsis is a subset of maternal sepsis.
- Various tools to pick sepsis early have been developed over years like qSOFA, NEWS, MEWS, MEOWS, and Carle's OEWS.
- Management of sepsis should start as early as the diagnosis is made with the key management steps initiated within first hour of diagnosis which constitutes the 1 hour bundle (Surviving Sepsis Campaign).
- SEPSIS 6 consists of: *S*enior obstetrician for help, *E*nsure saturation >95%, *P*arenteral access and IV fluids, *S*amples, *I*nfection control, *S*ee (monitor).
- Most commonly used empirical drug combinations are injection ampicillin + gentamicin + metronidazole for endometritis and injection ampicillin + gentamicin for urinary tract infection. These are one of the commonest reasons for postpartum sepsis.
- Most antibiotics have been seen to be safe and compatible with lactation.

REFERENCES

1. Daniels D, Nutbeam T. The Yellow Manual, 6th edition. United Kingdom: Sepsis Trust; 2022.
2. Evans L, Rhodes A, Alhazzani W, Antonelli M, Coopersmith CM, French C, et al. Surviving sepsis campaign: international guidelines for management of sepsis and septic shock 2021. Intensive Care Med. 2021;47(11):1181-247.
3. World Health Organization. Statement on Maternal Sepsis. Geneva: World Health Organization; 2017.
4. Khergade M, Suri J, Bharti R, Pandey D, Bachani S, Mittal P. Obstetric Early Warning Score for Prognostication of Critically Ill Obstetric Patient. Indian J Crit Care Med. 2020;24(6):398-403.
5. Plante LA, Pacheco LD, Louis JM; Society for Maternal-Fetal Medicine (SMFM). SMFM Consult Series #47: Sepsis during pregnancy and the puerperium. Am J Obstet Gynecol. 2019;220(4):B2-10.
6. French LM, Smaill FM. Antibiotic regimens for endometritis after delivery. Cochrane Database Syst Rev. 2004;(4):CD001067.
7. Scheeren TWL, Bakker J, De Backer D, Annane D, Asfar P, Boerma EC, et al. Current use of vasopressors in septic shock. *Ann Intensive Care.* 2019;9:20.
8. Al-Zidan RN. Drugs in Pregnancy: A Handbook for Pharmacists and Physicians. New York: Apple Academic Press; 2020.
9. Briggs GG, Freeman RK, Towers CV, Forinash AB. Drugs in Pregnancy and Lactation, 11th edition. Philadelphia (PA): Wolters Kluwer; 2017.

Chapter 17

Postpartum Hemorrhage

Renuka Malik, Meghna Reddy

Postpartum hemorrhage (PPH) is a major cause of maternal mortality in developing countries. Its incidence is 2% of all livebirths worldwide, but its effect is concentrated in the developing countries. National Health Mission of India attributes 38% of maternal deaths in India are due to PPH.[1] The classical definition of PPH, blood loss >500 mL after a vaginal delivery or a blood loss of >1,000 mL following a cesarean delivery, limits the spectrum of the maternal effects due to PPH, thus, hindering the ability to early recognition and treatment of the hemodynamic compromise due to PPH. This definition was later changed by World Health Organization (WHO) (2012), International Federation of Gynecology and Obstetrics (FIGO) (2015), and Royal College of Obstetricians and Gynaecologists (RCOG) (2017) to a blood loss of >500 mL irrespective of the mode of delivery. However, the qualitative and quantitative aspects of blood loss were taken into consideration by American College of Obstetricians and Gynecologists (ACOG) (2017) and defined PPH as blood loss >1,000 mL or any blood loss accompanied by signs or symptoms of hypovolemia, regardless of route of delivery. Primary PPH is defined as occurring within 24 hours of delivery. Secondary PPH is defined as within 24 hours of delivery and 6 weeks following delivery. The severity of PPH is defined on the basis of blood loss as minor (500–1,000 mL) or major (>1,000 mL) and major can be divided into moderate (1,000–2,000 mL) and severe (>2,000 mL).[2]

▪ ETIOLOGY

Uterine atony is the leading cause of PPH, accounting for 70–80% of cases. Factors causing uterine overdistension during pregnancy are risk factors for atonic PPH. The overdistended uterus may be due to multiple fetal gestations, fetal macrosomia, or polyhydramnios. Other factors that interfere with myometrial contraction are anemia, chorioamnionitis, and general anesthesia. Ongoing hemorrhage despite a well-toned uterus warrants an exploration of the cervix, vagina, and perineum for lacerations, especially in the setting of precipitate labor, abnormal labor, or an instrumental delivery. The *4 Ts* are used to classify the etiology of PPH **(Box 1)**.

▪ DRUGS IN POSTPARTUM HEMORRHAGE

Medical management is the first-line therapy for postpartum hemorrhage. Various drugs used can be categorized as shown in **Flowchart 1** and **Table 1**.

BOX 1: Etiology of postpartum hemorrhage.

Primary:
- Uterine atony (Tone)
- Genital tears, uterine rupture (Trauma)
- Retained placenta, placenta accreta (Tissue)
- Defects of coagulation (Thrombin*)
- Uterine inversion

Secondary:
- Infection (endometritis)
- Subinvolution of uterus
- Retained products of conception
- Coagulation defects

*4 Ts: These include inherited coagulation defects as well as acute coagulopathies that may develop from events such as amniotic fluid embolism, placental abruption, or severe preeclampsia.

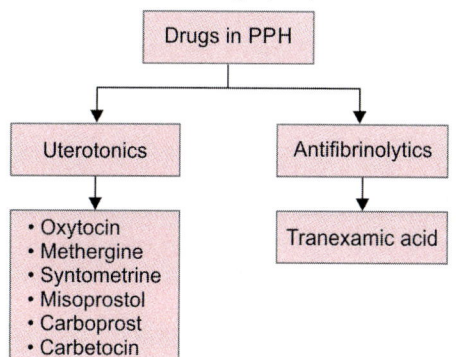

Flowchart 1: Classification of drugs in postpartum hemorrhage (PPH).

Uterotonics

Uterotonics augment the physiological uterine myometrial contractions and enhance their living ligature property to decrease the blood loss. The various drugs are described in the following text and summarized in **Table 1**.

Oxytocin

It is a synthetic cyclic peptide form of the naturally occurring posterior pituitary hormone. It is the first-line agent used in prevention and treatment of PPH.

Mechanism of action: It acts on the oxytocin GPCR (G protein-coupled receptor receptors) in the myometrium which activates phospholipase C, leading to IP3 (inositol triphosphate) which releases calcium from sarcoplasmic reticulum and causing myometrial contraction. Half-life is short 1–6 minutes. The onset of action through intravenous (IV) route is in 1–2 minutes and lasts for 15 minutes.

Dose and route: 10 IU, intramuscular (IM)/IV bolus for prevention; for treatment oxytocin infusion is given and a maximum of 2 L fluid containing oxytocin is prescribed

Advantages: It is easily available, cheap, and cost-effective.

Disadvantages: It is heat labile, needs refrigeration, and is stored at 2–8°C. It loses its efficacy when cold chain is interrupted.

Methergine

Methergine is a plant ergot derivative. It is a second-line agent used in the management of PPH.

Mechanism of action: It inhibits adenyl cyclase leading to decrease cyclic adenosine monophosphate (AMP), which causes release of calcium. It increases uterine muscle tone by causing sustained uterine contractions. It causes vasoconstriction and tonic contractions of smooth muscles of both upper and lower segments of the uterus with an advantage to control bleeding from lower segment. Onset is in 2–7 minutes after IV and lasts for 2–4 hours.

Dose and route: 200 µg, IM/IV for prevention; a maximum of five doses at 15-minute interval is used in treatment of PPH. Oral tablets 200 mg can be given for treatment thrice daily for 5 days.

TABLE 1: Drugs for prevention and treatment of postpartum hemorrhage (PPH).

Drug	Mechanism of action	Pharmacokinetics	Storage and transport	Dose	Contraindications	Side effects	Availability in India	Recommendation by WHO
First-line drug								
Oxytocin	Stimulates the upper segment of the myometrium to contract rhythmically, constricting spiral arteries and decreasing blood flow throughout	• IV: Almost immediate action with peak action concentration after 30 minutes • IM: Slower onset of action, taking 3–7 minutes, but produces a long-lasting action up to 1 hour; half-life: 1–6 minutes	Requires protection from light, and storage at 2–8°C to prolong shelf life	5 IU slow IV × 2 (may have repeat dose) or 40 IU/500 mL of Ringer lactate at 125 mL/h	Rare, hypersensitivity to drug	Overdose or prolonged use can cause water intoxication and hyponatremia IV push dosing may cause hypotension	Available	Listed as essential drug for prevention and treatment both
Second-line drug								
Ergometrine (ergot alkaloid)	Causes vasoconstriction and contracts smooth muscles and upper and lower segments of the uterus tetanically	• IM: Onset of action within 2–3 minutes, lasting for about 3 hours • IV: Onset of action within 1 minute, lasting 45 minutes • Half-life: 30–120 minutes	Requires protection from light, and storage at 2–8°C to prolong shelf life	• 0.2 mg slow IV/IM • Can be repeated at 20-minute interval, maximum up to five times	Hypertension (HTN), preeclampsia, cardiovascular disease, severe anemia, Rh-negative pregnancy vascular disease	Nausea, vomiting and severe HTN	Available	Listed as essential drug for prevention and treatment both
Carboprost (PGF2-α analog)	Improves uterine contractility by increasing the number of oxytocin receptors and cause vasoconstriction	• IM: 15–60 minutes to peak plasma concentration • Half-life: 8 minutes	Requires storage at 2–8°C to prolong shelf life	• 250 µg IM every 15 minutes up to 8 times • Direct intramyo-metrial inj. (off-label use)	Active or history of pulmonary disease (asthma), hepatic or cardiac disease	Nausea, vomiting, diarrhea, transient fever, headache, chills, shaking HTN, bronchospasm	Available	• Not listed as an essential drug • Used only for treatment

Contd...

Contd...

Drug	Mechanism of action	Pharmacokinetics	Storage and transport	Dose	Contraindications	Side effects	Availability in India	Recommendation by WHO
Misoprostol (PGE1 analog)	Causes generalized smooth muscle contraction	• Absorbed 9–15 minutes after sublingual, oral, vaginal or rectal use • Half-life: 20–40 minutes	• Does not have any special storage requirements • Tablets should be kept in tightly closed container and protected from humidity	600 or 800 g PO/sublingual/per rectal	Rare, hypersensitivity to drug	Nausea, vomiting, diarrhea, pyrexia, shivering	Available	• Listed as essential drug • Used for both prevention and treatment
Tranexamic acid	Inhibits breakdown of fibrin and fibrinogen by plasmin	IV: Apparent elimination half-life approximately 2 hours and mean terminal half-life approximately 11 hours	Stored at room temperature (15–30°C), with a shelf life of 3 years	• Slow IV bolus of 1 g (1 mL/min over 10 minutes) • Second dose of 1 g IV if bleeding continues after 30 minutes or if bleeding restarts within 24 hours	Hypersensitivity reactions, history of known thromboembolic event, history of coagulopathy	Rare	Available	• Listed as essential drug • Used only for treatment

Contd...

Contd...

Drug	Mechanism of action	Pharmacokinetics	Storage and transport	Dose	Contraindications	Side effects	Availability in India	Recommendation by WHO
Carbetocin	Binds to oxytocin receptors in the uterine smooth muscles, resulting in rhythmic contractions, increased frequency of existing contractions, and increased uterine tone	• IV: Sustained uterine contraction within 2 minutes, lasting for about 6 minutes and followed by rhythmic contraction for 60 minutes • IM: Sustained uterine contraction lasting for about 11 minutes and rhythmic contraction for 120 minutes • *Half-life:* 40 minutes	A heat-stable formulation of carbetocin is available	100 µg diluted in 10 mL NS and administered slowly IV (over 30–60 seconds)	Vascular disease, coronary artery disease, hypersensitivity to carbetocin	Nausea, flushing, abdominal pain, headache, tremors	Available	Listed as an essential drug
Syntometrine (oxytocin + ergometrine)	Fixed drug combination—oxytocin (5 IU) plus ergometrine (500 µg) in 1 ampoule for injection	• *IM:* Latent period for the uterine response is about 2.5 minutes, uterotonic effects last for around 3 hours • *Half-life:* 1–6 minutes (oxytocin) and 30–120 minutes (ergometrine)	Stored at 2–8°C. It may be stored up to 25°C for 2 months when protected from light	1 mL as a single IM dose Maximum of 1 dose used	HTN, heart disease, vascular disorders, severe sepsis, impaired pulmonary functions	Nausea, vomiting, diarrhea, coldness, extreme thirst	Not available in India	• Oxytocin and ergometrine are listed separately; fixed dose combination • Syntometrine is not listed

(IV: intravenous; IM: intramuscular; NS: normal saline; PGF2α: prostaglandin F2-alpha; PO: per oral; WHO: World Health Organization)

Contraindications: It is a potent vasoconstrictor and must be avoided in patients with hypertension, cardiovascular diseases, and peripheral vascular disease.

Side effects: These include nausea, vomiting, abdominal pain, headache, and increased blood pressure.

Syntometrine

It is a fixed dose combination of Syntocinon (5 IU) with ergometrine (500 µg) with the features of both the drugs. It is currently not available in India.

Mechanism of action: It combines both oxytocin and an ergot alkaloid, which stimulate contraction of uterine and vascular smooth muscle.

Dose and route: 5 IU/500 µg, IM.

Contraindication: These are severe kidney or liver disorder, vascular disease, hypertension, if allergic to any ingredient, in first and second stage of labor.

Side effects: These are nausea, vomiting, abdominal pain, headache, dizziness, and skin rashes.

Misoprostol

It is a prostaglandin E1 analog and acts on the prostaglandin receptors on the uterus and cervix.

Mechanism of action: It has oxytocic properties. It also inhibits gastric acid and pepsin secretion and enhances gastric mucosal resistance to injury.[3] Onset of action is in 3–5 minutes, peak at 20–30 minutes, and effect lasts for about 70 minutes.

Dose and route: 600 µg oral (PO) is approved for use as first-line agent to prevent PPH where resources for parenteral access are not available. Dose of 800 µg per rectal is used in the treatment of PPH.

Contraindications: Its use was previously limited in patients with heart diseases, but the European cardiac society safely recommends its use in PPH up to a dose of 1,000 µg.[4]

Side effects: These are nausea, abdominal pain, diarrhea, shivering, and pyrexia.

Methyl Prostaglandin F2-alpha (Carboprost)

It is a prostaglandin F2-alpha analog and causes effective uterine contractions.

Injectable prostaglandins are not recommended for the prevention of PPH. It is used as a second-line agent in the treatment of PPH. One ampoule contains carboprost tromethamine equivalent to 250 µg of carboprost. This product remains stable at 25°C for 15 days and at 40°C for 2 days.

Mechanism of action: It improves uterine contractility by increasing the number of oxytocin receptors and cause vasoconstriction. Onset of action is 1–2 minutes and effect lasts for 15–20 minutes. Storage is in refrigeration at 2–8°C.

Dose: 250 µg IM every 15 minutes till bleeding is controlled up to a maximum dose of 2 g (eight doses).

Contraindication: Bronchial asthma as it causes intense bronchospasm.

Side effects: These are nausea, vomiting, diarrhea, transient fever, headache, chills, shaking hypertension, and bronchospasm.

Carbetocin

It is a relatively newer drug. It is a heat-stable oxytocin analog designed to overcome the limitations of the traditional heat labile oxytocin. It has a shelf life of 48 months at 30°C.

The CHAMPION Trial concluded that heat-stable carbetocin was noninferior to oxytocin for the prevention of blood loss of at least 500 mL.[5] It was approved by Drugs Controller General of India (DCGI), for prevention of PPH in 2022. The use of carbetocin (100 µg, IM/IV) is recommended for the prevention of PPH for all births in contexts where its cost is comparable to other uterotonics. It has no role in induction of labor or augmentation and thus cannot entirely replace oxytocin.

Mechanism of action: It binds to oxytocin receptors in the uterine smooth muscle, resulting in rhythmic contractions, increased frequency of existing contractions, and increased uterine tone. It has rapid onset of action within 2 minutes. Half-life is 60 minutes for IV and 120 minutes for IM injection. The receptors remain blocked for 2 hours and in case of no response, oxytocin should not be used as second line. It is heat-stable and can be used at room temperature.

Dose: 100 µg, IM/slow IV.

Contraindications: These are epilepsy and renal and hepatic impairment.

Side effects: These are nausea, vomiting, abdominal pain, dizziness, and feeling of warmth.

Antifibrinolytic Drugs

Tranexamic Acid

It has been approved for the treatment, but not for prevention of PPH. The WOMAN Trial (World Maternal Antifibrinolytic Trial) has concluded that use of tranexamic acid (TXA) within 3 hours of PPH has reduced women bleeding to death by a third and overall maternal mortality by 1–2%.[5]

Mechanism of action: It is an antifibrinolytic drug. It prevents excessive blood loss by stabilizing the formed clot. Intact functioning of the coagulation system is a prerequisite for the action of TXA. It is of limited use when disseminated intravascular coagulation (DIC) has set in. The WHO recommends early use of IV TXA within 3 hours of birth in addition to standard care for women with clinically diagnosed PPH following vaginal birth or cesarean section.[6] TXA for PPH treatment should not be initiated >3 hours after birth. TXA should be used in all cases of PPH, regardless of whether the bleeding is due to genital tract trauma or other causes.

Dose and route: TXA should be administered at a fixed dose of 1 g in 10 mL (100 mg/mL) IV at 1 mL/min (i.e., administered over 10 minutes), with a second dose of 1 g IV if bleeding continues after 30 minutes. TXA should be administered via an IV route only for treatment of PPH.

Contraindication: Renal impairment.

Side effects: These include nausea, vomiting, diarrhea, abdominal pain, and muscle stiffness.

MANAGEMENT OF POSTPARTUM HEMORRHAGE

The management of postpartum hemorrhage starts with identification of risk factors and to have a high degree of suspicion to detect early signs of blood loss. The treatment approach should incorporate resuscitative measures alongside detection and correction of the cause of PPH. The steps in the management are shown in **Flowchart 2** and listed as follows:

- Call for HELP.
- Maintain ABC (evaluate and maintain Airway, Breathing and Circulation), 100% oxygen.
- Ascertain the cause of PPH. The corrective measures toward the cause must take place simultaneously with resuscitation. Look for the *4 Ts:* Tone, Tissue, Trauma, and Thrombin. The drugs used are described in **Table 1**.

Flowchart 2: Management of postpartum hemorrhage (PPH).

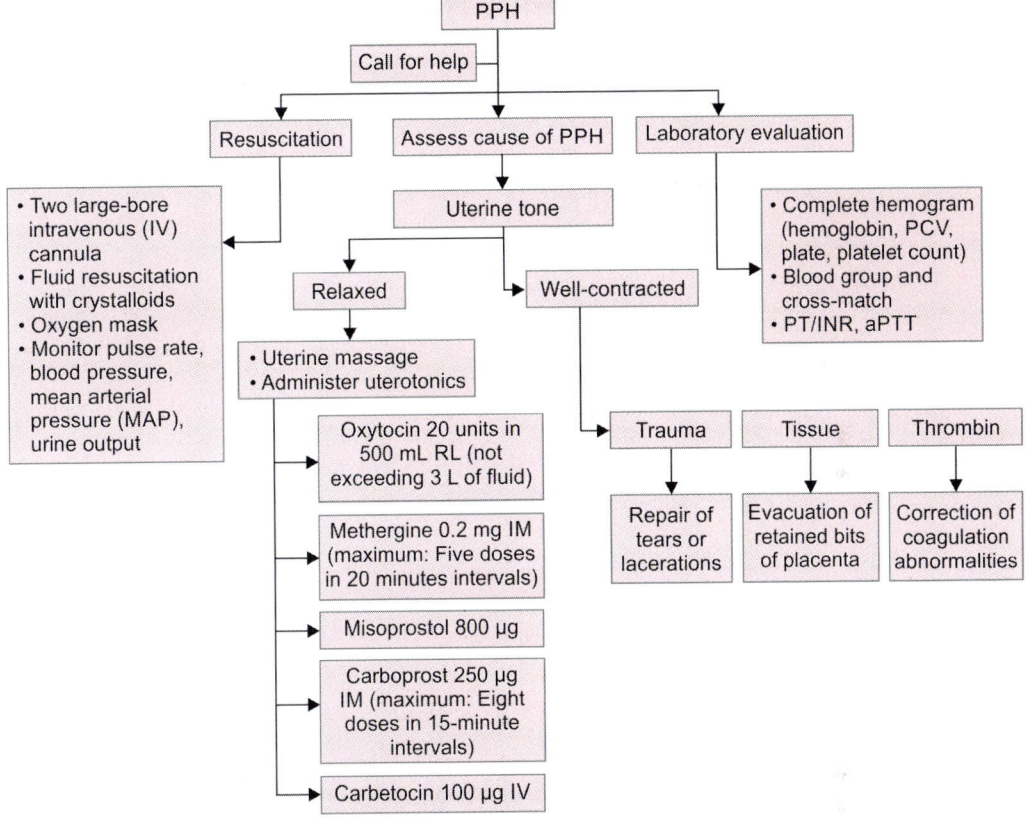

(aPTT: activated partial thromboplastin time; IM: intramuscular; INR: international normalized ratio; PCV: packed cell volume; PT: prothrombin time; RL: Ringer's lactate)

- Insert two IV large-bore IV cannula (14-gauge) and obtain blood samples for crossmatch and investigations [complete hemogram, baseline liver function test (LFT), kidney function test (KFT), prothrombin time (PT)/international normalized ratio (INR), fibrinogen if coagulopathy is suspected.]
- Monitor pulse rate, blood pressure, temperature, oxygen saturation, and respiratory rate every 15 minutes.
- *Fluid resuscitation:* (while awaiting blood components)
  - This forms the mainstay treatment to replace the lost blood volume.
  - Crystalloids are the fluid of choice and must be replace in the ratio of 3:1 for each unit of blood loss.
  - Infusion must be rapid bolus and care must be taken to not exceed 2.5 L of fluid without blood replacement.
- *Blood transfusion:*
  - Crossmatched and group-specific packed red blood cells (RBCs) are to be transfused.
  - If unavailable: Non-crossmatched group-specific blood OR give "O RhD negative" blood if required.
  - If massive transfusion is needed (massive transfusion is defined as

transfusion of 4 units of packed RBCs within 1 hour or transfusion of 10 or more units of packed RBCs within 24 hours or replacement of the complete blood volume) the transfusion of packed RBCs, platelets, and fresh frozen plasma is to be given in the ratio of 1:1:1.
- Fresh frozen plasma 4 units for every 4 units of red cells or PT/activated partial thromboplastin time >1.5 × normal (12–15 mL/kg or total 1 L)
- Transfuse platelets concentrates if platelet count <75,000.
- Cryoprecipitate is given if fibrinogen <2 g/L or if very low fibrinogen level is suspected, such as in case of disseminated intravascular coagulopathy and placental abruption.

■ KEY POINTS

- Postpartum hemorrhage is any blood loss accompanied by signs and symptoms of hypovolemia, regardless of mode of delivery.
- The aim of treatment of PPH is to find and stop the cause of the bleeding as soon as possible.
- Treatment of women having PPH has two components: resuscitation and management of obstetric hemorrhage.
- Medical management is the first-line therapy for atonic PPH.
- Uterotonics are considered the first-line treatment for uterine atony.
- Oxytocin is the uterotonic of choice for PPH prevention.

■ REFERENCES

1. Maternal Health Division, Ministry of Health and Family Welfare. (2015). Guidance Note on Prevention and Management of Postpartum Haemorrhage. [online] Available from: https://nhm.gov.in/images/pdf/programmes/maternal-health/guidelines/Guidance_Note_on_Prevention_&_Management_of_Postpartum_Haemorrhage.pdf [Last accessed December, 2023].
2. Mavrides E, Allard S, Chandraharan E, Collins P, Green L, Hunt BJ, et al. Prevention and Management of Postpartum Hemorrhage. BJOG. 2016;124:e106-e149.
3. Allen R, O'Brien BM. Uses of misoprostol in obstetrics and gynecology. Rev Obstet Gynecol. 2009;2(3):159-68.
4. Regitz-Zagrosek V, Roos-Hesselink JW, Bauersachs J, Blomström-Lundqvist C, Cífková R, De Bonis M, et al; ESC Scientific Document Group. 2018 ESC Guidelines for the management of cardiovascular diseases during pregnancy. Eur Heart J. 2018;39(34):3165-241.
5. Widmer M, Piaggio G, Nguyen TMH, Osoti A, Owa OO, Misra S, et al. WHO CHAMPION Trial Group. Heat-Stable Carbetocin versus Oxytocin to Prevent Hemorrhage after Vaginal Birth. N Engl J Med. 2018;379(8):743-52.
6. World Health Organization. (2017). Updated WHO Recommendation on Tranexamic Acid for the Treatment of Postpartum Haemorrhage. [online] Available from: https://iris.who.int/bitstream/handle/10665/259379/WHO-RHR-17.21-eng.pdf?sequence=1 [Last accessed December, 2023].

Section 7

Medical Management of Infections in Pregnancy

- **Human Immunodeficiency Viruses: Antiretroviral Drugs**
  Bharti Uppal Nayyar, Vandana Agarwal

- **Tuberculosis: Antitubercular Drugs**
  Namita Chopra, Kamal Chopra

Chapter 18

Human Immunodeficiency Viruses: Antiretroviral Drugs

Bharti Uppal Nayyar, Vandana Agarwal

India has the third highest burden of human immunodeficiency virus (HIV) in the world with an estimated 23.19 lakh people living with HIV in 2020 and around 57,000 estimated annual new infections in 2020 according to the latest surveillance data. In 2004, antiretroviral therapy (ART) drugs for treatment of patients living with HIV (PLHIV) were introduced under the National AIDS Control Programme.[1] ART comprises at least three antiretroviral drugs belonging to at least three different classes of drugs in order to inhibit viral replication and thereby reduce viremia to minimal levels. It has a wide network of coverage including 682 ART centers as well as 1,270 link ART centers, providing treatment to about 14 lakh PLHIV across India.[1] Greater than 90% of all new pediatric HIV infections are as a result of vertical transmission from mother to fetus, which can occur anytime during pregnancy, delivery, or through breastfeeding. However, efforts to increase the access to suppressive ART have led to a marked decrease in HIV transmission rates in resource-limited settings.[2]

According to the latest data, it has been seen that all over India, approximately 2,093,000 (1,533,000–2,908,000) pregnant women need ART for prevention of parent to child transmission (PPTCT) of HIV.[3]

Table 1 shows that the risk of HIV transmission from mother to child dramatically reduces with the introduction of ART.

Antiretroviral therapy works for prevention of transmission of HIV from parent to infant by:
- Decreasing the maternal viremia

TABLE 1: Risk of transmission of HIV from mother to child with or without interventions.[4]

ART intervention	Risk of fetomaternal transmission of HIV
No ARV; with breastfeeding	30–45%
No ARV; no breastfeeding	20–25%
Short course with one ARV and breastfeeding	15–25%
Short course with one ARV and no breastfeeding	5–15%
Short course with two ARVs along with breastfeeding	5%
Three ARVs with breastfeeding	2%
Three ARVs with no breastfeeding	1%

(ART: antiretroviral therapy; ARV: antiretroviral; HIV: human immunodeficiency virus)

- Loading the fetus with antiretroviral drugs which prevent the further replication of transmitted virions
- Decreasing the risk of transmission to infants exposed to HIV
- Causing improvement in the overall health of the mother.

Owing to the suppression of virus, there is reduction in the destruction of CD4 lymphocyte cells which in turn leads to an increase in the CD4 cell count. This causes partial restoration of pathogen-specific immune function. This further leads to decreased incidence of opportunistic infections, thereby reducing morbidity and mortality.

The mechanism of action of these drugs is that they act on various stages of the replication of the HIV virus thereby interrupting viral replication in the human body. **Figure 1** shows the various enzymes involved in the replication of virus and the sites where the antiretroviral drugs attack the virus. The ART drugs are categorized based on the site of their action as shown in **Table 2**.

- Drugs which block the binding or fusion of HIV to the host cells *(fusion inhibitors and CCR-5 coreceptor blockers)*
- Drugs which block the viral ribonucleic acid (RNA) cleavage and inhibit reverse transcriptase enzyme *(reverse transcriptase inhibitors)* by competitive

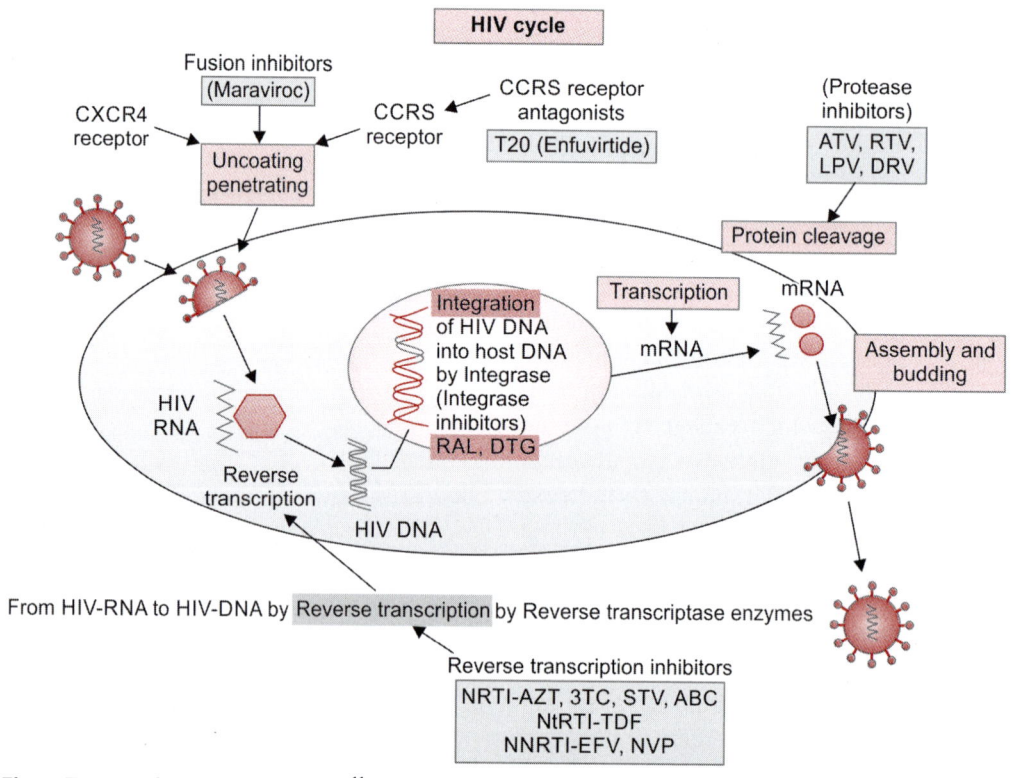

Fig. 1: Targets of antiretroviral drugs.[11] (DNA: deoxyribonucleic acid; HIV: human immunodeficiency virus; mRNA: messenger ribonucleic acid; RNA: ribonucleic acid)

TABLE 2: Classes of antiretroviral (ARV) drugs.[4]

Nucleoside reverse transcriptase inhibitors (NsRTIs)	Non-nucleoside reverse transcriptase inhibitors (NNRTIs)	Protease inhibitors (PIs)
Zidovudine (AZT/ZDV)*	Nevirapine (NVP)*	Saquinavir (SQV)
Stavudine (d4T)	Efavirenz (EFV)*	Ritonavir (RTV)*
Lamivudine (3TC)*	Delavirdine (DLV)	Nelfinavir (NFV)
Abacavir (ABC)*	Rilpivirine (RPV)	Amprenavir (APV)
Didanosine (ddI)	Etravirine (ETV)	Indinavir (INV)
Zalcitabine (ddC)	Doravirine (DOR)	Lopinavir (LPV)*
Emtricitabine (FTC)		• Fosamprenavir (FPV)
	Integrase inhibitors	• Atazanavir (ATV)*
Nucleotide reverse transcriptase inhibitors (NtRTIs)	• Dolutegravir (DTG)* • Raltegravir (RGV)* • Elvitegravir (EVG)	• Tipranavir (TPV) • Darunavir (DRV)*
Tenofovir disoproxil fumarate (TDF)*	Bictegravir (BIC)	
Tenofovir alafenamide (TAF)	Cabotegravir (CAB)	
Fusion inhibitors (FIs)	CCR5 entry inhibitor	Post attachment maturation inhibitor
Enfuvirtide (T-20)	Maraviroc (MVC)	Ibalizumab (IBA)

*Available in the National Program

inhibition. These drugs stop the building process of new viruses by incorporating themselves into the deoxyribonucleic acid (DNA) of the virus. This new DNA is incomplete and hence cannot form new viruses. These are of three types:
1. Nucleoside analogs need three intracellular phosphorylation steps in order to form the triphosphate nucleoside which is the active drug moiety.
2. Nucleotide analogs have a non-peptide structure, containing a monophosphate component attached to the adenine base. They require only two phosphorylation steps to form the active moiety.
3. Non-nucleotide reverse transcriptase inhibitors directly bind with reverse transcriptase enzyme and prevent conversion of RNA to DNA.

- Block the enzyme integrase, which catalyzes the two-step process of incorporation of HIV DNA into the genome of the host cell. This halts further replication of the virus *[integrase inhibitors/integrase strand-transfer inhibitor (INSTI)]*.
- Drugs which block the RNA thereby preventing viral protein production.
- Drugs which block the enzyme protease required at the last step of viral reproduction cycle *[protease inhibitors (PIs)]*. This prevents the successful assembly and release of HIV from infected CD4 cell.
- Drugs which inhibit the budding of HIV from host cells.

All pregnant women, when diagnosed to be HIV positive, should be referred to the ART center for registration into care, counseling, and rapid ART initiation in the PPTCT program. As per the National Program, it is recommended to provide lifelong ART for all pregnant and lactating women living with HIV, wherein they receive a "fixed drug combination (FDC)" triple-drug ART regimen irrespective of CD4 count or clinical stage (treat all). This is for their own health benefit as well as for prevention of vertical transmission.[1,5] Presently, as per National Guidelines, tenofovir, lamivudine, and dolutegravir (TLD) is the preferred regimen of treatment during pregnancy and is started after taking informed consent.

In order to decide regarding ART during pregnancy, additional considerations must be borne in mind that due to altered pharmacokinetics (owing to physiological changes of pregnancy), some toxicities may be magnified during pregnancy, making it potentially toxic to the fetus-in-utero. In addition to considering safety and efficacy of the drugs in mother and fetus, while selecting the most suitable ART regime, one should consider the resistance profile of the virus, and possibilities of drug interactions with other medications.

It can be started in the first trimester provided the mother is not experiencing nausea and vomiting. Most medications used to treat HIV/acquired immunodeficiency syndrome (AIDS) have thus far proven to be safe in pregnancy with an acceptable risk/benefit ratio as elaborated in **Table 3**.

■ REGIMEN MANAGEMENT

- *Patients already on ART prior to pregnancy*:
  - *Virally suppressed while on ART*: Such patients have a low risk of transmitting HIV to their infant. These women who are already taking and tolerating an acceptable antiretroviral regimen do not have to discontinue it in the first trimester. However, it is advised to change her present regime to TLD regimen[1] after explaining the benefits of DTG in achieving faster viral suppression (reduction in viral copies to <50 copies/mL within 4 weeks has been noted). Moreover, DTG-based regimens are expected to have fewer side effects, allergic reactions and neuropsychiatric events compared to non-nucleoside reverse transcriptase inhibitor (NNRTI)-regimens. DTG-based regimens can be prescribed for HIV-2 or combined HIV-1 and HIV-2 infection. Before the availability of DTG in the program, patients infected with HIV-2 were being initiated with two NRTIs plus boosted PI regimen. However, the availability of DTG in the program will now bring further harmonization amongst the patient population. Furthermore, there is no need for substitution of DTG-based ART regimen in PLHIV in case of coinfection with tuberculosis (TB), hepatitis B virus (HBV), or hepatitis C virus (HCV).
- *Not virally suppressed:* These patients should be provided adequate counseling and enhanced adherence interventions should be tried in order to achieve viral suppression as quickly as possible. It is advised to transition her present regime to TLD regimen. If viral suppression is not achieved within 8 weeks following these interventions, the patient should be switched to the next-in-line ART regimen. Also, these patients should undergo frequent assessment of viral load throughout pregnancy.

TABLE 3: Antiretroviral (ARV) drugs along with their side effects and ways of monitoring therapy.[6]

	Drug	Dosing recommendations[a]	Common side effects	Monitoring
A	*Nucleoside analogs (NsRTIs)*			
1.	Zidovudine (AZT)	• 600 mg orally daily in 2–3 divided doses without regard to food • Patients in active labor should receive ZDV 2 mg/kg IV as loading dose, followed by 1 mg/kg/h continuous infusion from beginning of active labor until delivery	High placental transfer to fetus.[b] Anemia, neutropenia, bone marrow suppression, gastrointestinal disturbance, myopathy and lactic acidosis.[7] These side effects are mainly due to mitochondrial toxicity (as these agents inhibit mitochondrial DNA polymerase gamma)	Complete blood count (CBC) with differential leukocyte count (DLC) every 3 months once stable
2.	Didanosine (ddI)	300 mg orally once daily	Peripheral neuropathy, pancreatitis, dry mouth, hepatitis	CBC with differential leukocyte count, aminotransferases, serum potassium, amylase, and triglycerides. Bimonthly neurologic questionnaire for neuropathy
3.	Zalcitabine (ddC)	0.375–0.75 mg orally thrice daily	Peripheral neuropathy, aphthous ulcer, hepatitis	Monthly neurologic questionnaire, aminotransferases
4.	Stavudine (d4T)	30 mg orally twice daily	Peripheral neuropathy, hepatitis, pancreatitis	Monthly neurologic questionnaire, aminotransferases, amylase
5.	Lamivudine (3TC) 3TC drugs which were specifically made for treatment of HBV contain a lower dose of 3TC which is inadequate for HIV treatment	150 mg orally twice daily, without regard to food	• High placental transfer to fetus.[b] Minimal toxicity, rash (very rare) • In case of hepatitis B virus/human immuno-deficiency virus (HBV/HIV) • coinfection, it is possible that a HBV flare may occur on the discontinuation of the drug	No extra monitoring

Contd...

Contd...

	Drug	Dosing recommendations[a]	Common side effects	Monitoring
6.	Abacavir (ABC)	300 mg orally twice daily, without regard to food	• High placental transfer to fetus.[b] Hypersensitivity reaction in 3–5% (can be fatal), fever, rash, fatigue, nausea, vomiting, anorexia, respiratory symptoms (sore throat, cough, shortness of breath) • Testing for HLA-B 57:01 (immunogenetic marker) identifies patients who are at risk of reactions, and a patient's negative status should be documented before starting ABC[8] (Grade 1A)	No specific monitoring
B	**Nucleotide analogs (NRTIs)**			
1.	Tenofovir disoproxil fumarate (TDF)	300 mg orally once a day without regard to food	• High placental transfer to fetus[b] • In presence of HBV/HIV coinfection, HBV flare may occur if the drug is discontinued. Nephrotoxicity, bone demineralization, GI distress	Kidney function test (KFT) in acute settings
C	**Protease inhibitors**			
1.	Saquinavir (SQV)	600 mg orally thrice daily	Gastrointestinal distress, headache	No extra monitoring
2.	Ritonavir (RTV)	600 mg twice daily or 400 mg twice daily with food (to improve tolerability) in combination with other PIs	Gastrointestinal distress, peripheral paresthesia	Bimonthly aminotransferases, uric acid, triglycerides
3.	Indinavir (IDV)	800 mg orally thrice daily	Renal calculi	Bimonthly aminotransferases, bilirubin level
4.	Nelfinavir (NLF)	750 mg orally thrice daily	Diarrhea	No additional monitoring
5.	Amprenavir (APV)	1,200 mg orally twice daily	Gastrointestinal distress, rash	Cholesterol levels, triglycerides

Contd...

Contd...

	Drug	Dosing recommendations[a]	Common side effects	Monitoring
6.	Lopinavir/ritonavir (LPV-r) (heat-stable tablet)	400 mg/100 mg orally twice daily	Diarrhea, glucose intolerance	Cholesterol levels, triglycerides, every other month aminotransferases
D	Non-nucleoside reverse transcriptase inhibitors (NNRTIs)			
1.	Nevirapine (NVP)	200 mg once daily for 2 weeks; thereafter 200 mg twice daily without regard to food	High placental transfer to fetus.[b] If started in patients with CD4 counts $\geq 250/mm^3$, there is an increased risk of hepatitis (usually within 12 weeks); sometimes life-threatening hepatotoxicity often associated with a skin rash occasionally progressing to severe conditions, including Stevens–Johnson syndrome (SJS) and toxic epidermal necrolysis (TEN). Patients who develop severe hepatotoxicity or grade 4 skin rashes should not be rechallenged	No additional monitoring. It should be started during pregnancy with CD4 counts $\geq 250/mm^3$ only if benefit clearly outweighs risk. Elevated baseline transaminase levels may increase the risk of nevirapine (NVP) toxicity. Patients who become pregnant while on NVP containing regime and are tolerating well, can continue taking that regime, regardless of their CD4 count
2.	Delavirdine	400 mg orally thrice a day	Rash	No additional monitoring
3.	Efavirenz (EFV)	600 mg orally daily Avoid after high-fat meals. [Also, bedtime administration is suggested to decrease central nervous system (CNS) side effects]	Moderate placental transfer to fetus.[b] Neurological disturbances like (dizziness, insomnia, somnolence, confusion, hallucinations, agitation) and personality changes. Rash occurs, but less common as compared to NVP	No additional monitoring
E	Integrase inhibitors			
1.	Raltegravir (RAL)	400 mg twice daily without regard to food	High placental transfer to fetus.[b] Rhabdomyolysis, myopathy, myalgia, insomnia, diarrhea, fever, rash, SJS, TEN, hepatitis, and hepatic failure	No additional monitoring

Contd...

Contd...

	Drug	Dosing recommendations[a]	Common side effects	Monitoring
2.	Dolutegravir (DTG) It is the preferred antiretroviral drug for use in pregnancy, irrespective of trimester, and for women who are trying to conceive	50 mg once daily without regard to food	High placental transfer to fetus.[b] Insomnia, headache, and weight gain. Also, can cause serious life-threatening side effects including hypersensitivity (allergic reactions and liver problems)	No additional monitoring (to maximize DTG absorption, doses should not be administered within 2 hours of ingesting any preparation that contains minerals such as iron/calcium/prenatal vitamins)

[a]Individual ARV drug doses may need to be adjusted in patients with renal or hepatic insufficiency
[b]Placental transfer categories are determined by mean or median cord blood/maternal delivery plasma drug ratio:
- High: >0.6
- Moderate: 0.3–0.6
- Low: <0.3

- *Patients not on ART prior to pregnancy:* The WHO recommends dolutegravir + TDF and lamivudine as the preferred first-line regimen for treatment of HIV in pregnant women.[5] Women not taking any ART medication, should be offered combination ART (commonly a dual nucleoside reverse transcriptase inhibitor combination and a ritonavir-boosted PI or an integrase strand transfer inhibitor) after counseling regarding the potential impact of therapy on both mother and fetus. As compared to the Efavirenz-based ART, Dolutegravir-containing regimens are associated with higher and faster viral suppression along with good maternal and fetal outcomes.[9]

  Alongside above measures and linking her to PPTCT program, they are also advised regarding regular antenatal care (ANC) visits, ART adherence (also checked by pill count), nutritional advice, iron, folic acid, calcium supplementation, and encouraged for institutional delivery.

  It has been reported that pregnant women receiving ART with a combined regimen of integrase inhibitors and tenofovir have increased risk of excess gestational weight gain.[10]

PRINCIPLES AND TECHNICAL GUIDELINES FOR ARV THERAPY IN INDIA

- In consideration of the WHO guidelines and inputs from the National AIDS Control Organisation (NACO) Technical Resource Group, following points have been recommended:
  - First-line ART[3] (ART naïve patient) recommends a triple drug combination therapy from two different classes of drugs, which constitutes an NRTI backbone (preferably tenofovir and lamivudine) + one INSTI (preferably DTG), i.e., tenofovir (TDF 300 mg) + lamivudine (3TC 300 mg) + dolutegravir

(DTG 50 mg) regimen. (TLD) as FDC in a single pill once daily (at a fixed time daily as per patient's convenience).

The following ART regimens have been designated as "national ART regimens" by National AIDS Control Organization **(Table 4)**.

In patients where preferred first-line ARV regimen of TDF + 3TC + DTG cannot be used, the alternative regimens are stated in **Table 5**.

- Dolutegravir is known to have some important interactions with certain drugs if coadministered, as detailed in **Table 6**.
- After beginning ART for a patient, she is advised to return for a visit within 3–15 days so that her general wellbeing can be assessed. On subsequent monthly follow-up visits, along with routine ANC examination, the caregiver should note any toxicity of ART, look for immune

TABLE 4: Recommended ART regimen in pregnant and lactating women with HIV by NACO.[1]

Preferred ART regimen	Remarks
Tenofovir + lamivudine + dolutegravir TDF + 3TC + DTG (TLD)	• FDC of TDF (300 mg) + 3TC (300 mg) + DTG (50 mg) • To be given once daily • Including HIV-1, HIV-2, HIV-1 and 2, women exposed to single-dose NVP in the past and coinfected with TB or hepatitis • Pregnant women with HIV should be educated about the risks and advantages of DTG in order to make informed choice

(ART: antiretroviral therapy; HIV: human immunodeficiency virus; NACO: National AIDS Control Organisation; NVP: nevirapine)

TABLE 5: Alternate first-line ART in special situations.[1]

Condition	Alternate first-line regimen
Patient on rifampicin-containing ATT regimen	• Tenofovir (300 mg) + lamivudine (300 mg) + dolutegravir (50 mg), i.e., FDC one tablet once daily (on any fixed time daily as per convenience) + • Additional dose of DTG 50 mg to be provided (12 hours after taking their regular dose) until 2 weeks after completion of ATT
Women who do not wish to take DTG-based ART after adequate counseling	• Tenofovir (300 mg) + lamivudine (300 mg) + Efavirenz (600 mg) • If efavirenz is contraindicated • (HIV-2/HIV-1 and 2/prior NNRTI exposure) then tenofovir (300 mg) + lamivudine (300 mg) + [lopinavir (200 mg) + ritonavir (50 mg) twice a day]

(ART: antiretroviral therapy; ATT: antitubercular treatment; HIV: human immunodeficiency virus NNRTI: non-nucleoside reverse transcriptase inhibitor)

TABLE 6: Drug interactions with dolutegravir.[1]

Key drug interaction	Suggested management
Carbamazepine	Use DTG twice a day or substitute it with another anticonvulsant
Metformin	Limit daily dose of metformin to 1,000 mg along with glycemic control monitoring
Polyvalent cation products containing Al, Ca, Fe, Mg, and Zn (e.g., antacids, multivitamins, and supplements)	Use 2 hours prior or 6 hours after DTG
Rifampicin	Use DTG 50 mg twice a day (as bioavailability of DTG is suppressed) or substitute with rifabutin

reconstitution inflammatory syndrome (IRIS) and also counsel her regarding adherence to ART.
- Caregivers should be able to promptly recognize the drug toxicities of PLHIV during their visits to ART centers and be able to treat them as described in **Table 7**.
- IRIS is a life-threatening condition characterized by worsening of signs and symptoms due to known infections, or development of disease owing to occult infections within a period of 6 weeks to 6 months after the initiation of ART. It is associated with an increase in CD4 count. It occurs in about 10–30% of patients, usually within the first 4–8 weeks of starting ART. However, late IRIS can be seen up to 6 months of starting ART. IRIS should be considered only when the symptoms cannot be explained by a new infection, drug toxicity or as an expected course of an already known infection. It is important for the clinician to differentiate any new clinical event post ART initiation from IRIS.

  Patients who are at maximum risk of developing IRIS are the ones who already have severe immunosuppression before the initiation of ART. Some clinical features of this condition include appearance/enlargement or suppuration of lymph nodes, pleural effusion, high-grade fever (with exclusion of other causes), cerebral cryptococcosis or toxoplasmosis, and pneumonitis. It is self-limiting in nature usually and requires observation. Interruption of ART is required rarely. However, patients have to be reassured in case of protracted symptoms so that discontinuation of ART can be prevented. Short-term therapy with corticosteroids or nonsteroidal anti-inflammatory drugs can be given to reduce the inflammation—prednisolone at 1.5 mg/kg orally for 2 weeks followed by 0.75 mg/kg orally for 2 weeks and then tapered off. Temporary cessation of ART must be considered, only if potentially life-threatening features develop.
- It is imperative to monitor ART in order to look for toxicity and to measure efficacy using objective markers to determine whether to maintain or change regimens. Single drug replacement (substitution) of ARV drug(s) in a PLHIV due to drug toxicity, intolerance or drug-drug interactions does not mean that a second-line regimen is being used.
- Failure of treatment leads to the loss of efficacy to the current antiviral regimen and the entire regimen has to be switched from first to second line. It is identified by clinical and/or immunological criteria and confirmed by the virological criteria (plasma viral load value of ≥1,000 copies/mL at or after 6 months of ART with >95% treatment adherence). Plasma viral load testing is recommended for all HIV-positive pregnant women during 32–36 weeks of pregnancy (regardless of duration of ART) to determine the risk of HIV transmission to the baby.
- Second-line ART[3] (after first-line therapy have failed) recommend use of ritonavir-boosted PIs supported by two agents from NRTI class, of which at least one should be new, as shown in **Table 8**.
- Standard guidelines have been issued for those pregnant patients who present in active labor, and have no history of prior ART **(Table 9)**.

Good adherence to treatment ensures success of ART as well as prevention of drug resistance. In order to achieve this, counseling must begin from the first point of contact with the patient. It should involve

TABLE 7: Adverse effects of antiretroviral therapy (ART) drugs and their management.[1]

Adverse effect	Possible offending drug(s)	Management
Acute hepatitis	• Nevirapine and PI/r • Less common with efavirenz	• Monitor serum transaminases, bilirubin • If ALT >5 times baseline level, stop ARVs till resolution of symptoms • NVP should be permanently stopped
Acute pancreatitis	• Stavudine • Infrequent with lamivudine	• Monitor serum pancreatic amylase, lipase • All ARVs should be stopped till symptoms resolve restart ART with change to different NRTI, preferably one without pancreatic toxicity (e.g., AZT, TDF, and ABC)
Lactic acidosis	All NRTI, especially stavudine	Discontinue ART; resume ART by replacing it with either ABC or TDF
Hypersensitivity reaction	Abacavir, nevirapine	Discontinue ART until symptoms resolve. Do not rechallenge with ABC (or NVP), as anaphylaxis and death have been reported. On resolution of symptoms, ART to be restarted with a change to different NRTI if ABC-associated or to PI- or NNRTI-based regimen if NVP associated
Rash/drug eruptions including Stevens–Johnson's syndrome or toxic epidermal necrolysis (TEN)	Nevirapine, efavirenz Rarely: Dolutegravir, lamivudine	• In mild cases, antihistaminics can be given • If rash is moderate, nonprogressive and without mucosal or systemic symptoms, consider substituting NVP to EFV after resolution of rash • In moderate and severe cases, discontinue all ARVs till resolution of symptoms and give supportive treatment • For rashes with systemic symptoms such as fever, mucosal lesions, urticaria, Stevens–Johnson's syndrome or TEN, permanently discontinue NVP. Once resolved, switch ART regimen to different ARV class (e.g., two NRTIs and PI)
Peripheral neuropathy	Stavudine	• Stop suspected NRTI early and change to different NRTI without neurotoxicity (e.g., AZT and ABC) • Symptoms resolve in 2–3 weeks usually
Diarrhea	Lopinavir/ritonavir (LPV/r)	Usually self-limited
Dyslipidemia, insulin resistance, and hyperglycemia	PIs, EFV	Replace suspected PI by drugs with lesser risk of metabolic toxicity
Gastrointestinal disturbance	All ARVs	Self-limited, symptomatic treatment is offered
Hematological toxicities	Zidovudine	Consider blood transfusion in severe anemia and replace with an NRTI with less effect on bone marrow, e.g., d4T, ABC, and TDF
Lipoatrophy/lipodystrophy	All NRTIs; particularly stavudine	Early replacement of suspected ARV drugs (e.g., d4T) with TDF or ABC
Neuropsychiatric changes	Efavirenz (EFV)	Usually self-limited. Counsel to take EFV before bedtime
Renal toxicity (renal tubular dysfunction)	TDF	Discontinue TD. After resolution, replace with another ARV

TABLE 8: Recommended antiretroviral therapy (ART) regimens for patients failed to first-line ART.[1]

Failing first-line antiretroviral treatment	Recommended regimens
TDF + 3TC + DTG	• Hemoglobin (Hb) ≥9 g/dL • AZT (300 mg) + 3TC (150 mg) BD + LPV (300 mg)/r (100 mg) fixed-dose combination OD • Hb <9g/dL • DTG 50 mg BD + LPV (300 mg)/r (100 mg) OD + existing NRTI backbone

TABLE 9: Recommended ART regimen during pregnancy in women with HIV presenting in active labor by NACO.[3]

Maternal status	Intrapartum	Postpartum
Presenting in active labor, no prior ART	TDF (300 mg) + 3TC (300mg) + DTG (50 mg)	• TDF (300 mg) + 3TC (300 mg) + DTG (50 mg)

(ART: antiretroviral therapy; HIV: human immunodeficiency virus; NACO: National AIDS Control Organisation)

preparing the patient for treatment as well as providing adequate psychosocial support by an identified caregiver and support networks. Patients should have two to three counseling sessions before starting ART. The time period of undergoing investigations and waiting for the results should be utilized for counseling.

Rapid initiation of effective lifelong ART at the time of diagnosis of HIV infection, scheduling regular antenatal visits for ART adherence counseling, and monitoring toxicity of ART along with routine pregnancy care followed by prompt initiation of ART prophylaxis for the neonate should be the goal of all obstetricians taking care of HIV patients.

Fixed-dose combinations (FDCs) of antiretroviral drugs are preferred since they are easy to prescribe as well as convenient for the patients to take. This facilitates improved treatment adherence. This is very important for PLHIV since the treatment is lifelong and drug-resistant mutants as well as the resultant treatment failure needs to be minimized. Moreover, FDCs have a distinct advantage when it comes to drug procurement as well as distribution. National experience shows that FDC regimens have better compliance, are well tolerated, and hence more acceptable.

It is important to repeatedly counsel mothers regarding the adherence to ART throughout their pregnancy and thereafter. All efforts should be undertaken to trace the PLHIV registered at the ART centers who have missed their visits or are lost to follow-up.

Long-term data on the safety of in utero drug exposure in humans are not available for any antiretroviral drug; however, short-term data about the same is reassuring. It is also important that information regarding in utero ART drug exposure should be entered in the child's medical record, in case any problem, that could be one of the long-term complications are identified in future.

■ **KEY POINTS**

- Use of ART drastically decreases fetomaternal transmission of HIV from 30–45 to 1%.
- FDC of TLD is the preferred regimen of ART in pregnancy.
- ART must be administered lifelong with timely monitoring of patient compliance and any drug toxicities.
- IRIS is a life-threatening complication occurring mainly in severely immunocompromised patients.
- Good adherence to treatment ensures success of ART as well as prevention of drug resistance.

REFERENCES

1. National AIDS Control Organisation. National Guidelines for HIV Care and Treatment. New Delhi: NACO, Ministry of Health and Family Welfare, Government of India; 2021.
2. UNICEF. (2023). Elimination of mother-to-child transmission. [online] Available from: https://data.unicef.org/topic/hivaids/emtct/. [Last accessed December, 2023].
3. National AIDS Control Organisation, ICMR-National Institute of Medical Statistics. India HIV Estimates 2020: Technical Brief. New Delhi: NACO, Ministry of Health and Family Welfare, Government of India; 2021.
4. World Health Organization. Antiretroviral drugs for treating pregnant women and preventing HIV infection in infants: towards universal access: recommendations for a public health approach—2006 version. Geneva: World Health Organization; 2006.
5. World Health Organization. Consolidated HIV guidelines for prevention, treatment, service delivery and monitoring. Geneva: World Health Organization; 2021.
6. Clinicalinfo. Table 14. Antiretroviral Drug Use in Pregnant People With HIV: Pharmacokinetic and Toxicity Data in Human Pregnancy and Recommendations for Use in Pregnancy. [online] Available from: https://clinicalinfo.hiv.gov/guidelines/perinatal/safety-toxicity-arv-agents-drug-use-pregnant-full. [Last accessed December, 2023].
7. Bolhaar MG, Karstaedt AS. A high incidence of lactic acidosis and symptomatic hyper-lactatemia in women receiving highly active antiretroviral therapy in Soweto, South Africa. Clin Infect Dis. 2007;45:254.
8. Saag MS, Gandhi RT, Hoy JF, Landovitz RJ, Thompson MA, Sax PE, et al. Antiretroviral Drugs for Treatment and Prevention of HIV Infection in Adults: 2020 Recommendations of the International Antiviral Society-USA Panel. JAMA. 2020;324:1651-69.
9. Kintu K, Malaba TR, Nakibuka J, Papamichael C, Colbers A, Byrne K, et al. Dolutegravir versus efavirenz in women starting HIV therapy in late pregnancy (DOLPHIN-2): an open-label, randomised controlled trial. Lancet HIV. 2020;7:e332-9.
10. Joseph NT, Satten GA, Williams RE, Haddad LB, Jamieson DJ, Sheth AN, et al. The Effect of Antiretroviral Therapy for the Treatment of Human Immunodeficiency Virus (HIV)-1 in Pregnancy on Gestational Weight Gain. Clin Infect Dis. 2022;75(4):665-72.
11. Zash R, Holmes K, Diseko M, Jacobson D, Mayondi G, Mabuta J, et al. Update on neural tube defects with antiretroviral exposure in the Tsepamo study, Botswana. Montreal, Canada: Presented at the 24th International AIDS Conference; 2022.

Chapter 19

Tuberculosis: Antitubercular Drugs

Namita Chopra, Kamal Chopra

Females of children-bearing age, when diagnosed with tuberculosis (TB), should be informed about the possible effects of anti-TB drugs on pregnancy and counseled about planned pregnancy. If a patient is already pregnant, effective treatment is important for maintaining pregnancy.[1] Although, few precautions need to be taken in the management of such cases.[2]

If not initiated on anti-TB treatment, it poses a great threat not only to the patient but also to the fetus. It can lead to lower birth weight and rarely some can have congenital TB in infants. Proper treatment of TB does not have much effect on pregnant patients or fetus if required precautions are taken. Some drugs cross the placental barrier, but except for aminoglycosides, no other drug has harmful effects on the fetus.

Tuberculosis control program has prepared guidelines for the management of TB during pregnancy to ensure adequate treatment and precautions to be taken for the successful outcome of both TB and pregnancy.[3]

TREATMENT OF DRUG SENSITIVE TB IN PREGNANCY

The treatment regimen consists of a 2-month intensive phase with a combination of four drugs [Isoniazid (INH), rifampicin, pyrazinamide, and ethambutol)], followed by a 4-month continuation phase (INH, rifampicin, and ethambutol) with all drugs administered daily **(Table 1)**.

2 HRZE/4 HRE

As per present guidelines for the management of TB, universal Drug Susceptibility Testing (DST) is done to prove or rule out rifampicin resistance. If the patient is suffering from drug-sensitive TB, this standard drug regimen is given. All the four drugs are safe in pregnancy. Sometimes injection streptomycin is used in certain situations like TB meningitis or if any first-line drug needs to be replaced due to adverse reactions. Streptomycin crosses the placental barrier and can cause ototoxicity in the fetus.

If a mother suffering from TB is lactating, it should be continued. Breastfeeding should never be discouraged. Mother should cover her mouth while feeding. If the mother is in the infective stage, the infant can be given TB preventive treatment after ruling out active TB.

Under the National Tuberculosis Program, drugs are given in fixed drug combination (FDC). The number of FDC tablets depends on weight of patient like two tablets for a person weighing 25–35 kg and six tablets for a person weighing >75 kg. If patient gains weight during treatment, the number of tablets is increased accordingly.

TABLE 1: Drug dosage for first-line drugs.

Drug	Mode of activity	Mechanism of action	Daily dose/kg body weight	Common side effects
Isoniazid (INH)	Bactericidal	Blocks mycolic acid synthesis in cell wall of bacteria	5	• Hepatotoxicity • Peripheral neuropathy • Lethargy
Rifampicin (R)	Bactericidal	Suppresses RNA synthesis in bacteria by inhibiting DNA dependent RNA polymerase	10	• Orange discoloration of urine and body fluids • Hepatotoxicity • Cutaneous syndrome • Flu-like syndrome
Pyrazinamide (Z)	Bactericidal	Inhibits plasma membrane synthesis	25	• Gouty arthralgia • Hepatotoxicity
Ethambutol (E)	Bacteriostatic	Inhibits polymerization reactors of arabinoglycan, essential component of cell wall	15	• Retrobulbar optic neuritis • Red and green color blindness
Streptomycin (S)	Bacteriostatic	Inhibits protein synthesis in cell wall	15	• Vestibular and cochlear nerve damage • Renal toxicity • Skin reactions

TREATMENT OF DRUG-RESISTANT TB IN PREGNANCY

Treatment of multidrug-resistant (MDR)-TB is as such very challenging but if associated with pregnancy, it is still a big challenge to manage. This is due to the second-line drug used for MDR-TB being very toxic and often causes vomiting, which is already a concern in pregnancy. So, it is better to counsel a presumptive MDR-TB to avoid pregnancy till MDR treatment is complete. But, if the patient is already pregnant, advise her to get medical termination of pregnancy (MTP) as permitted in law (up to 24 weeks of pregnancy).

If the patient is not willing for MTP or the period of gestation is more than permissible limit for MTP, treatment should be started with adequate precautions (like streptomycin to be avoided during first trimester and ethionamide up to 32 weeks because of suspected teratogenic effects. Newer drugs bedaquiline and delamanid are avoided as their safety profile in pregnancy is still not clear.

Flowchart 1 presents the management of MDR-TB case during pregnancy.

To conclude, in pregnant women, strict counseling needs to be done for MTP, especially regarding the risk of delaying treatment, the potential effects of new drugs on the fetus including fetal abnormalities (if MTP is not opted) and the need for more intense maternal-fetal-neonatal follow-up. Appropriate counseling and an informed decision-making process for consent need to be undertaken in each case.

Pregnant women initiated on bedaquiline must be encouraged to provide formula feed

Flowchart 1: Management of multidrug-resistant (MDR)-TB case during pregnancy.

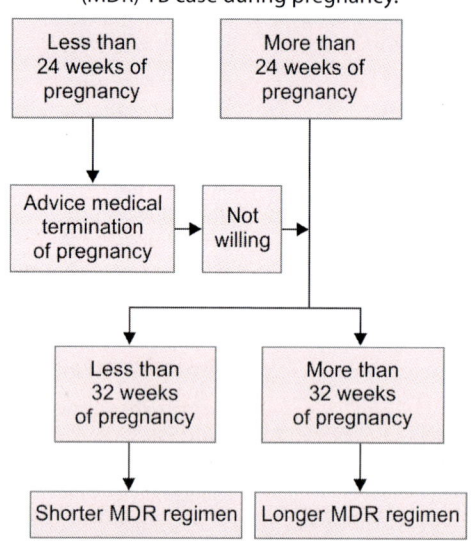

to their newborn child, till further evidence on the safety of this drug during lactation is available.

These are two drug regimens used for such cases.

1. Shorter regimen: Consisting of 4 months intensive phase with seven drugs [Bedaquiline, levofloxacin, clofazimine, pyrazinamide, and ethambutol followed by 5 months of levofloxacin, clofazimine, pyrazinamide, and ethambutol **(Table 2)**].

   (4–6) bedaquiline (Bdq) (6 m), levofloxacin (Lfx), clofazimine (Cfz), Z, E, Hh, Eto/(5) Lfx + cfz + Z + E

2. *Longer regimen:*

   (18–20) levofloxacin (Lfx), bedaquiline (Bdq) (6 m or longer) linezolid (LZD), clofazimine (Cfz.), cycloserine (Cs.)

A high rate of treatment success and favorable pregnancy outcomes can be achieved when pregnant patients with MDR-TB are treated with effective regimens.[4]

TREATMENT FOR LATENT TB INFECTION DURING PREGNANCY[5]

Management of latent TB is an important component of the National TB Elimination Strategy. We cannot achieve our goal of TB elimination without taking care of latent infected persons, as they are the source of future diseased cases.

If pregnant female is at the high risk of progression of infection to diseases like recent contacts or with any comorbidity or immune-suppressed condition. TB preventive therapy may be started even in the first trimester, otherwise, it can be delayed till delivery.

DRUG CONTRAINDICATED IN PREGNANCY[6]

- Streptomycin
- Kanamycin
- Amikacin
- Capreomycin
- Fluoroquinolones

If a pregnant female is diagnosed to be suffering from tuberculosis, effective treatment is important for maintaining the pregnancy. If not initiated on anti-TB treatment, it poses a great threat not only to the patient but also to the fetus. Treatment for drug-sensitive TB is for 6 months. During treatment, breastfeeding should be continued, but the mother should cover her mouth while feeding. Treatment of multi-drug resistant TB is challenging when associated with pregnancy. It is advised to counsel a presumptive MDR-TB case to avoid pregnancy until the treatment is complete. If the patient is already pregnant, termination of pregnancy, as permitted by the law, is advised. Tuberculosis preventive treatment is safe during pregnancy.

TABLE 2: Dose for second-line drugs.

Drug	Mode of action	Mechanism of action	Daily dose/kg bodyweight	Common side effects
Aminoglycosides (Kanamycin, amikacin	Bactericidal	Inhibits initiation of protein synthesis	25	• Vestibular and cochlear nerve damage • Renal toxicity • Skin reactions
Ethionamide	Bacteriostatic	Disruption of mycolic acid	25	• Metallic taste • Severe nausea vomiting • Hypothyroidism • Photosensitivity
Fluoroquinolones (Levofloxacin, moxifloxacin)	Weak bactericidal	Binds to two nuclear enzymes inhibiting DNA replication	15	• Gastroenteritis • Hypersensitivity reaction • Tenosynovitis
Cycloserine	Bacteriostatic	Inhibits cytosolic stages of peptidoglycan synthesis	25	• Headache • Depression • Seizures • Suicidal tendencies • Sideroblastic anemia
Para-aminosalicylic	Bacteriostatic	Inhibits folic acid and iron metabolism in bacteria	150	• Gastroenteritis • Hepatotoxicity • Hypersensitivity reactions • Hypothyroidism • Hypokalemia
Bedaquiline	Bactericidal	Adenosine triphosphate synthetase inhibition	• Loading dose 400 mg for 2 weeks • Maintenance dose 200 mg thrice a week × 22 weeks	• QTC interval prolongation • Elevated transaminases • Pruritus
Delamanid	Bactericidal	Inhibits synthesis of mycobacterial cell wall	• 100 mg in children • 200 in adults	• Nausea • Vomiting • Dyspepsia

■ KEY POINTS

- A successful outcome of pregnancy relies on the successful treatment of TB.
- Treating TB during pregnancy is safer for both the mother and the fetus compared to leaving it untreated.
- Except for streptomycin, first-line anti-TB medications are safe during pregnancy.
- While receiving TB drug treatment, breastfeeding should continue, and the mother should follow cough etiquette.
- Treating drug-resistant TB during pregnancy is not contraindicated but carries significant risks for both the mother and the fetus.
- If a pregnant woman is diagnosed with drug-resistant TB and is <24 weeks into her

pregnancy, she should be advised to consider a medical termination of pregnancy (MTP).
- For the majority of pregnant women, treatment for latent TB infection can be postponed until after delivery.

◼ REFERENCES

1. Division of Tuberculosis Elimination, National Centre for HIV, Viral Hepatitis, STD and TB Prevention, Centers for Disease Control and Prevention. (2020). Treatment of TB Drug Pregnancy. [online] Available from: https://www.cdc.gov/tb/topic/treatment/pregnancy.htm [Last accessed December, 2023].
2. National TB Elimination Programme, Central TB Division, Ministry of Health & Family Welfare, Government of India, New Delhi. (2019). Training Modules (1-4) for programme Managers and Medical officers. [online] Available from: https://tbcindia.gov.in/WriteReadData/NTEPTrainingModules1to4.pdf. [Last accessed December, 2023].
3. Ministry of Health and Family Welfare, Government of India. (2021). Collaborative Framework for Management of Tuberculosis in Pregnant Women, Feb 2021. [online] Available from: www.mohfw.gov.in/ and www.mohfw.nin.in Developed with Technical Support from: USAID-NISHTHA/Jhpiego. [Last accessed December, 2023].
4. National TB Elimination Programme, Central TB Division, Ministry of Health and Family Welfare, Govt. of India, New Delhi. (2021). Guidelines for Programmatic Management of Drug Resistant Tuberculosis in India, pp. 70-2. [online] Available from: https://tbcindia.gov.in/showfile.php?lid=3590 [Last accessed December, 2023].
5. Treatment for TB during pregnancy. Center for Disease Control and Prevention. Available at: https://www.cdc.gov/tb/topic/treatment/pregnancy.htm.
6. Alene KA, Murray MB, an de water BJ, Atalell K, Nicol M, Clements A, et al. Treatment Outcomes Among Pregnant Patients With Multidrug-Resistant Tuberculosis: A Systematic Review and Meta-analysis. JAMA Netw Open. 2022;5(6):e2216527.

Section 8

Medical Management of Miscellaneous Disorders in Pregnancy

▲ **Gestational Diabetes and Overt Diabetes Mellitus**
Geetanjali Nabiyal, Madhav Bahadur

▲ **Thyroid Disorders**
Indu Chawla, Seema Sheokand, Paridhi Gupta

▲ **Seizure Disorders**
Preeti Sainia

▲ **Hyperemesis Gravidarum**
Kavita Kumari

▲ **Constipation and Diarrhea**
Sandhya Jain, Pijush Kanti Nandi, Priyanka Shanker

Chapter 20

Gestational Diabetes and Overt Diabetes Mellitus

Geetanjali Nabiyal, Madhav Bahadur

Hyperglycemia is one of the common medical conditions encountered during pregnancy. It can be separated into pregestational/overt diabetes (diabetes before pregnancy) and gestational diabetes mellitus (GDM) (diagnosed during pregnancy). Hyperglycemia, specifically uncontrolled hyperglycemia, bestows a significantly higher maternal and fetal risk with accompanying chronic complications of diabetes.[1]

The worldwide prevalence of hyperglycemia in pregnancy in the 20–49 years age group was estimated to be 20.4 million or 15.8% of live births in 2019 of which 83.6% were due to GDM.[2] A community-based screening study for GDM performed in 2009 in Tamil Nadu on 12,056 pregnant women, funded by the World Diabetes Foundation, found a prevalence of 17.8% urban, 13.8% semi-urban, while 9.9% rural areas.[3] Almost 50% of women with GDM develop type 2 diabetes mellitus (T2DM) over the course of the next 5–20 years.[4]

Gestational diabetes mellitus is defined "as any degree of glucose intolerance with onset or first recognition during pregnancy" while overt diabetes is when a woman with known diabetes becomes pregnant or when hyperglycemia diagnosed for the first time in pregnancy meets the World Health Organization (WHO) criteria for DM in the nonpregnant state.[5] A detailed discussion of the pathophysiology, diagnosis, and complications of hyperglycemia in pregnancy is beyond the scope of this chapter. However, because it is essential for management, some important points will be mentioned.

The placenta and its hormones create an insulin resistance most marked in the last trimester. The Hyperglycemia and Adverse Pregnancy Outcome (HAPO) study,[6] a multinational cohort study including more than 23,000 pregnant individuals, demonstrated that risk of maternal, fetal, and neonatal adverse outcomes continuously increased in proportion with maternal hyperglycemia. Hence, all pregnant women, even in the absence of symptoms, should be screened for GDM. Assessment for hyperglycemia is advised at the very first prenatal visit.

DIAGNOSIS OF GESTATIONAL DIABETES MELLITUS

Diabetes in Pregnancy Study Group India (DIPSI): This is a "Single Test Procedure" and is approved by the Ministry of Health and Family Welfare (MoHFW), Government of India.[7] It is based on a prospective study, which was performed in India; it established that GDM could be diagnosed by a value of ≥140 mg/dL of the 2 hours postprandial plasma glucose (PPPG) level after 75 g oral glucose is administered to a pregnant women in the nonfasting state, irrespective of the last meal timing.[8] This has been endorsed by the WHO,[9] International Diabetes Federation (IDF),[10] and International Federation of Gynecologists and Obstetricians Society (FIGO).[11] National Institute of Clinical Excellence (NICE) guidelines have also recommended a 2-hour PPPG >140 mg/dL as diagnostic for GDM.[12] The advantages of this procedure include (1) A pregnant woman need not fast, (2) causes least disturbance in a pregnant woman's activities, (3) it serves both as a screening and diagnostic procedure making widespread testing promising. A comparison with other diagnostic tests including Carpenter and Coustan, National Diabetes Data Group (NDDG), International Association of Diabetes and Pregnancy Study Groups (IADPSG)[15] is given in **Table 1**.

■ MANAGEMENT

Due to the close association between maternal glycemic control and maternal and neonatal complications, efforts to achieve plasma glucose targets should be aggressive during pregnancy. Unfortunately, quite a few pregnancies may be unplanned; and women may begin their pregnancy with poor glycemic control. Consequently, management preferably should begin before pregnancy.

Guiding Principles of Management

- To maintain the glucose level as near the physiological level as possible by careful antenatal supervision and glycemic control.
- All women detected with GDM for the first time should be started on medical nutrition therapy (MNT) and physical exercise for 30 minutes daily for the first 2 weeks. If after 2 weeks, 2 hours PPPG >120 mg/dL, despite lifestyle changes and MNT, oral hypoglycemic agents (OHA) and/or insulin therapy is recommended **(Flowchart 1)**.
- In a pregnant patient, with overt diabetes, insulin should be continued and titrated according to point number 1.

Glucose Monitoring

Diabetes in Pregnancy Study Group India recommends the following targets[7] for pregnant women with overt diabetes and GDM:
- Fasting glucose value of 80–90 mg/dL

TABLE 1: Criteria for diagnosis of gestational diabetes mellitus (GDM).

	Oral glucose tolerance test (GTT): Venous plasma (mg/dL)				
Time/Criteria	DIPSI[7]	Carpenter and Coustan[13]	NDDG[14]	IADPSG[15]	WHO[9]
Glucose load	75 g	100 g	100 g	75 g	75 g
Fasting	—	95	105	92	126
1 hour	—	180	190	180	HBA1c: 6.5%
2 hours	≥140	155	165	153	200
3 hours	—	140	145	—	Overt diabetes mellitus criteria
Diagnosis	Single test	Any two met or elevated		Any one met or elevated	
(DIPSI: Diabetes in Pregnancy Study Group India; NDDG: National Diabetes Data Group; IADPSG: International Association of Diabetes and Pregnancy Study Groups; WHO: World Health Organization)					

Flowchart 1: Guiding principles of management of gestational diabetes mellitus (GDM).

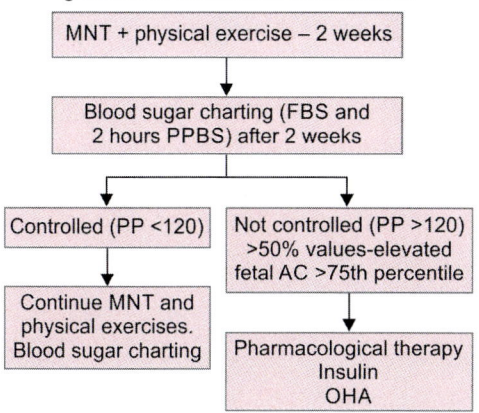

(FBS: fasting blood sugar; MNT: Medical Nutrition Therapy; OHA: oral hypoglycemic agents; PPBS: postprandial blood sugar)

- Two-hour postprandial glucose value of 110–120 mg/dL.

The above are similar to the American College of Obstetricians and Gynecologists (ACOG) and the American Diabetes Association (ADA) recommended targets[16] for pregnant women with overt diabetes and GDM:
- Fasting glucose 70–95 mg/dL (3.9–5.3 mmol/L) and either
- 1-hour postprandial glucose 110–140 mg/dL (6.1–7.8 mmol/L) or
- 2-hour postprandial glucose 100–120 mg/dL (5.6–6.7 mmol/L).

Monitoring should be performed every 2 weeks between 24th and 28th week of gestation and thereafter weekly for those on MNT and metformin. The goal of target blood glucose is to obtain newborn birthweight appropriate for gestational age between 2.5 and 3.5 kg and prevent the offspring from developing diabetes.[7]

Pregnant women with type 1 diabetes mellitus (T1DM) or T2DM on a multiple daily insulin injection regimen are advised to test their fasting, premeal, 1-hour postmeal, and bedtime blood glucose levels daily.

Management of Gestational Diabetes Mellitus

Medical Nutrition Therapy

- Medical nutrition therapy (MNT) should be individualized to each pregnant woman, preferably in consultation with a qualified medical dietician conversant with GDM.
- The diet plan should provide: (1) Sufficient calorie intake to encourage fetal/neonatal and maternal health, (2) achieve glycemic targets while avoiding ketosis, and (3) adequate weight gain, (2009 Institute of Medicine recommendations).[17]
- *Carbohydrates:* 175 g or around 35–55% of a 2,000-calorie diet is recommended. High quality, nutrient-rich carbohydrates like whole-grain cereals (bajra, jowar, and ragi), whole pulses, vegetables, and fruits with skins should be preferred over simple carbohydrates. They result in a better control of fasting/postprandial glucose, reduced free fatty acids, reduced insulin resistance, vascular benefits, and may decrease excess infant adiposity.
- *Fats:* The diet plan should emphasize monounsaturated and polyunsaturated fats while limiting saturated fats and completely avoiding transfats. The total calorie intake from fat should be around 25–30% of total calorie intake of which <10% is saturated fat.[17] Fat is essential as substituting it for carbohydrates, enhances lipolysis, promoting free fatty acids formation, worsening maternal insulin resistance.[18]
- *Protein*: The recommended intake for a pregnant woman is at least 71 g of

protein or 20–25% of total calorie intake.[17] Rich sources of protein are milk, milk products, egg, fish, chicken, pulses (dal), nuts, etc.
- *Fiber:* The recommended amount is a minimum of 28 g of fiber.[17] Soluble fiber may help by delaying gastric emptying, decreasing the absorption of glucose its postprandial rise. Soluble fiber in rich in flax seed, psyllium husk, oat bran, legumes (dried beans, peas, and lentils), and pectin (apples), and in root vegetables (carrots).

Physical Activity

The ACOG (2020) recommends regular physical activity integrating aerobic and strength-conditioning exercises during pregnancy. This also extends to women with GDM. Two recent meta-analyses demonstrated that planned exercise programs during pregnancy diminish excess weight gain and even reduce the development of GDM.[19] It also lowers glucose levels.[20]

Pharmacological Therapy

Insulin is the first-line drug recommended by both ACOG and ADA. While ACOG supports use of metformin and glyburide as second-line treatment for GDM, they are not cleared for use in GDM by the Food and Drug Administration (FDA) as they cross the placenta and long-term safety data for the neonate is not yet known.[16]

Metformin: It may be used in women with GDM not willing for insulin therapy after discussing the risks and the limited knowledge of long-term effects on the neonate. If glycemic targets are not met, then the need for insulin should be emphasized profusely.

Mechanism of action: A complete elucidation of the mechanism of action remains obscure, but their prime consequence is to lessen hepatic gluconeogenesis.

Pharmacokinetics: Twice-daily administration at doses of 0.5–2.0 g is recommended. A sustained-release preparation may be administered for once-daily dosing initiated at 500 mg daily, with titration up to a maximum of 2,000 mg as required. It is absorbed primarily from the small intestine with a bioavailability of 70–80%. Concentrations reach a peak at about 2 hours after an oral dose. The plasma $t_{1/2}$ (half-life) is 4–5 hours. It does not bind to plasma proteins and is excreted unchanged in the urine.

Dose and route: It is started at a dose of 500 mg twice daily up to a maximum dose of 2 g/day **(Table 2)**.

Side effects: Due to the potential for acidosis, it should not be used in pregnancy with risk of placental insufficiency like hypertension or preeclampsia and also those at risk for intrauterine growth restriction.[21] The most common adverse effects are gastrointestinal (anorexia, nausea, vomiting, abdominal discomfort, and diarrhea), occurring in up to 20% of patients. These effects are dose-related, transpire at the onset of therapy, and are often transient. Extended-release formulations have decreased gastrointestinal (GI) side effects and can be substituted for the immediate-release drug. Metformin should not be administered at creatinine clearance below 30 mL/min.

Safety profile: No clear association has been reported with any major birth defects, miscarriage, and adverse maternal or fetal outcomes. Poorly controlled diabetes during pregnancy have reported increased maternal and fetal risk as already mentioned.

TABLE 2: Summary of drugs used in gestational diabetes mellitus.

Drug	Mode of action	Pharmacokinetics	Dose	Duration	Adverse effects
I. Insulins	Activate insulin receptor	Parenteral (SQ or IV)	Refer to content	Table 3	• Hypoglycemia • Weight gain • Fluid retention • Lipodystrophy • Lipohypertrophy
II. Biguanides					
Metformin	Reduces hepatic and renal gluconeogenesis	• Oral • Bioavailability 70–80% • Peak 2 hours • $t_{1/2}$ 4–5 hours • Renal excretion	1–2 g	2–3 hours	• *GI:* Nausea, vomiting, abdominal cramps, bloating, and diarrhea • Reduced vitamin B_{12} GI absorption • Lactic acidosis (rare)
III. Sulfonylureas (Secretagogues)					
Glyburide (micronized)	Increase insulin release from pancreas	• Oral • Good absorption • Protein-bound • High Vd • Liver metabolism • Renal excretion	• 1.25–20 mg • Before meals	10–24 hours	• Maternal and neonatal hypoglycemia • Weight gain • Nausea, vomiting • Cholestatic jaundice • Agranulocytosis • Aplastic/Hemolytic anemia • Hypersensitivity
IV. α-glucosidase inhibitors					
Acarbose	• Reduces GI absorption • Increase release of GLP-1	• Oral • GI absorption minimal • Rapid onset • Renal excretion	25–100 mg before meals		• *GI:* Malabsorption, flatulence, diarrhea, abdominal bloating • Malabsorption • Raised ALT/AST • Cutaneous hypersensitivity • Hypoglycemia • *C/I:* Hepatic/renal/intestinal dysfunction

(ALT: alanine aminotransferase; AST: aspartate aminotransferase; GLP-1: glucagon-like peptide 1)

TABLE 3: Characteristics of insulin.

Type	Insulin preparation	Onset	Peak	Duration	Route
Short-acting	• Lispro • Aspart • Glulisine	5–15 minutes	0.5–1.5 h	3–5 h	Subcutaneous
Intermediate-acting	Regular insulin	30–60 minutes	2–3 h	4–8 h	
Long-acting	• NPH insulin • Insulin glargine • Insulin detemir • Insulin degludec	2–4 h 2–4 h 0.5–4 h 0.5–9 h	6–10 h Flat Flat Flat	10–20 h ~24 h 12–24 h ~42h	
Inhaled insulin		<0.5 h	1–2 h	3 h	Inhaled
Premixed insulins	70 NPH/30 regular	Dual action	Dual action	Dual action	Subcutaneous

(NPH: neutral protamine Hagedorn)

Sulfonylureas
Mechanism of action: The key action is to increase insulin release from the pancreas. They bind to a 140-kDa high-affinity sulfonylurea receptor that is associated with a β-cell inward rectifier adenosine triphosphate (ATP)-sensitive potassium channel. Its binding inhibits the efflux of potassium ions through the channel and results in depolarization of the β-cell of pancreas. Depolarization opens a voltage-gated calcium channel and results in calcium influx and the release of preformed insulin in the portal system.

Pharmacokinetics: They are effectively absorbed from the GI tract but absorption is reduced by food and hyperglycemia. In plasma, they are mainly (90-99%) protein-bound, especially albumin. The volumes of distribution of most of the sulfonylureas are about 0.2 L/kg. Although they have short half-lives (3–5 hours), their hypoglycemic effects last for 12-24 hours, hence, they can be prescribed once daily. They are metabolized by the liver and the end-products are excreted in the urine. Thus, administration in renal or hepatic insufficiency should be done with caution.

Dose and route: Treatment is started at the lower dose and titrated based on the patient's glycemic response. Glyburide (micronized) may be started at 1.25 mg and increased to a maximum of 20 mg.

Side effects: Glyburide (see **Table 2**) has been linked with more neonatal hypoglycemia, increased macrosomia, and higher neonatal abdominal circumference than insulin or metformin in meta-analyses.[22]

Safety profile: Pregnancy category C drug. Although, ACOG supports use of glyburide as second-line treatment for GDM,[16] neither DIPSI nor FDA have approved it for similar use.

Alpha-glucosidase inhibitors
Mechanism of action: They decrease GI absorption of starch, dextrin, and disaccharides by inhibiting the action of α-glucosidase in the intestinal brush border. They also increase the release of the glucoregulatory hormone GLP-1 into the circulation, which may also contribute to their glucose-lowering effects. The drugs in this class are acarbose, miglitol, and voglibose. Acarbose is ACOG approved but is not recommended in the Indian setting. Voglibose is currently being investigated in GDM.

Pharmacokinetics: Acarbose is negligibly absorbed in the GI; the small amount of drug reaching the systemic circulation is cleared by the kidney. They are not given in patients with creatinine clearance <30 mL/min.

Dose and route: Acarbose is provided as 25, 50 or 100-mg tablets taken before meals. Treatment should start with a lower dose and titrated by corresponding postprandial glucose, A1c, and GI symptoms.

Side effects: Malabsorption, flatulence, diarrhea, and abdominal bloating are the most prominent. Mild-to-moderate elevated hepatic transaminases are noted but symptomatic liver disease is very rare. Cutaneous hypersensitivity has also been described but is rare. Hypoglycemia occurs when they are added to insulin or an insulin secretagogue. Acarbose can decrease the absorption of various drugs. The α-glucosidase inhibitors are contraindicated in patients with stage 4 renal disease, hepatic dysfunction, and intestinal disorders.

Safety profile: Pregnancy category B drug. They are not currently recommended in the Indian setting.

Insulin: Insulin is started in GDM when glycemic control is not achieved through nutrition and exercise. Its advantages are (1) does not cross the placenta and (2) gives tight glycemic control.

Mechanism of action: The insulin receptor is expressed on practically all mammalian cell types. The tissues, which are critical for regulation of blood glucose, include liver, skeletal muscle, fat specific regions of the brain, and the pancreatic islet. The actions of insulin are largely anabolic, and insulin signaling promotes the uptake, use, and storage of glucose, lipids, and amino acids. Insulin stimulates glycogenesis, lipogenesis, and protein synthesis; conversely, it inhibits the catabolism of these compounds. Some effects of insulin (e.g., activation of glucose and ion transport systems, phosphorylation or dephosphorylation of specific enzymes) manifest in seconds or minutes; other effects (e.g., those promoting protein synthesis and regulating gene transcription and cell proliferation) occur over minutes to hours to days. The effects of insulin on cell proliferation and differentiation transpire over an even longer period of time.

Pharmacokinetics: Subcutaneous administration of insulin provides insulin delivery into the peripheral circulation. It can lead to near-normal glycemia but differs from physiological secretion of insulin: (1) The absorption kinetics do not replicate the rapid rise and subsequent decline of endogenous insulin in response to changes in blood glucose values; (2) Injected insulin is not released into the portal circulation, thus, the portal/peripheral insulin concentration is not physiological, and this may alter hepatic metabolism.

Dose and route: The starting dose is usually 0.1 unit/kilogram body weight/day. Dose can be increased on follow-up till 2 hours PG is around 120 mg/dL. If a GDM woman requires >20 units insulin/day, a physician's opinion should be taken. It is given in divided doses in a combination of intermediate-acting and short-acting insulin. **Table 3** lists the profiles of common rapid-, short-, intermediate-, and long-acting insulins. Dose adjustments should be done according to glucose levels at particular times of the day.

Self-monitoring of blood glucose (SMBG): Levels should be taught to pregnant women and charting should be advised. The proper technique of SMBG should be reinforced on every visit. Charts should be checked and insulin titrated accordingly every 3 days till adequate control is achieved. Once adequate control is achieved, charts may be reviewed and insulin titrated once a week.

Side-effects:
- Hypoglycemia is the foremost risk weighed against the benefit of glucose control
- Modest weight gain
- Though infrequent, allergic reactions to recombinant human insulin may occur due to small quantities of aggregated or denatured insulin, or due to minor contaminants, or because of sensitivity to a constituent added to insulin (protamine, Zn^{2+}, etc.)
- Lipoatrophy of subcutaneous fat at the site of insulin injection was a rare side effect of older insulin preparations
- Lipohypertrophy (enlargement of subcutaneous fat depots) has been attributed to the lipogenic action of insulin.

The various regimens are as follows **(Fig. 1)**:
- *Continuous subcutaneous infusion:* Some healthcare professionals in better equipped centers prefer insulin pumps in pregnancy to multiple daily injections. Insulin pumps administer rapid-acting insulin analog subcutaneously at a basal level and prandial excursions of glucose are managed with meal-time boluses decided by sensor attached to the pumps. A subcutaneous insulin infusion regimen by a calibrated pump is not known to yield better pregnancy outcomes compared with the multiple daily injections regimen.[23]
- *Mixtard 30/70 (Flowchart 2):* Contains 30% regular or a rapid-acting analog and 70% intermediate-acting neutral protamine Hagedorn (NPH) insulin. The total dose calculated is usually administered in two doses: two-thirds of total dose 30 minutes before breakfast and one-third of total dose 30 minutes before dinner. NPH insulin provides a basal level while mealtime hyperglycemia is managed by the regular insulin. Two doses a day makes it more convenient for most pregnant women.
- *Basal + Bolus:* It is preferred for tighter control. A long-acting peak-less insulin, glargine, is administered at night-time, which provides a basal insulin level. A rapidly acting insulin is administered according to premeal glucose level before the major three meals of the day.
- *Basal only:* A single dose of long-acting insulin is administered.

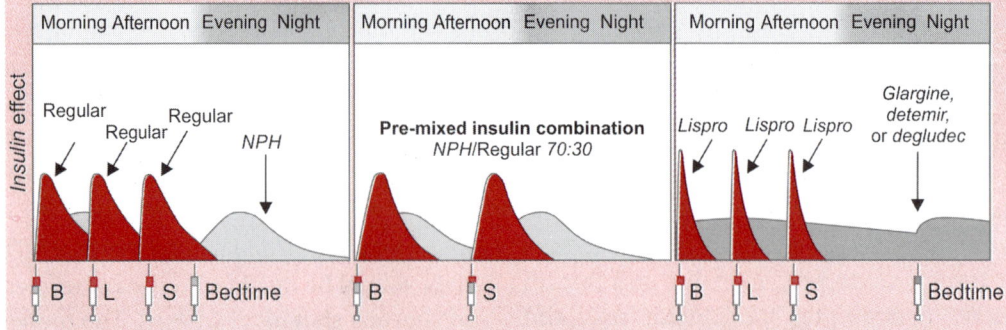

Fig. 1: Insulin regimens commonly followed. (X-axis: insulin effect; Y: time; B: breakfast; L: lunch; NPH: neutral protamine Hagedorn; S: supper/dinner)

Flowchart 2: Scheme for using Mixtard for management for gestational diabetes mellitus (GDM).

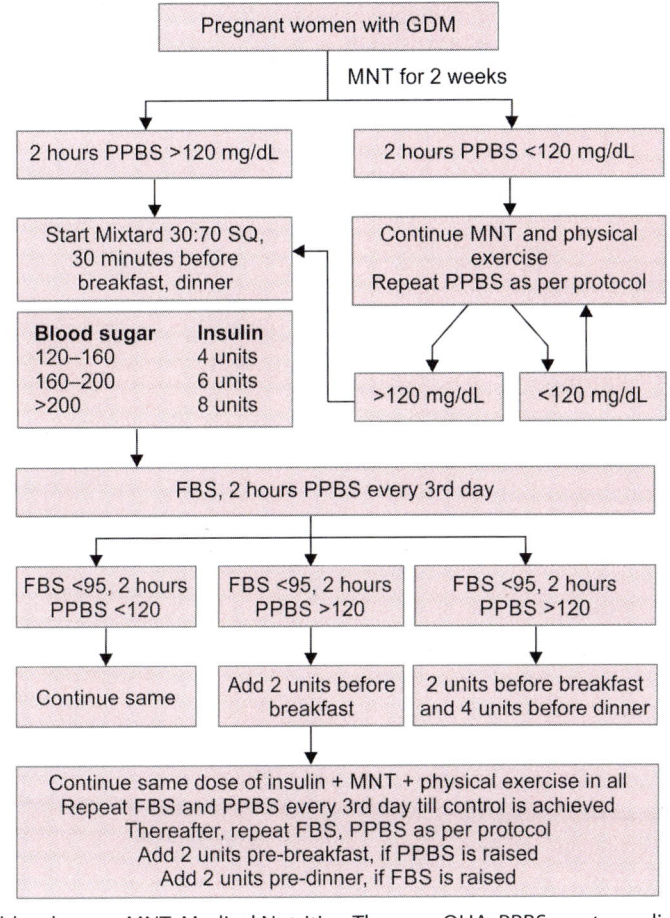

(FBS: fasting blood sugar; MNT: Medical Nutrition Therapy; OHA: PPBS: postprandial blood sugar)

MANAGEMENT OF OVERT DIABETES MELLITUS

Preconception Counseling

Its importance for pregnant women is highlighted by the American College of Obstetricians and Gynecologists (ACOG) Committee Opinion 762, "Pre-pregnancy Counseling."[24] This is essential to reduce early pregnancy loss and congenital malformations. It enables women to make informed decisions about themselves and their family.

- It should start at puberty and continue in all women with diabetes and reproductive potential; and should be included in routine diabetes care.
- Family planning with effective contraception should be discussed and used until optimum glycemic control. Diabetic women should be taught self-monitoring of blood glucose.
- It should address the significance of achieving adequate glycemic control: preferably A1C <6.5% (48 mmol/mol) to cut the risk of congenital abnormalities,

preeclampsia, macrosomia, preterm birth, and other complications.[25]
- It should include all the standard screenings and care that is given to any pregnant woman.
- Counseling should include details of the risks to the mother and fetus and the methods to reduce risk, emphasizing on glycemic goal, lifestyle management and MNT.
- Diabetes-specific testing should comprise A1C, serum creatinine, urine albumin-creatinine ratio and a complete eye examination and to provide treatment, if indicated.
- The medication list should be reviewed for potentially teratogenic drugs.

Insulin Therapy

Pregnant women with overt diabetes are treated with insulin similarly as in GDM but oral hypoglycemic agents are not currently recommended for overt diabetes.[26]

First Trimester

- For careful monitoring of glucose control, routine hospitalization of pregnant women with overt diabetes may be recommended to begin individualized glucose control and offer awareness.
- Hospitalization is also used to assess the presence of diabetic complications using a checklist of the Society for Maternal-Fetal Medicine (2020). This includes assessment of 24-hour urine protein excretion, serum creatinine, retinal examination and blood pressure (BP) monitoring.[27]
- Screening for aneuploidy may be done by measurement of maternal serum pregnancy-associated plasma protein A (PAPP-A), β-human chorionic gonadotropin (hCG) and ultrasound measurement of fetal nuchal translucency.

Second Trimester

Sonographic assessment with maternal serum α-fetoprotein level should be used at 16–20 weeks gestation to detect neural-tube defects and other anomalies. Fetal echocardiography is an important aspect of this evaluation as the incidence of congenital cardiac malformations is increased fivefold in mothers with overt diabetes.[27]

Third Trimester

- An institutional protocol should be formulated, which should include fetal movement count, biophysical profile and nonstress test. Pregnant women should be instructed to routinely perform fetal kick counts.
- Delivery should be planned for 39 weeks' gestation in women with good glycemic control and encouraging antenatal test. Earlier delivery should be planned for women with poor glycemic control or significant comorbidities.

Preeclampsia

Overt diabetes causes an enhanced risk of preeclampsia. The US Preventive Services Task Force recommends low-dose aspirin as prophylaxis at 12 weeks of gestation in pregnant women at increased risk of preeclampsia.[28]

MANAGEMENT OF HYPOGLYCEMIA

Hypoglycemia is defined at <70 mg/dL and a pregnant woman on insulin can develop it at any time. Recognition of the symptoms is important and may be masked by β-blockers. Symptoms are usually divided into:
- *Early:* Tremors, sweating, palpitations, hunger, easy fatigability, headache,

irritability, drowsiness, and perioral tingling
- *Severe:* Confusion, abnormal behavior, blurring of vision, and anxiety
- *Uncommon:* Seizures and loss of consciousness.

A fast-acting form of oral glucose-like glucose powder should be readily available at home. If a woman does not recover with glucose or develops more than one episode of hypoglycemia, she should be taken to the nearest healthcare center. Blood glucose levels are unstable in pregnancy with overt diabetes mellitus, especially in the first trimester. Tight control, defined by fasting values <90 mg/dL, also shows no benefit in a Cochrane database review.[29]

MANAGEMENT OF DIABETIC KETOACIDOSIS (DKA)

- Pregnancy is a ketogenic state, women with T1DM and to some extent those with T2DM and even GDM are at risk.
- DKA can occur at lower blood glucose levels than in the nonpregnant women. Euglycemic ketoacidosis is also possible in pregnancy.[30]
- Urine ketone strips should be prescribed and its use should be adequately explained.
- Women should be educated about DKA prevention and detection.
- DKA usually develops with hyperemesis gravidarum, infections, insulin non-compliance, β-agonists administered for tocolysis and corticosteroids used to induce fetal lung maturation.
- The maternal mortality is <1% but perinatal mortality rates reach about 35%.[31]
- The management of DKA is given in **Box 1**.[31]

BOX 1: Management of diabetic ketoacidosis.[31]

- Confirm diagnosis using plasma glucose, positive serum and urine ketones, metabolic acidosis (HCO_3^-: 15 mmol/L with increased anion gap)
- Admit to ICU and assess clinical condition: Manage serious complications and initiate treatment of underlying precipitating factors
- Assess and monitor regularly vitals, serum electrolytes (Na, K, Mg, Cl, phosphate), acid base status, renal function (urine output and creatinine) every 1–4 hours for first 24 hours
- *Replace fluids:*
  - 2–3 L over 1–3 h (10–20 mL/kg/h) of 0.9% saline
  - Then 0.45% saline at 250–500 mL/h (Total 4–6 L in 12 hours)
  - Change to 5% dextrose at 150–250 mL/h when glucose reaches 250 mg/dL
  - Saline should be changed to Ringer's lactate to reduce hyperchloremia
- *Potassium:*
  - Do not administer insulin if K <3.3 mEq/L
  - Give 10 mEq/h if K <5.0–5.2 mEq/L after documenting normal ECG, urine flow and creatinine
  - Give 40–80 mEq/h if K <3.5 mEq/L
  - If K >5.2 mEq/L, stop potassium supplementation
- *Regular insulin:*
  - 0.1 unit/kg IV STAT
  - 0.1 unit/kg/h by continuous infusion, increase to 0.2–0.3 units/kg/h if no response in 2–4 hours
  - 0.02–0.1 units/kg/h after acidosis is resolved and a glucose goal of 150–200 mg/dL is achieved
  - Long-acting insulin is given when patient starts taking orally
  - Long-acting insulin is overlapped with insulin infusion for 2–4 hours after which infusion may be stopped
- *Glucose:* Begin 5% dextrose once glucose reaches 250 mg/dL
- *Bicarbonate:* Add one ampule (44 mEq) to 1 L of 0.45% saline if serum pH is <7.1
- Continue above till acidosis is resolved and a glucose goal of 150–200 mg/dL is achieved

MANAGEMENT OF LABOR

- Induction may be attempted for vaginal delivery when the cervix is favorable and the fetus is not very large.
- Cesarean delivery at or near term should be done only for obstetric indications but some obstetricians use it to circumvent traumatic birth of a large fetus. When vascular disease is present, the likelihood of successful labor induction is reduced.
- On day of labor or scheduled cesarean delivery:
  - Give evening dose of insulin the day earlier but withhold long-acting insulin.
  - Withhold morning dose of insulin.
  - Regular insulin should be used as insulin requirements characteristically decrease after delivery.
  - Intravenous saline at 100–125 mL/h should be used to maintain adequate hydration.
  - Regular insulin should be infused at 1–1.25 units/h if glucose >100 mg/dL.
  - If glucose is 70–100 mg/dL and during active labor, replace saline with 5% dextrose at 100–150 mL/h.
  - Glucose should be measured hourly an insulin titrated with a target of ~100 mg/dL.

POSTPARTUM CARE

- Early breastfeeding should be initiated within to prevent neonatal hypoglycemia along with assessment of clinical signs of hypoglycemia, blood glucose levels, and initiation of IV dextrose. Regular breastfeeding at 2 hours intervals also prevents neonatal hypoglycemia.
- Mothers should be explained that they are at risk of hypoglycemia in the postnatal period, so they should have a meal or snack before breastfeeding.
- Insulin should be stopped after birth and monitoring is advised to find the new appropriate dose.
- For women with overt diabetes, routine diabetes care should be restarted. Metformin may be used during breastfeeding, but other OHA are not advised.
- For GDM mothers, persisting hyperglycemia should be ruled out. ACOG recommends either fasting glucose estimation or 75 g, 2-hour OGTT at 4–12 weeks postpartum for the diagnosis of DM.[16] The ADA endorses testing every 1–3 years in women with history of GDM with normal postpartum glucose screening. Breastfeeding is known to decrease the risk of development of DM after GDM in the mother and has multiple benefits for the child.[32]
- Lifestyle modification, contraception, and risks during future pregnancies should be emphasized.

KEY POINTS

- Gestational diabetes mellitus (GDM) is defined "as any degree of glucose intolerance with onset or first recognition during pregnancy".
- Overt diabetes is when a woman with known diabetes becomes pregnant or when hyperglycemia diagnosed for the first time in pregnancy meets the WHO criteria for DM in the nonpregnant state.
- GDM can be easily controlled by diet (Medical Nutrition Therapy) and exercise.
- When blood sugar is not controlled by above, oral medicines or insulin injections are required in GDM.
- In overt diabetes, insulin is the only approved treatment during pregnancy.
- Regular antenatal fetal monitoring is advised.
- Self-monitoring of capillary blood glucose is best for optimum glycemic control
- Timing of delivery should be with fetal maturation keeping in mind maternal and fetal complications.

- Mode of delivery depends on the level of glycemic control, fetal size, associated complication, and pelvic adequacy.
- GDM women should be screened in postpartum period for persistence of hyperglycemia.

■ REFERENCES

1. Barker DJ. The developmental origins of adult disease. J Am Coll Nutr. 2004;23(6 Suppl):588S-95S.
2. International Diabetes Federation (IDF). (2019). Atlas Ninth edition 2019. Online version of IDF Diabetes Atlas. [online] Available from: www.diabetesatlas.org [Last accessed December, 2021].
3. Seshiah V, Balaji V, Balaji MS, Panneerselvam A, Kapur A. Pregnancy and Diabetes Scenario around the World: India. Int J Gynecol Obstet. 2009;104(suppl 1):S35-8.
4. Bellamy L, Casas JP, Hingorani AD, Williams D. Type 2 diabetes mellitus after gestational diabetes: a systematic review and meta-analysis. Lancet. 2009;373(9677):1773-9.
5. Wilmot EG, Mansell P. Diabetes and pregnancy. Clin Med (Lond). 2014;14(6):677-80.
6. HAPO Study Cooperative Research Group; Metzger BE, Lowe LP, Dyer AR, Trimble ER, Chaovarindr U, Coustan DR, et al.; Hyperglycemia and adverse pregnancy outcomes. N Engl J Med. 2008;358:1991-2002.
7. Mishra S, Bhadoria AS, Kishore S, Kumar R. Gestational diabetes mellitus 2018 guidelines: an update. J Family Med Prim Care. 2018;7(6):1169-72.
8. Balaji CA, Balaji MS, Ashalatha S, Suganthi S, Arthi T, Thamizharasi M, et al. A single Test procedure to diagnose Gestational Diabetes Mellitus. Acta Diabetol. 2008;46:52-4.
9. Colagiuri S, Falavigna M, Agarwal MM, Boulvain M, Coetzee E, Hod M, et al. Strategies for Implementing the WHO Diagnostic Criteria and Classification of Hyperglycaemia First Detected in Pregnancy. DRCP. 2014;103:364-72.
10. Hod M, Kapur A, Sacks DA, Hadar E, Agarwal M, Di Renzo GC, et al. The International Federation of Gynecology and Obstetrics (FIGO) initiative on gestational diabetes mellitus; a pragmatic guide for diagnosis, management and care. Int J Gynaecol Obstet. 2015;131(Suppl 3):S173-211.
11. Purandare CN, Sadikot S, Han NC, Hod M. (2017). FIGO-IDF Joint Statement and Declaration on Hyperglycemia in Pregnancy. IDF Congress. Abu Dhabi, 6th December 2017. [online] Available from: www.diabetesatlas.org/atlas@idf.org. [Last accessed December, 2023].
12. National Institute for Health and Care Excellence (NICE) guidelines. (2015). Diabetes in pregnancy: management from preconception to the postnatal period. [online] Available from: nice.org.uk/guidance/ng3 [Last accessed December, 2023].
13. O'Sullivan JB, Mahan CM. Criteria for the oral glucose tolerance test in pregnancy. Diabetes. 1964;13:278-85.
14. Sacks DA, Hadden DR, Maresh M, Deerochanawong C, Dyer AR, Metzger BE, et al.; HAPO Study Cooperative Research Group. Frequency of gestational diabetes mellitus at collaborating centers based on IADPSG consensus panel-recommended criteria: the Hyperglycemia and Adverse Pregnancy Outcome (HAPO) Study. Diabetes Care. 2012;35:526-8.
15. McIntyre HD, Sacks DA, Barbour LA, Feig DS, Catalano PM, Damm P, et al. Issues with the diagnosis and classification of hyperglycemia in early pregnancy. Diabetes Care. 2016;39:53-4.
16. ACOG Practice Bulletin No. 190: Gestational diabetes mellitus. Obstet Gynecol. 2018;131:e49-e64. Reaffirmed 2019.
17. Weight GDP. Reexamining the Guidelines. Washington, D.C.: National Academies Press; 2009.
18. Hernandez TL, Mande A, Barbour LA. Nutrition therapy within and beyond gestational diabetes. Diabetes Res Clin Pract. 2018;145:39-50.
19. American College of Obstetricians and Gynecologists. Physical activity and exercise during pregnancy and the postpartum

period. Committee Opinion No. 804. 2020; 135(4):e178-88.
20. Jovanovic-Peterson L, Durak EP, Peterson CM. Randomized trial of diet versus diet plus cardiovascular conditioning on glucose levels in gestational diabetes. Am J Obstet Gynecol. 1989;161(2):415-9.
21. Barbour LA, Feig DS. Metformin for gestational diabetes mellitus: progeny, perspective, and a personalized approach. Diabetes Care. 2019;42:396-9.
22. Balsells M, Garcıa-Patterson A, Sola I, Roque M, Gich I, Corcoy R. Glibenclamide, metformin, and insulin for the treatment of gestational diabetes: a systematic review and meta-analysis. BMJ. 2015;350:h102.
23. Farrar D, Tufnell DJ, West J. Continuous subcutaneous insulin infusion versus multiple daily injections of insulin for pregnant women with diabetes. Cochrane Database Syst Rev. 2016;6:CD005542.
24. ACOG Committee Opinion No. 762: Prepregnancy counseling. Obstet Gynecol. 2019; 133:e78-89.
25. Guerin A, Nisenbaum R, Ray JG. Use of maternal GHb concentration to estimate the risk of congenital anomalies in the offspring of women with prepregnancy diabetes. Diabetes Care. 2007;30:1920-5.
26. American College of Obstetricians and Gynecologists' Committee on Practice Bulletins—Obstetrics. ACOG Practice Bulletin No. 201: Pregestational Diabetes Mellitus. Obstet Gynecol. 2018;132(6):e228-48.
27. Patient Safety and Quality Committee. Society for Maternal-Fetal Medicine: Special statement: updated checklist for antenatal care of pregestational diabetes mellitus. Am J Obstet Gynecol. 2020;223:82.
28. Henderson JT, Whitlock EP, O'Conner E, Senger CA, Thompson JH, Rowland MG. Low dose aspirin for the prevention of morbidity and mortality from preeclampsia: a systematic evidence review for the U.S. Preventive Services Task Force. Rockville, MD, Agency for Healthcare Research and Quality, 2014.
29. Middleton P, Crowther CA, Simmonds L. Different intensities of glycaemic control for pregnant women with pre-existing diabetes. Cochrane Database Syst Rev. 2016;5: CD008540.
30. Sibai BM, Viteri OA. Diabetic ketoacidosis in pregnancy. Obstet Gynecol. 2014;123(1):167.
31. Bryant SN, Herrera CL, Nelson DB, Cunningham FG. Diabetic ketoacidosis complicating pregnancy. J Neonatal Perinatal Med. 2017;10:17-23.
32. American Diabetes Association. Management of diabetes in pregnancy: standards of medical care in diabetes-2019. Diabetes Care. 2019;42(Suppl 1):S165.

Chapter 21

Thyroid Disorders

Indu Chawla, Seema Sheokand, Paridhi Gupta

PHYSIOLOGY OF THYROID IN PREGNANCY

Pregnancy has a profound impact on the functioning of the thyroid gland and thyroid hormone **(Table 1)**. The two major causes of enlargement in the thyroid gland during pregnancy are glandular hyperplasia and increased blood supply. The major hormones responsible for these changes are human chorionic gonadotropin (hCG) and estrogen.[1]

The iodine requirement also increases for maternal and fetal thyroid hormone production during pregnancy. The reference value for the recommended dietary allowance for iodine in pregnancy by the World Health Organization is 250 µg/day.[3] The thyroid gland increases by 10% in size in iodine-replete areas and 30–40% in iodine-deficient areas. Production of thyroid hormones increases approximately by 50%, hence resulting in a further increase in the daily iodine requirement.[4]

The thyroid dysfunction spectrum during pregnancy and postpartum varies from hypothyroidism (overt or subclinical) to hyperthyroidism (Graves' disease, gestational transient thyroiditis, thyroid nodular disease, etc.), or postpartum thyroiditis.

INCIDENCE AND PREVALENCE OF THYROID DISORDERS

Overt hypothyroidism is reported in pregnancy in 0.2–2.5%, while subclinical hypothyroidism (SCH) is seen in 2–7%.[5] In 60% of the fertile women antithyroid antibodies are detected.[6]

The incidence of hyperthyroidism in pregnancy has been found to be around 0.2% with Graves' disease being the most common cause.[7]

Postpartum thyroiditis seen in 1.1–16% women,[8] with a higher prevalence (10–25%) reported in type 1 diabetics.[8] These patients have an increased likelihood (10–20%) of developing permanent hypothyroidism in the following 5–10 years.[4]

TABLE 1: Physiological changes of thyroid hormone in pregnancy.[2]

Test	Normal pregnancy
TSH	Decreased or no change
T3	Increased
FT3	No change/slight decrease
T4	Increased
FT4	No change/slight decrease
TGB	Increased

(FT3: free T3; FT4: free T4; TGB: thyroxine-binding globulin; TSH: thyroid-stimulating hormone; T3: triiodothyronine; T4: thyroxine)

Hypothyroidism in Pregnancy

Clinical/overt hypothyroidism is confirmed when the thyroid-stimulating hormone (TSH) is increased and the T4 level is low.[8] Subclinical hypothyroidism is also commonly encountered in antenatal women. It is defined as a high TSH level above the pregnancy reference range with a normal serum thyroxine level. Prepregnancy hypothyroidism should be adequately optimized prior to conception to prevent maternal and fetal complications.[9]

Maternal and fetal risks associated with it are abortions, preeclampsia, preterm birth, abruption, low birth weight, stillbirth, fetal hypothyroidism, and abnormal neuropsychological development in offspring.

Universal screening for thyroid disorders is recommended in the first trimester.[3] Anti-thyroid peroxidase (anti-TPO) testing should be done in cases with TSH value >2.5 mIU/mL.[4] Trimester-specific TSH cutoffs to make a diagnosis of hypothyroidism during pregnancy as per different guidelines have been provided in **Table 2**.

Management of Overt Hypothyroidism

The recommended treatment for hypothyroidism is oral levothyroxine (T4). The fetal central nervous system (CNS) is relatively impermeable to T3; therefore, any T3-containing preparation should be avoided.[4]

In new cases, levothyroxine is to be started at a dose of 1.6–2.0 µg/kg/day to achieve TSH levels ≤2.5 mIU/L.[3] While, in overt cases after confirmation of pregnancy, levothyroxine dose is escalated by 25–30%.[4] For adequate optimization, TSH levels are regularly checked antenatally every 4 weeks in the initial half of pregnancy and repeated once in the third trimester at 28 weeks followed by testing at 6 weeks postpartum period. The dose titration is done to achieve the target TSH pregnancy levels of 2.5 mIU/L or less to prevent any fluctuating levels of thyroid hormones.

If levothyroxine therapy was started during pregnancy and the dose was ≤50 µg/day, then it can be discontinued in the postpartum period. The TSH should be checked 6 weeks later.[3] If a woman was already taking levothyroxine, then it can be reduced to a prepregnancy dose.[4]

Pregnant women should be advised to take prenatal vitamins and iron supplements at least 4 hours apart from levothyroxine.

Management of Subclinical Hypothyroidism

- Levothyroxine 50–100 µg/day should be started for the following indications,[3] as depicted in **Flowchart 1**.

TABLE 2: TSH cut-off as recommended by various guidelines.

Guidelines	Country	Trimester-specific recommended TSH reference range
ITA Guidelines 2019	India	• First trimester: 2.5 mIU/L • Second trimester: 3.0 mIU/L • Third trimester: 3.0 mIU/L
ATA Guidelines 2019[4]	American	• First trimester: 4.0 mIU/L • Second trimester: Nonpregnant levels • Third trimester: Nonpregnant levels
ETA Guidelines 2014	European	• First trimester: 2.5 mIU/L • Second trimester: 3.0 mIU/L • Third trimester: 3.0 mIU/L

(ATA: American Thyroid Association; ETA: European Thyroid Association; ITA: Indian Thyroid Society; TSH: thyroid-stimulating hormone)

Flowchart 1: Indications of treatment in subclinical hypothyroidism in pregnancy as per ATA 2019.[10]

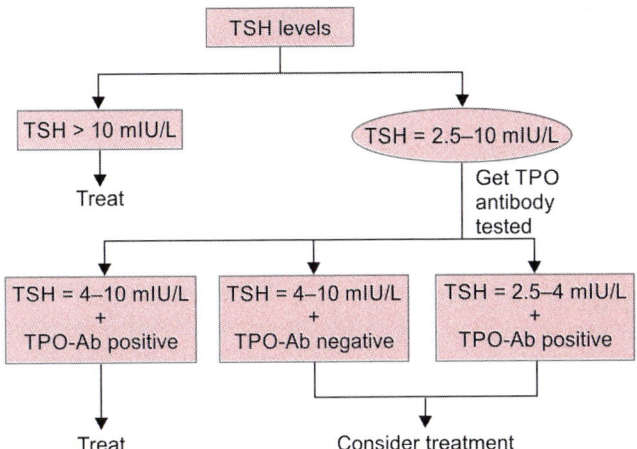

(ATA: American Thyroid Association; TPO: thyroid peroxidase antibodies; TSH: thyroid-stimulating hormone)

- In women with antithyroid peroxidase antibody (TPO-Ab) positive, treatment with levothyroxine is started preconceptionally to achieve the target range.

When thyroxine level is low with a normal TSH level it is termed isolated hypothyroxinemia. Levothyroxine therapy is not recommended for isolated hypothyroxinemia.[4,11]

Hyperthyroidism in Pregnancy

Overt hyperthyroidism during pregnancy is characterized by elevated thyroid hormone levels than the normal range for pregnancy and suppressed/undetectable (<0.01) serum TSH levels.[12] The most common cause, Graves' disease is an autoimmune condition associated with the presence of thyroid-stimulating hormone receptor antibody (TRAb) that binds to thyroid receptors and increases the production of thyroid hormone. Graves' hyperthyroidism is different from gestational transient thyrotoxicosis (GTT) which is a transient increase in free T4 due to hCG stimulation of TSHs.

Other nonautoimmune causes of hyperthyroidism in pregnancy are hyperemesis gravidarum, hydatidiform mole, multigravidae and single toxic adenoma or toxic multinodular goiter, thyroid nodule, subacute thyroiditis, and iatrogenic hyperthyroidism.[3]

Maternal risks associated with hyperthyroidism include preeclampsia, preterm delivery, pregnancy loss, thyroid storm, and congestive heart failure. Fetal complications include fetal growth retardation, small for gestational age, fetal tachycardia, fetal or neonatal hyperthyroidism, and fetal demise.

Management of Hyperthyroidism in Pregnancy

Serum blood testing is confirmatory; TSH levels are significantly depressed while serum-free T4 levels are elevated. Thyroid-stimulating hormone receptor antibody levels are measured to differentiate between Graves' disease from GTT.

The treatment options available are antithyroid drugs (ATDs), radioactive iodine, and thyroidectomy. Most commonly used are thionamide drugs namely propylthiouracil

(PTU), methimazole (MMZ), and carbimazole[13] **(Table 3)**. ATDs should be avoided in the first trimester of pregnancy, due to increased risks of congenital malformations, but when necessary PTU is generally favored. The ATDs should be used in the lowest possible dose whenever possible, maintaining T4 levels at the upper limit of the reference range.

The recommended therapeutic targets are:
- TT4 is 12–18 µg/dL
- fT4 2–2.5 ng/dL
- TSH 0.1–0.4 mIU/L

Clinical improvement is seen within 1 week of initiating treatment, but biochemical response is achieved only after 4–6 weeks of therapy as they prevent the synthesis of thyroid hormones, not their release. Switching of drugs has the disadvantage of poor control of thyroid function; hence there are no specific recommendations for it. If switching is required, it is recommended in the dosage of 1:20 for MMI:PTU. As there are risks of inducing fetal goiter and or fetal hypothyroidism, therefore overtreatment is usually avoided.

In newly pregnant women who are euthyroid on low dose PTU (<100–200 mg/day) or MMI (<5–10 mg/day), discontinuation of drugs can be considered to avoid teratogenic effects followed by 1–2 weekly monitoring.[4] The patient treated with ATDs should be monitored clinically by pulse rate, weight gain, thyroid size, and T4 and TSH levels every 4 weeks.[3] Thyroid-stimulating hormone receptor antibody testing is recommended in all patients taking antithyroid medications. If it becomes undetectable, ATD therapy can be stopped.[4]

Gestational transient thyrotoxicosis is managed conservatively with symptomatic treatment and rarely needs hospitalization or ATD therapy commencement.[4]

Due to the associated risk of fetal goiter, oral potassium iodide (6–40 mg/day) is not advised.

Indications of subtotal or total thyroidectomy in pregnancy are when women are not compliant with therapy or when there is toxicity to antithyroid drugs. The best time to operate is the second trimester of pregnancy. Radioactive iodine therapy is contraindicated in pregnancy due to its teratogenic effect on the fetus. Postpone pregnancy for at least 3 months (preferably 6 months as per ATA) after I-131 ablative therapy.[3]

- *Subclinical hyperthyroidism:* Normal serum fT4 level and low serum TSH level. The reference range is 0.1–0.45 mIU/L. Studies have not demonstrated any adverse effect of subclinical hyperthyroidism on pregnancy; therefore no treatment is recommended.
- *Fetal hyperthyroidism:* When TRAb serum concentration >5 IU/L which is three times the above range of normal levels) in the later half of pregnancy, predicts neonatal hyperthyroidism with 100% sensitivity and 43% specificity.[15] A fetal ultrasound can be considered in women with positive TRAb or those who received ATD to detect fetal thyroid dysfunction along with fetal heart rate, intrauterine growth restriction, fetal nonimmune hydrops, and the presence of goiter.
- *Postpartum:* ATDs can be continued postdelivery as there is less secretion of these drugs in breast milk.

■ THYROID STORM

It is a medical emergency arising from an underlying hypermetabolic state and can lead to preeclampsia, anemia, cardiac arrhythmias, heart failure, and CNS abnormalities.

It is treated with:
- PTU 1,000 mg loading dose PO then 200 mg 6 hourly.

TABLE 3: List of antithyroid drugs with their dosing, mechanism of action, and adverse effects.

Drug	MOA	Dose	Trimester in which it is recommended	Adverse effects
PTU	Blocks the conversion of T4 to T3	• Initiated at 50–150 mg/8 h, PO • Then decreased to 50 mg 6–8 hourly once the levels are normal	First trimester (through 16 weeks)	• Hepatotoxicity, 0.1% • Transient leukopenia • Allergic rash • Rare birth defects involving the face or neck (preauricular and branchial sinus/fistula/cysts) or urinary system (single cyst of kidney and hydronephrosis)[13]
MMI	Reduce iodine organification and coupling of monoiodotyrosine and diiodotyrosine, therefore inhibiting thyroid hormone synthesis (ATA 2017)	10–20 mg in a divided dose	Second/third trimester	• Allergic rash • Cutis aplasia, choanal atresia, gastrointestinal (esophageal atresia), and facial anomalies, mental retardation[14]
CM	Same as MMI	15 mg in a divided dose	Second/third trimester	Same as MMI
Propranolol or atenolol	Beta-adrenergic blockers inhibit the conversion of T4 to T3	20–40 mg orally every 8–12 hours, 50–100 mg/day (atenolol)	Any trimester	Placental insufficiency, FGR, neonatal respiratory distress, postnatal, bradycardia, hypothermia, and hypoglycemia

(CM: carbimazole; FGR: fetal growth restriction; MMI: methimazole; PTU: propylthiouracil)

- Iodine forms sodium iodide, potassium iodide, or Lugol's iodine
- Dexamethasone 2 mg IV 6 hourly, total four doses, or hydrocortisone 100 mg IV 8 hourly, total three doses
- Propranolol, labetalol, or esmolol can be used to treat associated tachycardia and preeclampsia.

▪ POSTPARTUM THYROIDITIS

Postpartum thyroiditis is defined as thyroid dysfunction (hypothyroidism/hyperthyroidism or both), in the first-year postdelivery in those females who had normal thyroid function before conception.[16] It is an autoimmune condition characterized by two phases, the initial one of destruction-induced thyrotoxicosis followed by the phase of hypothyroidism, later thyroid function becomes normal by the end of the initial first year. At-risk women are those with type 1 diabetes or TPO positivity during the first trimester. More severe cases will need treatment with beta blockers. ATDs are not recommended in postpartum thyroiditis; hence, their TSH levels are monitored at

3 and 6 months postpartum. Treatment with levothyroxine is recommended if a woman is symptomatic or she is planning conception.

An association has been proposed between postpartum depression and postpartum thyroiditis, therefore, patients with the former should be screened for hypothyroidism.[3]

Annually screening should be done with TSH testing to detect permanent hypothyroidism.[3]

■ KEY POINTS

- All patients should be screened for thyroid functions in the first trimester.
- Levothyroxine is the drug of choice for hypothyroidism in pregnancy.
- All pregnant women with TSH concentrations >2.5 mIU/L should be evaluated for TPOAb status.
- Treatment of choice for hyperthyroidism in pregnancy is antithyroid drugs, i.e., PTU, MMI, or CM.
- Methimazole and carbimazole are avoided in the first trimester due to their teratogenic effects in pregnancy.
- Women with postpartum depression should be screened for thyroid function and those with PPT should be evaluated annually for permanent postpartum hypothyroidism.

■ REFERENCES

1. Gaberšček S, Zaletel K. Thyroid physiology and autoimmunity in pregnancy and after delivery. Expert Rev Clin Immunol. 2011;7(5):697-706;quiz 707.
2. Moleti M, Trimarchi F, Vermiglio F. Thyroid physiology in pregnancy. Endocr Pract. 2014; 20(6):589-96.
3. Indian Thyroid Society. (2019). 2019 Recommendations for the Management of Thyroid Dysfunction in Pregnancy. [online] Available from: https://www.indianthyroidsociety.in/pdf/ITS_FOGSI_Recommendations.pdf [Last accessed December, 2023].
4. Alexander EK, Pearce EN, Brent GA, Brown RS, Chen H, Dosiou C, et al. 2017 Guidelines of the American Thyroid Association for the Diagnosis and Management of Thyroid Disease During Pregnancy and the Postpartum. Thyroid. 2017;27(3):315-89.
5. Nambiar V, Jagtap VS, Sarathi V, Lila AR, Kamalanathan S, Bandgar TR, et al. Prevalence and impact of thyroid disorders on maternal outcome in Asian-Indian Pregnant Women. J Thyroid Res. 2011;429097.
6. Gayathri R, Lavanya S, Raghavan K. Subclinical hypothyroidism and autoimmune thyroiditis in pregnancy—A study in south Indian subjects. JAPI. 2009;57:691-3.
7. Marx H, Amin P, Lazarus JH. Hyperthyroidism and pregnancy. BMJ. 2008;336(7645):663-7.
8. Gallas PR, Stolk RP, Bakker K, Endert E, Wiersinga WM. Thyroid dysfunction during pregnancy and in the first postpartum year in women with diabetes mellitus type 1. Eur J Endocrinol. 2002;147(4):443-51.
9. Maraka S, Mwangi R, McCoy RG, Yao X, Sangaralingham LR, Singh Ospina NM, et al. Thyroid hormone treatment among pregnant women with subclinical hypothyroidism: US national assessment. BMJ. 2017;356:i6865.
10. American Thyroid Association. (2019). Hypothyroidism in pregnancy (patient brochure). [online] Available from: https://www.thyroid.org/wp-content/uploads/patients/brochures/hypothyroidism_pregnancy_brochure.pdf [Last accessed December, 2023].
11. Lazarus J, Brown RS, Daumerie C, Hubalewska-Dydejczyk A, Negro R, Vaidya B. 2014 European thyroid association guidelines for the management of subclinical hypothyroidism in pregnancy and in children. Eur Thyroid J. 2014;3(2):76-94.
12. Ross DS, Cooper DS, Lockwood CJ, Mulder JE. (2023). Hyperthyroidism during pregnancy: Treatment. [online] Available from: https://www.uptodate.com/contents/hyperthyroidism-during-pregnancy-treatment?search=hyperthyroidism%20in%20pregnancy&source=search_result&selectedTitle=1~150&usage_type=default&display_rank=1 [Last accessed December, 2023].

13. Andersen SL, Knøsgaard L, Olsen J, Vestergaard P, Andersen S. Maternal thyroid function, use of antithyroid drugs in early pregnancy, and birth defects. J Clin Endocrinology Metab. 2019;104(12):6040-8.
14. Inoue M, Arata N, Koren G, Ito S. Hyperthyroidism during pregnancy. Can Fam Physician. 2009;55(7):701-3.
15. Besancon A, Beltrand J, Le Gac I, Luton D, Polak M. Management of neonates born to women with Graves' disease: a cohort study. Eur J Endocrinol. 2014;170(6):855-62.
16. Amino N, Mori H, Iwatani Y, Tanizawa O, Kawashima M, Tsuge I, et al. High prevalence of transient post-partum thyrotoxicosis and hypothyroidism. N Engl J Med. 1982;306(14):849-52.

Chapter 22

Seizure Disorders

Preeti Sainia

Recurrent, spontaneous convulsions are the hallmark of epilepsy. The conventional treatment for epilepsy is the administration of a daily, long-term prescription of anti-epileptic drug (AED).[1] The majority of individuals diagnosed with epilepsy may anticipate the ability to conceive and engage in other facets of life, as long as their seizures are well managed and they maintain a state of overall well-being.

Nearly one-sixth of the world's 70 million epilepsy sufferers are thought to call India home. This equates to an estimated 12 million people. Although there are notable variations in demographic characteristics and research methodology, recent studies conducted in India have shown general population prevalence rates ranging from 3.0 to 11.9 per 1,000 individuals, as well as incidence rates ranging from 0.2 to 0.6 per 1,000 individuals per year.[2] These figures are similar to the rates seen in high-income countries (HICs).

Based on the prevailing estimates of the United States population and the documented prevalence of epilepsy, it is projected that around 500,000 women who are within the reproductive age range are affected by epilepsy. Three to five out of every thousand births are predicted to be women with epilepsy WWE.[3] Certain antiepileptic medicines (AEDs) have been associated with an elevated likelihood of major congenital malformations (MCMs) and other adverse outcomes, including birth abnormalities, neonatal complications, and developmental delays in the children. These dangers need to be evaluated against the possibility of the mother having more seizures and other problems if her AED therapy is altered or stopped.[4]

Using AEDs while pregnant has been linked to a higher risk of fetal malformations since at least the 1960s.[3] The increased likelihood of MCMs in offspring of WWE who had AED treatment during pregnancy has been well acknowledged, with a nearly two to threefold higher risk compared to the general population's incidence of 1-2%.[4] Recent studies have shown that valproate carries a unique danger.

Women with epilepsy may have an increased likelihood of experiencing certain complications, including cesarean section, preeclampsia, preterm contractions or early labor, and spontaneous abortion.[4]

Instances of small for gestational age (SGA), suboptimal Apgar scores, and the possibility for perinatal death are all indicative of probable perinatal and neonatal complications. Unfortunately, several potential essential contributing variables, such as variations between AEDs, amounts of in utero exposure, or types of epilepsy, have not been characterized by research.[4]

Concern about the effects of maternal AED use on a fetus's cognitive and behavioral development is relatively new. Prenatal exposure to some AEDs has been linked to cognitive impairment in WWE babies,[5] suggesting the need for more study in this area. Despite recent advances in building pregnancy registries, it remains challenging to evaluate and compare findings on AED teratogenicity, cognitive results, and behavioral consequences. There is a lack of final results data. Registries are observational studies with a wide range of differences in technique, population studied, definitions, standardized tests used (including cognitive assessments), and duration of follow-up. Different registries gather information at various points in time (such as MCMs at birth vs. 1 year old).[5]

PREVALENCE AND BURDEN

Globally, epilepsy affects around 70 million individuals, with nearly 12 million residing in India, contributing significantly to the overall burden. When compared to high-income nations, India has a relatively low prevalence and incidence of epilepsy, which highlights the need of paying attention to the disorder's effect on maternal health.

RISKS ASSOCIATED WITH ANTIEPILEPTIC DRUG DURING PREGNANCY

For pregnant WWE, the occurrence of certain MCMs, complications during pregnancy, difficulties in newborns, and worse cognitive and behavioral results in children was shown to be linked to prenatal exposure to particular AEDs. When making the choice to continue, alter, or terminate AED therapy during pregnancy, it is crucial to carefully evaluate the trade-off between effectively treating seizures in the mother and mitigating any adverse effects on the developing fetus.[6]

ANTIEPILEPTIC DRUG AND PREGNANCY

Several AEDs are commonly used during pregnancy, each carrying specific risks and benefits.

Notably:
- *Carbamazepine:* A sodium channel blocker, carbamazepine is considered relatively safe during pregnancy, with caution required to manage blood levels effectively. On the other hand, research has linked it to an increase in neural tube abnormalities.
- *Phenytoin:* This hydantoin derivative has been linked to fetal hydantoin syndrome, characterized by intrauterine growth restriction (IUGR), dysmorphic facies, orofacial clefts, and cardiac defects.
- *Valproic acid:* An increased risk of birth abnormalities including neural tube defects (NTDs), heart malformations, cognitive difficulties, low IQ, and behavioral issues has been linked to the use of valproic acid during pregnancy, a condition known as valproate syndrome.
- *Lamotrigine:* Although lamotrigine is generally considered to be safer than valproic acid, there is a potential association between greater dosages of lamotrigine and the occurrence of cleft lip and palate.
- *Levetiracetam:* A newer AED, levetiracetam's fetal safety profile is still being evaluated, but its use appears to carry lower risks compared to older AEDs.[7]

PRECOUNSELING (PRECONCEPTION COUNSELING)

All women of reproductive age who have been diagnosed with epilepsy should be provided preconception counseling to help reduce potential dangers to the unborn child. Medical experts should provide thorough explanations of the following essential problems related to pregnancy and epilepsy management:

- Regular consultations with a neurologist are necessary for patients in order to ascertain the diagnosis and, if applicable, determine the specific kind of seizures by a comprehensive evaluation of the patient's medical records, imaging studies, and electroencephalography (EEG) findings.
- Analyze AED levels in the blood and talk to your doctor about changing your dose or medicine while you are pregnant.
- Consultation with a group of medical experts from different fields, including neurologists, obstetricians, and maternal–fetal medicine specialists, is important.[8]

The inclusion of birth control information, the need of AEDs, and the selection of a suitable kind, as well as the importance of folic acid supplementation, are all integral components of preconception planning, as shown in **Figure 1**.[8]

Table 1 shows the commonly used antiepileptic drugs used in pregnancy.

ANTIEPILEPTIC DRUGS

Carbamazepine

Mechanism: It is a sodium channel blocker that reduces abnormal brain impulses.

Dosage: Typically 600–1,800 mg/day orally divided into two to three doses.

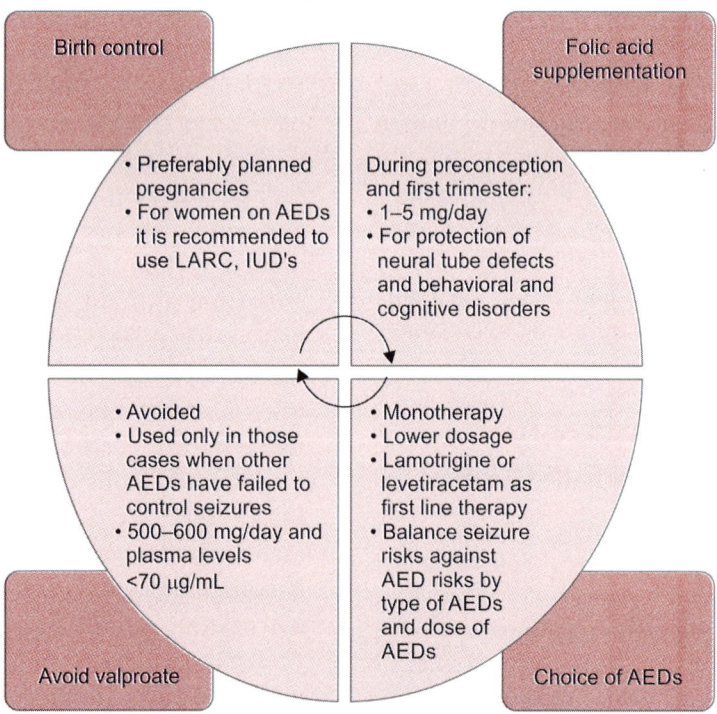

Fig. 1: Preconception planning. (AEDs: antiepileptic drugs; IUDs: intrauterine devices; LARC: long-acting reversible contraception)

TABLE 1: AEDs used in pregnancy.

Class	Drug
Sodium channel blocker	• Carbamazepine • Phenytoin
Sodium and T-type calcium channel blocker and blockade of GABA transaminase	Valproic acid
Sodium channel and high voltage-dependent calcium channel blocker	Lamotrigine
High affinity for synaptic vesicle protein	Levetiracetam
T-type calcium channel blocker	Ethosuximide
GABA analog	Gabapentin
Benzodiazepine	Lorazepam
Carbonic anhydrase inhibitor	Topiramate

(AEDs: antiepileptic drugs; GABA: gamma-aminobutyric acid)

Adverse effects: Gastrointestinal (GI) irritation, vertigo, dizziness, leukopenia, and aplastic anemia.

Drug interactions: Interacts with contraceptive steroids, macrolide antibiotics, and monoamine oxidase (MAO) inhibitors.

Pregnancy safety: Classified as a "category D" medicine because of its link to birth abnormalities of the nervous system, including spina bifida, NTD, hypospadias, cleft lip, cleft palate, and GI anomalies.

Recommendation: Use only if benefits outweigh risks, monitor plasma concentrations.

Phenytoin

Mechanism: Membrane stabilizer; blocks voltage-gated sodium channels. It promotes sodium efflux and decreases sodium influx from the membrane in motor cortex neurons.

Dosage: Loading dose and then maintenance dose orally or IV 100 mg TDS; can be increased to 600 mg/day in two to three divided doses.

Adverse effects: Arrhythmias, confusion, dizziness, osteomalacia, gum hyperplasia, and low blood pressure.

Pregnancy safety: Category D drug, associated with fetal hydantoin syndrome.

Fetal Hydantoin Syndrome

It is a characteristic pattern of mental and physical birth defect that results from maternal use of drug phenytoin during pregnancy. The range of severity varies greatly from one infant to another. The distinctive features are mid face hypoplasia, ocular hypertelorism, low nasal bridge, and accentuated cupid bow of upper lip. Hypoplastic nails of finger and toes are also seen. It may also be associated with cleft lip, cleft palate, and microcephaly. Prenatal onset of growth deficiency, poor gain of weight, and length and head circumference have also been seen. Chorionic villus sampling (CVS) anomalies and reduction in cognitive function has also been seen in fetal hydantoin syndrome. There may be bleeding disorder in a neonate.

Recommendation: Monitor total and free levels. Check before starting folate supplementation. Administer vitamin K injection to mother before delivery and to the neonate after delivery.

Valproic Acid

Mechanism: It blocks gamma-aminobutyric acid (GABA) transaminase which leads to decreased GABA metabolism and increased GABAergic neurotransmission. As GABA is an inhibitory neurotransmitter, it leads to increased inhibitory activity in the brain.

Dosage: Typically 750–2,000 mg/day in divided doses.

Adverse effects: Thrombocytopenia, sedation, GI side effects, hepatotoxicity, and tremors.

Drug interactions: Interacts with acetaminophens, warfarin, alcohol, oral contraceptive pills (OCPs), and others.

Pregnancy safety: Category D drug, associated with NTDs, cardiac malformations, learning disabilities, etc.

Fetal Valproate Syndrome

The use of valproic acid in the first trimester significantly increases the chances of major and minor malformations in the fetus. Almost a 20-fold increase is reported in NTD such as spina bifida. Cleft lip, cleft palate, genitourinary defect, and cardiovascular abnormalities are seen. Endocrine disorder, autism, and limb defect along with developmental delay have also been seen.

Recommendation: High risk of major malformations in the fetus. Its use should be avoided in women of reproductive age group and pregnant women.

Lamotrigine

Mechanism: Inhibits glutamate release by acting on sodium channels.

Dosage: Typically taken in daily divided doses, adjusted gradually.

Adverse effects: Sedation, diplopia, headache, ataxia, dizziness, tremors, hepatic and renal impairment.

Pregnancy safety: Category C drug, relatively safe compared to valproate.

Recommendation: Doses over 200 mg/day are linked to cleft lip and palate risk.

Levetiracetam

Mechanism: Modulates neurotransmitter release by binding synaptic vesicle glycoprotein 2A (SV2A).

Dosage: Starts at 1,000 mg/day and can be increased up to 3,000 mg/day.

Adverse effects: Somnolence, agitation, disturbed sleep, respiratory depression, and coma.

Pregnancy safety: Category C drug, and limited data available.

Recommendation: Watch for interactions with benzodiazepines, cetirizine, etc.

Phenobarbital

Mechanism: Increases time the chloride channels are open, reducing neuron excitability.

Dosage: 1–3 mg/kg/day in divided doses.

Adverse effects: Dizziness, drowsiness, headache, fatigue, irritability, nystagmus, and vertigo.

Pregnancy safety: Category D drug, crosses placental barrier, associated with fetal malformations. The use of phenobarbital in the first trimester of pregnancy has been seen with increased incidence of cleft palate, cardiac malformation, stunted growth, and fetal mortality.

Recommendation: Use is limited due to side effects and fetal risks.

Topiramide

Topiramate is an AED that is often used for the management of epilepsy and the prophylaxis of migraines.

Mechanism: It decreases the excitability of neuronal pathways by influencing GABA receptors, glutamate receptors, and voltage-dependent sodium channels. Topiramate exhibits inhibitory properties via augmenting GABA-A receptor activity at nonbenzodiazepine receptor sites within the brain and reducing excitatory activity at AMPA and kainate receptors.

Dosage: The recommended adult dosage for monotherapy of newly onset seizures is 100 mg/day.

The dosage has to be adjusted when taken in conjunction with other enzyme-inducing AEDs and may be raised to 400 mg/day.

No hepatic enzymes are stimulated by topiramate.

Adverse effects: Generally well tolerated, but adverse effects limit its use in around 25% of patients.

Possible adverse effects include cognitive dysfunction, problems with expressive speech, and impaired verbal memory.

Other potential effects include weight loss, renal stones, paresthesias, and various central nervous system (CNS) side effects.

Drug tolerability can be improved by starting with a low initial dose and titrating slowly based on the patient's response.

Pregnancy safety: Topiramate is a medication of concern during pregnancy, category D.

Fetal adverse effects: There is an increased chance of birth defects including cleft palate, heart defect, and ureter defect in infants whose mothers used topiramate during pregnancy.

Oxcarbazepine

Similar to carbamazepine, it is used to treat seizures.

Adverse effects: Include dizziness, drowsiness, nausea, vomiting, and more.

Pregnancy safety: Pregnancy category C.

Ethosuximide

Mechanism: Used for absence (petit mal) seizures.

Adverse effects: Can include nausea, vomiting, dizziness, and more.

Pregnancy safety: Pregnancy category C.

Sodium Divalproex

It is a form of valproic acid, used for seizures and mood disorders.

Similar adverse effects and pregnancy category to valproic acid.

Acetazolamide

It is used for various conditions including epilepsy.

Adverse effects: Can include drowsiness, tingling, taste alterations, and more.

Pregnancy safety: Pregnancy category C.

Gabapentin

It is effective for the treatment of epilepsy and neuropathic pain.

Adverse effects: Dizziness, sleepiness, and other side effects are possible.

Pregnancy safety: Pregnancy category C.

Pregabalin

Similar to gabapentin, it is used for epilepsy and neuropathic pain.

Adverse effects: Can include dizziness, drowsiness, and more.

Pregnancy safety: Pregnancy category C.

Vigabatrin

It is used for epilepsy, particularly for infantile spasms.

Adverse effects: Can include vision changes, dizziness, drowsiness, and more.

Pregnancy safety: Pregnancy category C.

Primidone

It gets converted to phenobarbital in the body. It is used for epilepsy.

It has similar adverse effects and pregnancy category to phenobarbital.

Diazepam and Lorazepam

These are benzodiazepines used for seizures, including status epilepticus.

Adverse effects: Can include drowsiness, sedation, and more.

Pregnancy safety: Pregnancy category D for diazepam and category D for lorazepam.[9]

FETAL RISKS OF BARBITURATE USE

Some barbiturates, such as phenobarbital, are able to enter the placenta and go throughout the fetal organs. There exists data suggesting that the use of these substances throughout the first and final trimesters of pregnancy heightens the probability of teratogenic effects and withdrawal symptoms in the offspring. Notably, they are associated with cardiac malformations and oral clefts. Hence, they are not recommended as first-line drugs.[10]

Phenobarbital, one of the earliest AEDs used across patient cohorts, had not been extensively studied for fetal effects until the 1970s. Fetal cleft palate was shown to be 4.3% more common in studies when pregnant mice were given phenobarbital.[8] Similarly, phenobarbital exposure during pregnancy led to increased fetal mortality, stunted growth, and a delay in motor development in rats. These neurological problems may be caused by oxidative stress caused by an increase in the formation of superoxide radicals and subsequent hydroxyl radicals due to an upregulation of cytochrome P450s of the 2B family. This cascade may cause GC to TA transversions, potentially contributing to developmental defects.

A Word about Levetiracetam

There has been a lot of research for an AED to search for an antiepileptic that is (1) effective in seizure control and (2) free from teratogenic side effects.

Levetiracetam has a relatively low risk associated with its use during pregnancy, with a reported rate of 2.3 for MCMs. A comprehensive review and meta-analysis of pregnancy registries and cohorts examined several AEDs such as carbamazepine, valproic acid, lamotrigine, phenytoin, gabapentin, and topiramate.[7]

Levetiracetam was first approved by the Food and Drug Administration as an AED in 1999. It has certain advantages over the conventional AEDs, namely twice-daily dosing, good oral bioavailability, linear bioavailability, excretion through kidneys, and relatively less drug-to-drug interaction.

A retrospective study done by Bansal et al. that included 99 WWE on monotherapy with different drugs concluded that although valproic acid had better control of seizure during pregnancy as compared to levetiracetam, its use was associated with a higher incidence of MCMs.[11]

Flowchart 1 shows the proposed mechanism of how AEDs may be causing fetal malformations.

Many theories attempt to shed light on why AEDs might cause birth defects. Ischemia, neural suppression, reduced folate absorption, neural apoptosis, and an increase in free radical production are all potential

Flowchart 1: Antiepileptic drugs.

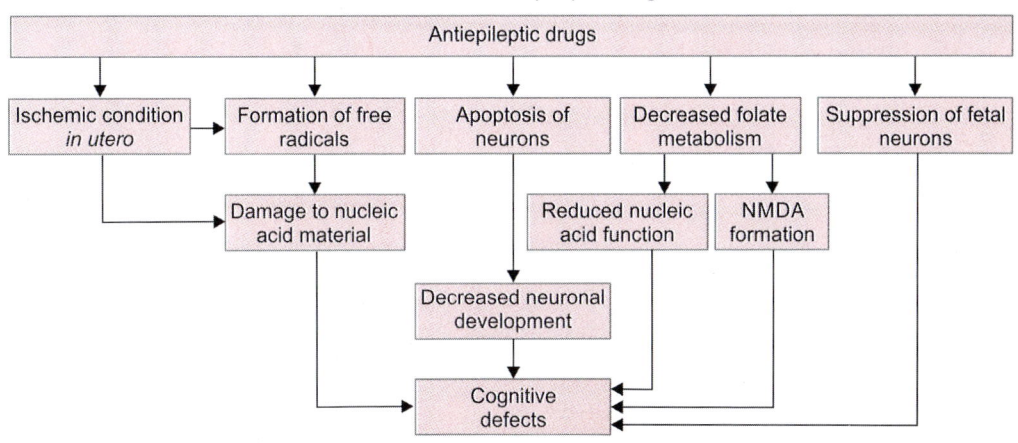

(NMDA: N-methyl-D-aspartic acid)

pathways that contribute to the development of cognitive impairments in fetuses.[5]

Prenatal exposure to AEDs is associated with a significantly increased occurrence of congenital abnormalities.

Figure 2 shows the trend of teratogenicity with commonly used drugs.

Table 2 shows concise information regarding commonly used drugs in pregnancy in WWE.

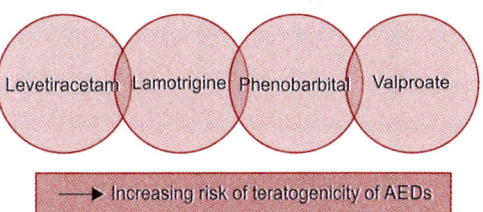

Fig. 2: Trend of teratogenicity with commonly used drugs.

STRATEGIES FOR WOMEN WITH EPILEPSY WHO WANT TO CONCEIVE OR HAVE ALREADY CONCEIVED

- If a WWE is planning a conception, she should consult her gynecologist and neurologist and immediately start folic acid supplementation at 5 mg/day.
- The AED being taken by the woman should neither be stopped nor be changed without the guidance of the neurologist.
- The risk of fetal malformation depends on the type of drug and dosage and increases if the patient is taking more than one drug for epilepsy.
- If the patient is on sodium valproate when she conceives, it should not be stopped immediately and the neurologist should take a call on change of treatment and dosage.
- Adequate rest and minimizing stress will be very helpful for the patient in prevention of seizure in both antenatal and postnatal periods.
- AEDs can pass through breast milk, but the amount is usually small and does not cause harm to the baby. Breast feeding is considered safe in patients on AED.

The management of pregnant woman on AED poses a great challenge for the treating clinician. Our goal should be to optimize the control of seizure with minimal exposure of the fetus to the AED in order to minimize the structural and neurodevelopmental teratogenic effects. The pharmacokinetics of AEDs are also altered due to physiological changes of pregnancy which may result

TABLE 2: Commonly used drugs in pregnancy in women with epilepsy (WWE).

Drug	Information/MOA	Dose	Side effects	Pregnancy category and teratogenic effects
Carbamazepine	It is a sodium channel blocker and helps in reducing the abnormal brain impulses	600–1,800 mg/day in 2–3 divided doses	Vertigo, GI side effects, dizziness, leukopenia, and aplastic anemia	• Pregnancy category D drug • It can cause CNS anomaly like spina bifida in fetus, hypospadias, renal anomaly, cleft lip, and cleft palate
Phenytoin	Membrane stabilizer—it blocks voltage-gated sodium channel	• 100 mg TDS can be increased to 600 mg/day in 2–3 divided doses. • To adjust the dose not sooner than 7–10 days	Arrythmias, confusion, dizziness, osteomalacia, gum hyperplasia, and low blood pressure	Pregnancy category D drug, orofacial clefts, cardiac defects, and fetal hydantoin syndrome
Phenobarbitone	It increases the time for which chlorine channels are open which leads to depression of CNS	• 1–3 mg/kg/day in 1–2 divided doses. • Maintain therapeutic steady level at 20 mg/day	Dizziness, drowsiness, headache, fatigue, and irritability, nystagmus	• Pregnancy category D, increased incidence of orofacial clefts • May increase incidence of impaired growth and delayed motor response withdrawal symptoms • May be seen in neonate
Valproic acid	It inhibits succinic semialdehyde dehydrogenase which inhibits GABA transaminase which leads to increase in GABAergic neurotransmission. As GABA is an inhibitory neurotransmitter, it leads to increased inhibitory activity in brain	750–2,000 mg/dL	Thrombocytopenia, sedation, GI side effects, hepatotoxicity, and tremors	• Pregnancy category D drug. 20-fold increase in incidence of NTDs, orofacial defects, and cardiac malformations • Fetal ECHO to be recommended
Levetiracetam	Modulation of synaptic neurotransmitter release by binding to synaptic vesicle protein SV2A in brain	Starts at 1,000 mg/day in 2 divided doses can go up to 3,000 mg/day	Somnolence, agitation, disturbed sleep, and respiratory depression	• Pregnancy category C. Increased incidence of minor fetal skeletal abnormality and growth retardation. • No major congenital malformation reported in humans

(CNS: central nervous system; GABA: gamma-aminobutyric acid; NTD: neural tube defect)

in lower levels of the drug in blood and seizure deterioration. Sometimes, this calls for regular monitoring of drug and dose adjustment during pregnancy and postpartum period.

■ KEY POINTS

- *Prepregnancy folic acid*: Taking a daily dose of 5 mg of folic acid before pregnancy can help reduce the risk of cognitive dysfunction associated with AED use.
- *Lowest approved dose*: Opt for the lowest approved dose of the most suitable AED when treating seizures during pregnancy.
- *Monotherapy preferred*: Monotherapy (using a single AED) is preferred over polytherapy (using multiple AEDs) to minimize potential risks.
- *Valproate exposure minimization*: Minimize exposure to sodium valproate and other AEDs by considering alternative medications before conception, especially due to the higher risks associated with valproate.
- *Abrupt changes during unexpected pregnancy*: In cases of unexpected pregnancy, it is not recommended to abruptly change or stop AEDs without medical consultation.
- *Seizures during labor*: Seizures during labor should be promptly terminated using intravenous benzodiazepines. This helps prevent fetal and maternal acidosis and associated complications.
- *Regular medical consultation*: To guarantee the best results for mother and child, it is crucial to continue frequent consultations with healthcare specialists who specialize in epilepsy treatment during pregnancy.

■ REFERENCES

1. Rosa FW. Spina bifida in infants of women treated with carbamazepine during pregnancy. N Engl J Med. 1991;324(10):674-7.
2. Morrow J, Russell A, Guthrie E, Parsons L, Robertson I, Waddell R, et al. Malformation risks of antiepileptic drugs in pregnancy: A prospective study from the UK Epilepsy and Pregnancy Register. J Neurol Neurosurg Psychiatry. 2006;77(2):193-8.
3. Craig JJ, Hunt SJ. Treating women with myoclonic epilepsy: A practical approach. Pract Neurol. 2009;9(5):268-77.
4. Hunt S, Russell A. Topiramate in pregnancy: Preliminary experience from the UK Epilepsy and Pregnancy Register. Neurology. 2008;71(4):272-6.
5. Meador KJ, Baker G, Cohen MJ, Gaily E, Westerve M. Cognitive/behavioral teratogenetic effects of antiepileptic drugs. Epilepsy Behav. 2007;11(3):292-302.
6. Meador K, Reynolds MW, Crean S, Fahrbach K, Probst C. Pregnancy outcomes in women with epilepsy: A systematic review and meta-analysis of published pregnancy registries and cohorts. Epilepsy Res. 2008;81:1-13.
7. Shank RP, Gardocki JF, Streeter AJ, Maryanoff BE. An overview of the preclinical aspects of topiramate: Pharmacology, pharmacokinetics, and mechanism of action. Epilepsia. 2000;41(Suppl 1):S3-S9.
8. Walker MC, Sander JW. Topiramate: A new antiepileptic drug for refractory epilepsy. Seizure. 1996;5(3):199-203.
9. Allen MJ, Sharma S, Sabir S. GABA Receptor. StatPearls [Internet]. Treasure Island (FL): StatPearls Publishing; 2023 Jan.
10. Ornoy A. Neuroteratogens in man: An overview with special emphasis on the teratogenicity of antiepileptic drugs in pregnancy. Reprod Toxicol. 2006;22:214-26.
11. Bansal R, Suri V, Chopra S, Aggarwal N, Sikka P, Saha SC, et al. Levetiracetam use during pregnancy in women with epilepsy: Preliminary observations from a tertiary care centre in Northern India. Indian J Pharmacol. 2018;50(1):39-43.

Chapter 23

Hyperemesis Gravidarum

Kavita Kumari

Nausea and vomiting in pregnancy are common symptoms that affect many women, especially in the first trimester. It is called as "morning sickness". Symptoms usually begin between the 4th and 7th weeks and resolved by 12th week of pregnancy and mostly by 20th week. Prevalence is 75-80% for nausea and 50% for vomiting.[1] Hyperemesis gravidarum (HG) is severe form of nausea and vomiting in pregnancy which is characterized by persistent vomiting, weight loss of more than 5%, ketonuria, electrolyte imbalance (hypokalemia), and dehydration. Incidence of HG is 0.3–1%.[2] It is a clinical diagnosis of exclusion. To stop the progression of HG, early treatment of nausea and vomiting in pregnancy may be beneficial.

A severity index, currently known as the mother risk pregnancy unique quantification of emesis and nausea, is used to measure the severity of nausea and vomiting during pregnancy during the first trimester.[3] Thus, PUQE scores are used to define the severity of symptoms and aggressiveness of treatment. Mild nausea and vomiting in pregnancy (score 6 or less), moderate nausea and vomiting in pregnancy (score 7 to 12), and severe nausea and vomiting in pregnancy (score more than 13).

■ RISK FACTOR

It was found that younger, primi gravida, nonsmoking, and obese women are more likely to have nausea and vomiting during pregnancy.[4] It has been shown that nausea and vomiting are more frequent in women who are carrying multiple pregnancy. An individual's prior experience with nausea and vomiting during pregnancy has been found to be a risk factor for the same symptoms during a subsequent pregnancy. The risk of experiencing nausea and vomiting during pregnancy is increased by a family history of the condition.

■ PATHOGENESIS

It is unknown what exactly causes nausea and vomiting during pregnancy. It is generally accepted that numerous metabolic and endocrine factors contribute to nausea and vomiting in pregnancy and HG. Since the peak of nausea and vomiting during pregnancy and the peak of hCG both occur between 12 and 14 weeks, hCG is the most common factor. In conditions with increased hCG, such as molar pregnancy and multiple gestations, nausea and vomiting in pregnancy and HG frequently get worse.[5]

■ DIFFERENTIAL DIAGNOSIS[6]

Differential diagnoses for nausea and vomiting in pregnancy and HG are:
- Peptic ulcer disease
- Gastroenteritis

- Cholecystitis
- Cholelithiasis
- Pancreatitis
- Appendicitis
- Pyelonephritis
- Hepatitis

■ INVESTIGATION

No specific investigations are required for the diagnosis of nausea and vomiting in pregnancy, but investigations should be done to exclude other causes of nausea and vomiting.
- Complete blood count (CBC): Leukocytosis indicates infectious or inflammatory causes.
- Urine routine microscopy: To rule out UTI
- Liver function test (LFT): To rule out hepatitis
- Kidney function test (KFT)
- *Thyroid profile:* Abnormal thyroid profile indicates either hyperthyroidism or hypothyroidism. In both conditions, nausea and vomiting in pregnancy occurs.
- *Blood sugar:* Fasting and postprandial
- *Serum electrolyte*
- *Ultrasound:* For confirmation of pregnancy and rule out molar pregnancy and twin pregnancy.

■ MANAGEMENT

As the etiology and pathogenesis of nausea and vomiting in pregnancy are not known, main aim of treatment is to reduce the symptoms and minimize the risk to pregnant women and their fetus. If nausea and vomiting in pregnancy left untreated, it may progress to severe form (HG) and may need hospitalization. There are different modalities of treatment like nonpharmacological and pharmacological. They are dietary changes, drug therapy, and nutritional therapy. PUQE scores are used to determine the severity of symptoms and aggressiveness of treatment. Mild case requires outpatient treatment with oral liquids antiemetics. Moderate cases may be treated as outpatient or may require hospitalization. Severe cases require hospitalization for correction of dehydration and electrolyte imbalance **(Flowchart 1)**.

Nonpharmacological Therapy

- *Dietary advice:*[7]
  - Avoid having an empty stomach. Eat little, frequently, and every 1–2 hours. Avoid large meals at one time.
  - Avoid fatty or spicy foods because fatty foods delay gastric emptying.
  - Took more protein than carbohydrate.
  - Early morning nausea may be helped by eating a dry biscuit or crackers before getting out of bed.
  - Salty food such as potato chips or salted crackers may help.
  - Drink small amount more frequently to maintain hydration.
- *Lifestyle modification:*[7]
  - Eat well when feeling the best or feeling hungry.
  - If the smell of hot food worsens nausea, try cold food instead.
  - Lie down when nauseated.
  - Avoid stress.
- *Emotional support:* Emotional support by family members and healthcare professional may improve symptoms by relieving the stress. Psychological counseling may be considered.[8]
- *Ginger:* It is recommended by the ACOG.[9]
  - By increasing gastrointestinal tract motility, salivary flow, bile and gastric secretion, it reduces nausea and vomiting in pregnancy. It shares similar properties with the 5HT3 antagonist.[10]
  - *Dose:* 250 mg 4 times a day

Flowchart 1: Therapeutic treatment of nausea and vomiting in pregnancy.[21]

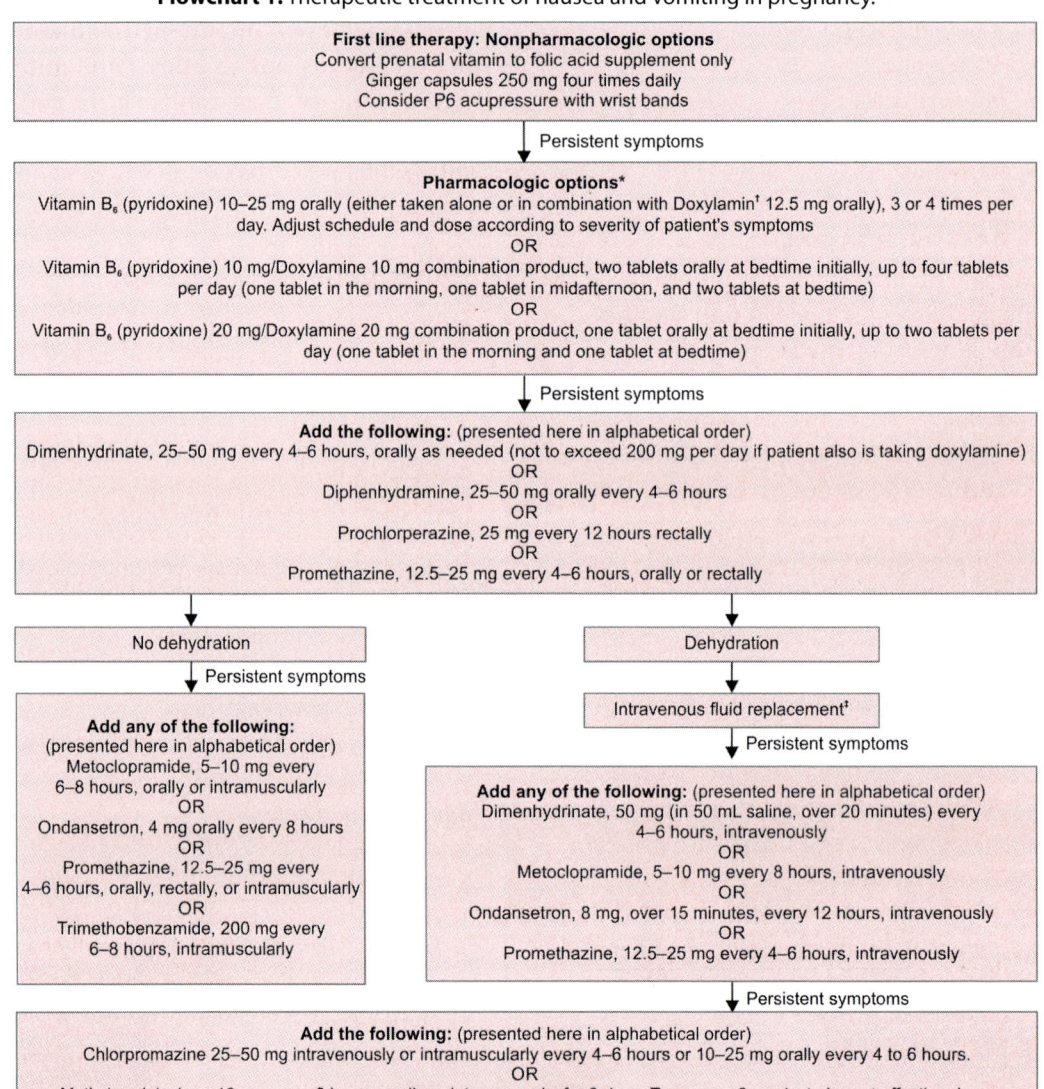

*Some antiemetic medications have only been approved by the US Food and Drug Administration for use in nonpregnant patients; however, off-label use is common. Obstetricians and other obstetric care providers should counsel patients and document such discussions accordingly. Care should be exercised if multiple antiemetic medications are used simultaneously. Parallel use of some medications (see text) may result in an increased risk of adverse effects.

†In the United States, doxylamine is available as the active ingredient in some over-the-counter sleep aids; one half of a scored 25-mg tablet can be used to provide a 12.5-mg dose of doxylamine.

‡Thiamine, intravenously, 100 mg with the initial rehydration fluid and 100 mg daily for the next 2–3 days (followed by intravenous multivitamins), is recommended for women who require intravenous hydration and have vomited for more than 3 weeks to prevent a rare but serious maternal complication, Wernicke encephalopathy.

- *Drug interaction:* It is not recommended to consume ginger and anticoagulants simultaneously
- *Acupressure/acupuncture:* Acupressure at point P6 blocks abnormal energy and relives the symptoms. Pressure may be applied by elastic bands or electrical nerve stimulators worn on the wrists.[11]

Pharmacological Therapy

- *Pyridoxine (vitamin B_6):* It is a water-soluble B-complex vitamin. It is a coenzyme in the metabolism of lipids, carbohydrates, and amino acids.

  Doses: 25 mg every 8 hours or 75 mg per day orally.[12]

  It can be used alone or in combination with doxylamine. It has a good safety profile with minimal adverse effects. It is easily available in the market. It is FDA Class A drugs. There is no risk of fetal anomalies with pyridoxine.
- *Doxylamine:* It is an anti-histaminic and it is usually used with pyridoxine.

  Doxylamine pyridoxine: It was used from very long time and only FDA approved drug for treating nausea and vomiting of pregnancy.

  Dose: Doxylamine 10 mg plus pyridoxine 10 mg two tablets at night for mild symptoms up to maximum four tablets per day.

  If symptoms not improved, then other anti-emetic drugs are added.
- *Promotility agents (metoclopramide):* It is frequently used to treat HG and pregnancy-related nausea and vomiting. It is a category B drug for pregnancy.

  Mechanism of action: It acts as an antiemetic by blocking dopamine receptor at chemoreceptor trigger zone (CTZ) of the CNS. It acts by increasing lower esophageal sphincter pressure and increasing gastric transit. It also stimulates antral contraction and promoting intraduodenal contraction.

  Dose: 5–10 mg 8 hourly either oral or IV or IM

  Side effects: Restlessness, dizziness, diarrhea, dystonia and somnolence. It also increases the risk of tardive dyskinesia with chronic use
- *Antihistamines and anticholinergics:* Antihistamines work by altering the vestibular system, which reduces stimulation of the vomiting center. In addition, muscarinic receptor inhibition may place a role in antihistamine antiemetic activity. The drugs in the group are dimenhydrinate, diphenhydramine, and meclizine. These antihistamines do not increase teratogenic risk.

  Doses:
  - *Diphenhydramine:* 25–50 mg every 4–6 hours/10–50 mg IV or IM every 4–6 hours
  - *Dimenhydrinate:* 50–100 mg orally or rectally every 4–6 hours as needed
  - *Meclizine:* It is pregnancy B drug. It is safe in pregnancy. Dose is 25 mg every 4–6 hours
- *Other agents:* Ondansetron (serotonin antagonist) is pregnancy category B drugs.

  Mechanism of action: It blocks the depolarizing action of serotonin through 5HT3 receptors on vagal afferents as well as CTZ. Thus, it works both centrally and peripherally. It is safe in pregnancy with no significant major congenital malformation.

  Dose: 4–8 mg 8 hourly IV oral

Side effects are drowsiness, headache, and fatigue. Ondansetron can prolong the QT interval especially in patient with cardiac disease, hypokalemia, hypomagnesemia.[13]

Caution: It should not be used with cardiac diseases.

It can be considered as a treatment option for women for refractory nausea and vomiting in pregnancy or HG.

- *Phenothiazines:* Drugs used are prochlorperazine, chlorpromazine, and promethazine.

Mechanism of action: These drugs act by blocking postsynaptic mesolimbic dopaminergic receptors in CNS and reduce stimulus to the brainstem reticular system.

- *Promethazine:* It can be used orally, intramuscular, or rectal route. Dose is 12.5–25 mg oral/IV/IM every 4–6 hours. Prominent side effects are sedation and dryness of mouth. It should not be used by subcutaneous or intra-arterial route.
- *Prochlorperazine:* Dosage 25 mg rectally every 12 hours

Side effects: Muscle dystonia and other extra paramedial side effects are seen. These drugs are used only in refractory nausea and vomiting. These drugs are pregnancy category C.

- *Corticosteroid:* This drug is used for treatment of severe nausea and vomiting in pregnancy and HG which is refractory to other treatment. It was thought that severe nausea and vomiting in pregnancy may be partially due to deficiency of corticotrophin leading to relative adrenal insufficiency.

Current recommendation is that corticosteroids should not be used before 10 weeks of gestation as has shown increased incidence of cleft palate in some studies.[14]

Doses: Oral or intravenous methylprednisolone 48 mg per day in three divided doses for 2–3 days. If no response is seen within 3 days, treatment should be stopped. Doses may be tapered over 1–2 weeks.[15]

- *Antacid:* Aluminum and calcium-containing antacids are first-line agents for acid reflux and heartburn and can be used to treat women with nausea and vomiting in pregnancy.
- *H2 blockers:* Ranitidine (150 mg BD) can be safely used to treat acid reflux or heart bun in women with nausea and vomiting in pregnancy.
- *Proton pump inhibitors:* Pantoprazole and omeprazole can be used safely to treat acid reflux or heartburn in women with nausea and vomiting in pregnancy.

TABLE 1: Safety classifications of agents used in the treatment of nausea and vomiting during pregnancy.[18]

Drug, product, or drug class	Pregnancy safety classification
Multivitamins	A
Ginger	Unknown
Pyridoxine	A
Doxylamine–pyridoxine	A
Antihistamines (meclizine, diphenhydramine, and dimenhydrinate)	B
Phenothiazines (chlorpromazine, prochlorperazine, and promethazine)	C
Metoclopramide	B
Ondansetron	B
Corticosteroids	C

CHAPTER 23: Hyperemesis Gravidarum

TABLE 2: Pharmacological agents used in nausea and vomiting of pregnancy.[19]

Drug name/category	Dosage and route	Mechanism of action	Side effects	Contraindications	Safety
Pyridoxine	25 mg po q8h or 75 mg PO daily	May treat underlying pyridoxine deficiency	Minimal side effects, fatigue	Hypervitaminosis B6, as toxic levels may cause sensory neuropathy	There is no risk of fetal anomalies
Doxylamine	Usually used with pyridoxine, 10 mg PO 2–4 tablets daily	Antihistaminic	Drowsiness	In patients with bronchial asthma, narrow angle glaucoma	Safer in pregnancy
Pyridoxine + doxylamine	10 mg + 10 mg 2–4 tablets PO daily	Treats pyridoxine deficiency and H1 antagonist	Drowsiness	–	Safer in pregnancy
Metoclopramide	5–10 mg 8 h PO IV/IM	Dopaminergic receptor blocker (central and peripheral)	Extrapyramidal side effects, dizziness, dystonia, neuroleptic malignant syndrome	Patients with pheochromocytoma, history of epilepsy and patients on other drugs with extrapyramidal side effects	There was no significant association between metoclopramide use and malformation overall
Antihistaminic: • Dimenhydrinate • Diphenhydramine	 • 25–50 mg PO 4–6 h/10–50 mg IV/IM 4–6 hourly • 50–100 mg PO and rectally 4–6 hourly	Peripheral H1 receptor antagonist	Drowsiness, dizziness, HA, and fatigue	Contraindicated in patients using other CNS depressants	They do not increase teratogenic risk
Ondansetron	4–8 mg every 8 hourly oral or IV	Serotonin receptor antagonist (central and peripheral)	Drowsiness, headache, fatigue, prolongs QT interval especially in cardiac patient	Contraindicated in patients with prolonged QT interval, heart failure, hypokalemia, hypomagnesemia	Teratogenic risk with ondansetron is low but it increases risk for cardiac septum defects

Contd...

Contd...

Drug name/category	Dosage and route	Mechanism of action	Side effects	Contraindications	Safety
Phenothiazines • Promethazine • Prochlorperazine	• 12.5–25 mg 4–6 hourly per orally, rectal or IM • 5–10 mg orally, 10–25 mg rectally every 4–6 hours	Central/peripheral dopamine antagonist	Drowsiness, decreased seizure threshold, akathisia	Hypersensitivity to phenothiazines, uncorrected hypokalemia, porphyria, patients with Torsade's de points	Slightly increased risk of birth defects
Corticosteroids	48 mg oral/IV in 3 divided doses for 3 days	May treat relative ACTH deficiency, inhibit central PG synthesis or decrease central 5-HT turnover	Hyperglycemia, possible increased risk of oral facial clefts with first trimester use	Not to be used before 10 weeks of pregnancy	Increased risk of fetal oral clefts
Ranitidine	150 mg PO q12 h or 50 mg IV q8h	Peripheral H2 antagonist	HA, drowsiness, dizziness, diarrhea, or constipation	In patients with acute porphyria	
Domperidone (used in refractory cases)[20]	10 mg orally every 8 hours	Dopamine antagonist	Dizziness, headache, on IV use, it causes arrhythmia, cardiac arrest, and sudden death	Not to be used in patients with cardiac disease	Limited safety data in pregnancy

(CNS: central nervous system)

- *Nutritional support:* The patient who is not responding to oral antiemetics and dietary modification with weight loss needs hospitalization for nutritional support. It is given by intravenous fluid therapy, enteral nutrition, or parenteral nutrition.
    - *Intravenous fluid therapy:* Main aim of this therapy is to maintain hydration and correct calorie deficit and electrolyte imbalance. IV fluid of choice is normal saline and lactated Ringers' solution. Amount of fluid infused will depend upon severity of dehydration and adjusted according to urine output. Dextrose-containing fluid can be given but prior thiamine infusion is required to prevent Werneck's encephalopathy.[16]
    - *Enteral tube feeding:* When intravenous fluid therapy is not successful in reducing symptoms and there is caloric deficit, then enteral tube feeding is required. This type of feeding can be given by nasogastric tube, nasojejunal tube or percutaneous endoscopic gastrojejunostomy.
    - *Parental nutrition:* The patient who does not tolerate enteral feeding, parental nutrition should be considered. This therapy has more complications such as infection and thrombosis.[17]

Pharmacological agents used in nausea and vomiting in pregnancy are given in **Tables 1 and 2**.

Nausea and vomiting of pregnancy is very common disorder in early pregnancy. It may be mild, moderate and severe (Hyperemesis gravidarum). Its pathogenesis is still not known, so treatment is mainly symptomatic like dietary modification, pharmacotherapy and even hospitalization.

■ KEY POINTS

- Treatment of pregnancy-induced nausea and vomiting with pyridoxine alone or in combination with (doxylamine) is safe and effective, and it ought to be used as the first line of pharmacotherapy.
- Treating nausea and vomiting early in pregnancy before it progresses can help control symptoms and prevent more serious complications including hospitalizations.
- Ginger has demonstrated some positive effects in lowering nausea sensations and might be thought of as a nonpharmacologic treatment for morning sickness and vomiting during pregnancy.
- Treatment of severe nausea and vomiting of pregnancy or HG with methylprednisolone may be efficacious in refractory cases; however, the risk profile of methylprednisolone suggests it should be a last-resort treatment.

■ REFERENCES

1. Niebyl JR. Nausea and vomiting in pregnancy. N Eng J Med. 2010;363(16):1544-50.
2. National Collaborating Centre for Women's and Children's Health (UK). Antenatal care: routine care for the healthy pregnant woman. [online] Available from: www.nice.org.uk. [Last accessed December, 2023].
3. Koren G, Piwko C, Ahn E, Boskovic R, Maltepe C, Einarson A, et al. Validation studies of the Pregnancy Unique-Quantification of Emesis (PUQE) scores. J Obstet Gynaecol. 2005;25(3):241-4.
4. Klebanoff MA, Koslowe PA, Kaslow RI, Rhoads GG. Epidemiology of vomiting in early pregnancy. Obstet Gynecol. 1985;66(5):612-6.
5. Davis M. Nausea and vomiting of pregnancy: an evidence-based review. J Perinat Neonatal Nurs. 2004;18(4):312-28.
6. Koch KL, Frissora CL. Nausea and vomiting during pregnancy. Gastroenterol Clin. 2003;32(1):201-34.
7. Sheehan P. Hyperemesis gravidarum: assessment and management. Aust Fam Physician. 2007;36(9):698-701.

8. Simon EP, Schwartz J. Medical hypnosis for hyperemesis gravidarum. Birth. 1999;26(4):248-54.
9. American College of Obstetricians and Gynecologists. Clinical management guidelines for obstetrician-gynecologists: Nausea and vomiting of pregnancy. ACOG Educ Bull. 2004;103:803-15.
10. Mahady G, Pendland S, Yun G, Lu ZZ, Stoia A. Ginger and the gingerols inhibits the growth of CagA+ strains of Helicobacter Pylori. Anticancer Res. 2003;23(5A):3699-702.
11. Rosen T, De Veciana M, Miller HS, Stewart L, Rebarber A, Slotnick RN. A randomized controlled trial of nerve stimulation for relief of nausea and vomiting in pregnancy. Obstet Gynecol. 2003;102(1):129-35.
12. Sahakian VI, Rouse DW, Sipes SU, Rose NA, Niebyl JE. Vitamin B_6 is effective therapy for nausea and vomiting of pregnancy: a randomized, double-blind placebo-controlled study. Obstet Gynecol. 1991;78(1):33-6.
13. Klauser CK, Fox NS, Istwan N, Rhea D, Rebarber A, Desch C, et al. Treatment of severe nausea and vomiting of pregnancy with subcutaneous medications. Am J Perinatol. 2011;28(09):715-22.
14. Goetzl LM. ACOG Committee on Practice Bulletins-Obstetrics. ACOG Practice Bulletin. Clinical Management Guideline for Obstetrician-Gynecologists Number 36, July 2002. Obstetric analgesia and anesthesia. Obstet Gynecol. 2002;100:177-91.
15. Badell ML, Ramin SM, Smith JA. Treatment options for nausea and vomiting during pregnancy. Pharmacotherapy. 2006;26(9):1273-87.
16. Giugale LE, Young OM, Streitman DC. Iatrogenic Wernicke encephalopathy in a patient with severe hyperemesis gravidarum. Obstet Gynecol. 2015;125(5):1150-2.
17. Katz VL, Farmer R, York J, Wilson JD. Mycobacterium chelonae sepsis associated with long-term use of an intravenous catheter for treatment of hyperemesis gravidarum. A case report. J Reprod Med. 2000;45(7):581-4.
18. Briggs GG, Freeman RK, Yaffe SJ. Drugs in pregnancy and lactation, 7th editon. Philadelphia: Lippincott Williams and Wilkins; 2005. pp. 493, 519, 1059, 1209, 1376.
19. Lee NM, Saha S. Nausea and vomiting of pregnancy. Gastroenterol Clin North Am. 2011;40(2):309-34,
20. Sumona S, Rosanna M. Domperidone for the treatment of severe hyperemesis gravidarum: 512. Am J Gastroenterol. 2007;102:S304.
21. Erick M, Cox JT, Mogensen KM. ACOG practice bulletin 189: nausea and vomiting of pregnancy. Obstet Gynecol. 2018;131(5): 935.

Chapter 24

Constipation and Diarrhea

Sandhya Jain, Pijush Kanti Nandi, Priyanka Shanker

Gastrointestinal (GI) disorders are a very common complaint in pregnancy. Gastrointestinal symptoms such as nausea, vomiting, gastroesophageal reflux, constipation, and diarrhea cause discomfort to the pregnant population at rates similar to or greater than the general nonpregnant population. The dramatic anatomic and physiologic (including hormonal) changes during pregnancy may induce or exacerbate these symptoms. The complaints of constipation and diarrhea can be a regular part of a healthy pregnancy and rarely cause long-term ill effects for the mother or infant or cause significant discomfort and distress.

■ CONSTIPATION IN PREGNANCY

Introduction

Constipation being the second most common GI complaint in pregnant women after nausea and vomiting, defined as dissatisfaction with defecation or as per Rome IV criteria (for functional constipation): ≥2 of the following six symptoms during the last 3-6 months during at least 25% of the defecations—lumpy/hard stools, straining, feeling of incomplete evacuation, a sensation of anorectal obstruction, manual maneuvers to facilitate defecation, and stool frequency <3 times/week.[1]

Constipation during pregnancy occurs in about 11-38%. The symptoms of constipation are seen mostly in the first and second trimesters as compared to the third trimester. Constipation is associated with several risk factors such as a sedentary lifestyle, bed rest, low fiber intake, inadequate intake of fluid, and use of medications, such as iron tablets during pregnancy.[2,3] For no apparent reason, subsequent pregnancies are more prone to develop constipation.[4]

Etiopathogenesis

In general, the etiologies of constipation could be either primary (slow colonic transit vs. pelvic floor dyssynergia) or secondary [such as (1) mechanical obstruction—malignancy, compression, rectocele, and strictures; (2) medications—opioids, tricyclic antidepressants, anticholinergics, calcium channel blockers (CCBs), nonsteroidal anti-inflammatory drugs (NSAIDs), diuretics, Ca^{2+}, Fe, low fiber diet; (3) metabolic/endocrinopathy—diabetes mellitus (DM), hypothyroid, uremia, pregnancy, panhypopituitarism, porphyria, hypercalcemia, hypokalemia, hypomagnesemia; and (4) myopathy/neuropathy—Parkinson's disease, Hirschsprung's disease, amyloid, multiple sclerosis, spinal injury, and dysautonomia].[3]

TABLE 1: Causes of constipation in pregnancy.[2,3,5,6]	
Hormonal factors	• Effect of progesterone on the gastrointestinal tract: – Inhibition of gastric smooth muscle – Decreased colonic smooth muscle contractility – Delayed colonic transit – Prolonged gastric emptying – ↓ Levels of motilin leading to reduced gastric activity – ↑ Aldosterone levels leading to increased colonic water absorption (facilitated by prolonged colonic transit time) • Increased levels of relaxin lead to decreased colonic smooth muscle contractility
Dietary factors	• Lack of fiber • Decreased fluid intake • Associated vomiting • Iron supplementation
Physical activity	• Strenuous exercise may exacerbate • ↓ Level of physical activity
Metabolic	• Diabetes mellitus • Hypothyroidism • Hypercalcemia • Hypokalemia and hypomagnesemia
Mechanical factors	• Fetal compression • Physical impedance due to uterine enlargement • Pregnancy-induced hemorrhoids • Pelvic floor muscle dysfunction • *Colonic disease:* Neoplasm/stricture

Constipation in pregnancy has multiple causes. The etiopathogenesis is summarized in **Table 1**.

Evaluation

It includes a detailed history and physical examination (including per rectal examination), laboratory parameters including complete blood count, blood glucose, electrolytes with Ca and thyroid-stimulating hormone (TSH), and colonoscopy if alarming symptoms. Special evaluation includes an anorectal manometry/balloon expulsion test (to test anorectal structure and function), colonic transit study, and defecography in appropriate situations.[3]

Management

Dietary and lifestyle modifications are the initial treatment of constipation in pregnancy which is similar to that of the general nonpregnant population.

Lifestyle Modifications

Increased fluid intake: It is recommended to increase intake of fluid (>8 glasses/day) to relieve constipation [but no randomized controlled trial (RCT) is available to support this]. Increasing water intake (1.5–2 L/day) may enhance the effects of fiber intake in patients with constipation.[2]

Dietary advice: Evidence supports high-fiber diet consumption (>20–35 g/day) to treat constipation. Dietary fiber can reduce constipation by stimulating the secretion of digestive juices, promoting intestinal peristalsis, and shortening the time of food in the digestive tract. Fiber-rich food such as green leaves and vegetables such as onion, bottle gourd, radish, and brinjal, and fruits such as banana and papaya will help maintain regular bowel movements in pregnancy.[2,3]

Regular use of probiotics during pregnancy increases the frequency of defecation, reduces abdominal tension and pain, and reduces bowel obstruction, and thus could help prevent constipation. Natural probiotics or indirect prebiotics such as yogurt, are both recommended as supplementation.[6]

Physical activity: Strenuous exercise may worsen constipation as compared to light physical activity which can be advised to promote regular bowel function during pregnancy. Swimming, walking, jogging, gymnastics, yoga, climbing stairs, and Kegel exercises can be suitable exercises during pregnancy. Proper activities promote the healthy development of the fetus and the intestinal peristalsis and strengthen the pelvic floor muscles in pregnant women.[2,3]

In addition, enough sleep and maintaining a good mood have beneficial effects on relieving constipation. Intermittent supplementation of iron can be as effective as daily dosing in treating anemia and reducing constipation.

Pharmacological Treatments

A second-line therapy after failure to treat with lifestyle modifications.

Bulk-forming agents: Bulk-forming agents play a role when lifestyle, as well as dietary modifications, do not provide adequate symptomatic relief. Fiber-containing bulk-forming agents such as Methylcellulose (1–4 g/day), ispaghula (psyllium) (3–4 g/day), guar gum, etc., are probably the safest laxatives used in pregnancy as they are not absorbed in the systemic circulation and so may be used for long durations in uncomplicated cases.[2] These agents act by holding water and changing stool consistency. They take several days to exert their effects and are unsuitable for acute symptom relief. They are also contraindicated in fecal impaction. Excessive gas, crampy pain, and abdominal bloating are the adverse effects of bulking agents.[3,6]

Osmotic laxatives: Lactulose and polyethylene glycol (PEG) are examples of osmotic laxatives that create an osmotic gradient, increasing electrolyte secretion and fluid accumulation in the GI lumen. In patients with constipation refractory to dietary fiber, PEG can improve defecation by accelerating colorectal transit and increasing the frequency of bowel movements. Osmotic laxatives have no known fetal risks as the body hardly absorbs these agents.

Stimulant laxatives: Stimulant laxatives [sennosides and bisacodyl (Dulcolax)] are used if patients do not respond to osmotic laxatives. These agents stimulate intestinal motility, induce water and electrolyte secretion, and increase prostaglandin release. They have minimal systemic absorption and appear to be safe in pregnancy.[2] However, side effects, such as abdominal pain and diarrhea limit its use.

In general, the short-term use of stimulating and osmotic laxatives is considered safe in pregnancy.[3] However, as with the general population, long-term use should be avoided as it can cause electrolyte abnormalities. An adequate amount of fluids should be taken along with these agents.[3,6]

Mineral oil (emollient), ricinoleic acid (castor oil), and saline osmotic agents are avoided in pregnancy as mineral oil can cause decreased maternal absorption of fat-soluble vitamins, leading to bleeding and neonatal hypoprothrombinemia.[2] Because of concerns for premature uterine contractions induced by ricinoleic acid and maternal fluid retention from osmotic saline agents (magnesium citrate and sodium phosphate), these agents are not usually recommended. Anthraquinones (senna and cascara sagrada), 5-hydroxytryptamine receptor 4 (5-HT4) agonist, and tegaserod are considered unsafe during pregnancy.[2]

Prosecretory stimulant laxatives: These newer agents increase ion and fluid secretion into the GI lumen. Insufficient data regarding the use of lubiprostone (chloride channel activator), linaclotide, and plecanatide (guanylate cyclase C agonist) in human pregnancies, and potential harmful effects in animal studies, limit its use with caution in pregnancy.

Role of enema: If fecal impaction happens, a glycerin enema is safely recommended. Finger auxiliary to defecate is also helpful. The enemas for pregnant women are not recommended unless there are exceptional circumstances because these agents will cause changes in maternal intra-abdominal pressure and affect the life safety of the fetus.

The commonly used medications for constipation and their safety profile in pregnancy are summarized in **Tables 2 and 3**.

In the case of secondary causes, detailed evaluation (to ascertain the cause) and appropriate management are considered in consultation with specialists.

■ DIARRHEA IN PREGNANCY

Introduction

As compared with constipation in pregnancy, there is less availability of literature on diarrhea in pregnancy. Diarrhea is loosely defined as the passage of abnormally liquid or unformed stools with stool weight >200 g/day (in Western countries) at an increased frequency of three or more/day.[2,3] During pregnancy, diarrheal episodes can be associated with fecal incontinence. Fecal incontinence is the involuntary discharge of rectal contents and is most often caused by structural anorectal problems or neuromuscular disorders.[9]

Types, Prevalence, and Risk Factors

Diarrhea may be classified as acute if <4 weeks and chronic if >4 weeks in duration.[3]

There are very few recent studies that have documented the prevalence of diarrhea in pregnancy. In a previous study in a tertiary care center in South Asia, the prevalence of diarrhea was more rampant in pregnancy (9.2%), especially in the third trimester (13.1%) than before pregnancy (1.6%).[10] Diarrhea that develops at or near term can act as a precursor to labor. The differential diagnosis of both acute as well as chronic diarrhea in pregnancy is similar to that in the general nonpregnant population.

Etiopathogenesis

Acute Infectious Diarrhea

Diarrhea in pregnancy is most commonly caused by acute infections. In developed countries, viruses (such as rotavirus and norovirus) are the most commonly associated with acute diarrhea. The second most common cause after viruses is bacteria: *Escherichia coli*, *Salmonella*, *Shigella* spp., *Vibrio* spp., and *Campylobacter*. *Clostridium difficile*-associated diarrhea (CDAD) should be considered if there is a history of recent usage of antibiotics.[1] In developing countries, the persistence of an acute diarrheal episode beyond 7 days increases the possibility of a protozoal cause, such as giardiasis, cryptosporidiosis, and amebiasis. Lastly, *Listeria* infection should be suspected when diarrhea is present along with flu-like symptoms with or without a recent outbreak of foodborne illness, and it is associated with pregnancy-associated listeriosis and its negative impact on the fetus.[3]

Other causes of acute diarrhea are medications, toxic ingestions, ischemia, food indiscretions, and other conditions.

Besides infectious and inflammatory pathologies, noninfectious, noninflammatory diarrhea may occur during pregnancy because of several causes.[3,9] The common causes of diarrhea in pregnancy are summarized in **Table 4**.

TABLE 2: Medical management of constipation and safety comments in pregnancy.[2,3,7]

Medications		FDA classification	Comments
Bulk-forming agents	Ispaghula (psyllium)	B	• It can be used during pregnancy; generally considered safe • On the basis of the data available, there is no negative impact on the fetus as there is no systemic absorption • It can lead to cramping, bloating, and abdominal discomfort
	Methylcellulose	B	• On the basis of data available, there is no negative impact on the fetus as there is no systemic absorption • It can lead to cramping, bloating, and abdominal discomfort
Osmotic laxatives	Lactulose	B	Animal studies are available with no adverse effects
	PEG	C	Limited data; good option for constipation in pregnancy
	Saline hyperosmotic	X	It can lead to the retention of fluid
Stimulant laxatives	Bisacodyl	C	• Short-term use is generally considered safe; avoid long-term use • Use limited by cramping
	Sennosides	C	Can be used in pregnancy as there is no evidence of negative impact on the fetus
	Ricinoleic acid (castor oil)	X	To be avoided in pregnancy as there is an increased risk of maternal uterine bleeding and spontaneous abortion
Emollient	Mineral oil	X	It can lead to a deficiency of fat-soluble vitamins in the mother, better to be avoided
Prosecretory stimulant laxatives	Lubiprostone	C	Insufficient studies available
	Linaclotide and plecanatide	C	• It assesses risk/benefit during pregnancy • On the basis of the data available, there is no negative impact on the fetus as there is no systemic absorption though some animal studies available showing the risk of fetal malformations
Enema/suppositories	Glycerin suppository	NA	• It can be prescribed during pregnancy • No human data available, though the risk of fetal harm is not expected (based on minimal systemic absorption)

(FDA: Food and Drug Administration; PEG: polyethylene glycol)

TABLE 3: Definition of Food and Drug Administration pregnancy categories.[8]

Food and Drug Administration pregnancy categories*	
Category A	No risk in human studies (studies in pregnant women have not demonstrated a risk to the fetus during the first trimester)
Category B	No risk in animal studies (there are no adequate studies in humans, but animal studies did not demonstrate a risk to the fetus)
Category C	Risk cannot be ruled out. There are no satisfactory studies in pregnant women, but animal studies demonstrated a risk to the fetus; the potential benefits of the drug may outweigh the risks
Category D	Evidence of risk (studies in pregnant women have demonstrated a risk to the fetus; potential benefits of the drug may outweigh the risks)
Category X	Contraindicated (studies in pregnant women have demonstrated a risk to the fetus, and/or human or animal studies have shown fetal abnormalities; risks of the drug outweigh the potential benefits)

*Discontinued June 30, 2015, for biological products and prescription drugs, replaced by the Pregnancy and Lactation Labeling Rule. The latter includes more comprehensive information discussing the potential risks and benefits to the mother and the fetus and how these risks may change during the course of pregnancy based on human and/or animal studies.

Noninfectious Chronic Diarrhea

Like in the general population, in the presence of chronic diarrhea in pregnancy, the clinician must consider noninfectious causes first. Chronic conditions include functional causes such as inflammatory bowel disease (IBD), irritable bowel syndrome (IBS), malabsorption syndromes like celiac disease, osmotic causes like lactose intolerance, and secretory causes like bile acid-induced diarrhea, hyperthyroidism, that can become unmasked or exacerbate during pregnancy.[3] Other pathologies like colorectal malignancy can also be considered in a patient presenting with a recent alteration in the pattern of bowel habit and fecal incontinence.[9]

Evaluation

A detailed history, physical examination, and laboratory investigations should be performed. In acute diarrhea, which is usually self-limiting, further evaluation is needed if any of the following symptoms are present—persistence of diarrhea, weight loss, malnutrition, fever, or signs of dehydration. The stool assessment should be done to rule out infectious causes, and additional workup may be needed to rule out noninfectious causes. The workup of diarrhea in pregnancy is summarized in **Table 5**.

Management

The treatment of diarrhea majorly depends on diagnosis targeting the underlying organic cause when present. Our discussion will focus mainly on treating acute diarrhea, functional causes of chronic diarrhea, and the safety profile of the drugs used in these conditions during pregnancy **(Table 6)**.

Acute Diarrhea

Acute diarrhea is mainly managed conservatively by adequate rehydration, dietary modification, and the judicious use of loperamide. *Clostridium difficile* and *Listeria* infections should be diagnosed early and treated effectively, as these infections carry

TABLE 4: Causes of diarrhea in pregnancy.[2,9,11]	
Acute infection	• Viral • Bacterial • Protozoal
Medications	• Antibiotics • Drugs causing accelerated gastrointestinal (GI) transit
Dietary indiscretion	• Raw food intake • Fiber-rich foods • Calcium-rich milk products • Sugar substitute intake – Mannitol, Sorbitol
Pregnancy-related	• Increased prostaglandins leading to accelerated GI transit • Constipation followed by overflow diarrhea • *Fecal incontinence*: Pelvic floor dysfunction or posterior pelvic floor trauma from a previous pregnancy-associated injury
New onset or exacerbation of preexisting disorders	• Irritable bowel syndrome • Inflammatory bowel disease • Malabsorption • Bile acid diarrhea (postcholecystectomy or ileocolonic resection)

significant morbidity in pregnant patients as well as hurt the fetus.

Fluid Replacement and Dietary Recommendations

Most acute diarrheal episodes are mild and self-limiting. However, the low threshold regarding medical care and fluid replacement should be considered due to the severe risk of dehydration in pregnancy. Mild cases can be managed conservatively with adequate oral rehydration therapy and careful monitoring of serum electrolytes and vitals monitoring of the patient as well as fetal well-being.[1] Oral rehydration solutions (ORS) containing glucose and electrolytes accelerate fluid absorption in the jejunum. However, ORS containing a microbially fermentable nonabsorbable starch (hypoosmolar high-amylose maize starch) is superior, as this allows delivery of a nonabsorbable fermentable starch into the colon, which is then fermented into short-chain fatty acids which further stimulates colonic sodium and fluid absorption.[3] If there is persistence of diarrhea leading to severe dehydration, intravenous (IV) hydration with the correction of electrolyte abnormalities may be required.

Dietary modifications include the intake of small, frequent meals such as salty soups, carbohydrates, fruit juices, and foods that are low in fat and fiber content and without artificial sweeteners.[3,9] Dairy products, except yogurt, should be avoided as enteritis can cause a secondary deficiency of lactase.[9]

Pharmacological Treatments

Role of Antidiarrheal Agents

Opioids: Loperamide is the preferred agent in persistent or severe cases where antidiarrheal agents are needed to decrease stool frequency. It is a peripheral opiate-receptor agonist (mu opiate receptor selective). Loperamide has been found to be associated with a moderate risk of infant malformations, placenta previa, and cesarean section in one registry trial, but in a prospective, controlled multicenter trial, no such association was found, except for lower birth weights. Diphenoxylate with atropine showed adverse events in animal and human studies and should be avoided during pregnancy.[2]

Racecadotril, a drug that inhibits enkephalinase and thereby increases the effects of endogenous opiates on the mu opiate

TABLE 5: Approach of diarrhea during pregnancy.[3,9]

History	• Stool frequency, urgency, incontinence, change in stool caliber, blood in stool, abdominal pain, duration of symptoms [~1 week for viral and bacterial (except *Clostridium difficile*), >1 week for parasitic], history of constipation, history of immunocompromised state, extraintestinal symptoms such as rash, joint pains, neurologic dysfunction, and urinary incontinence • *Diet:* Change in diet, sugar-free or fat-free products, and artificial sweeteners • History of medication use • Prior pregnancy and vaginal delivery with complications • *Risk of infection:* Children/working in daycare, history of travel, and antibiotic use • *History of surgeries:* Anorectal surgery, bowel resection, ileal pouch-anal anastomosis, and cholecystectomy • Prior diagnosis of a diarrheal disorder (irritable bowel syndrome, inflammatory bowel disease, and lactose intolerance)	
Physical examination	• *General physical examination:* Signs of volume depletion (vital status, urine output, axillae, skin turgor, mental status), fever, abdominal tenderness, ileus, and rash • *Perianal area examination:* Skin lesions, perianal sensation, pelvic descent with simulated defecation, and rectal prolapse • *Digital rectal examination:* Rectal mass, sphincter tone at rest, with a squeeze and with simulated defecation	
Laboratory investigations	Stool and blood workup (for infectious, inflammatory, or systemic causes)	• *Blood:* Electrolytes, C-reactive protein, thyroid function test, celiac serology, serologies, and blood culture if suspecting *Listeria* • *Stool:* Culture, Giardia antigen, ova, and parasites, *Clostridioides difficile* toxin, and fecal calprotectin
	Imaging	Flexible sigmoidoscopy and magnetic resonance imaging pelvis (consider if warning signs of fever, severe abdominal pain, blood, or pus in the stool, >6 stools/day, severe dehydration, immunosuppressed states, duration >7 days, hospital-acquired)

receptor (along with delta opiate receptor effects), is available for treating acute diarrhea in some countries.[2,3] Still, it should not be administered to pregnant women since no specific clinical studies are available.

Bismuth preparations: Bismuth subsalicylate works by reducing the number of unformed stools and symptoms in the general nonpregnant population, is not recommended during pregnancy, especially in the second and third trimesters, due to the potential teratogenic risks caused by subsalicylate, such as prolonged labor and gestation, decreased birth weight, neonatal hemorrhage, and increased perinatal mortality.[3,9]

Bile acid sequestrants: Bile acid sequestrants (colestipol or cholestyramine) can be used in the management of bile acid-induced diarrhea and irritable bowel syndrome-diarrhea (IBS-D). Bile acid sequestrants may cause fat-soluble vitamin deficiency as they interfere with the absorption of fat-soluble vitamins, leading to maternal coagulopathy.[3] Patients on regular therapy with these agents

TABLE 6: Commonly used drugs.

Name	Dosage	Route	Mechanism of action	Maximum dosage	Side effects	Contraindications
Ispaghula (psyllium)	5–10 g daily (single dose)	Oral	Psyllium husk is capable of absorbing 40 times of its own weight in water. GI tract motility and transit rate is capable of being modified by psyllium husk via mechanical stimulation of the gut wall as a result of an increase in intestinal bulk by water and a decrease in viscosity of luminal contents	No universal guideline	• Hives or rash • Wheezing • Sudden severe Diarrhea • Shortness of breath • Swelling of face, lips, tongue, or throat	• People who are allergic to psyllium • Phenylketonuria
Methylcellulose	Two tablets (1,000 mg)	Oral	Absorbs water in the GI lumen thereby increasing the bulk of stool and stimulation of peristalsis	Not to exceed 12 tablets/day	• Allergic reactions • Choking can lead to chest pains, trouble swallowing, and vomiting	• GI ulceration • Rectal bleeding • Symptoms of appendicitis or acute surgical abdomen
Lactulose	15–30 mL (1–2 tablespoons/day)	Oral	Causes retention of water through osmosis leading to softer, easier-to-pass stool	60 mL/day	• Diarrhea • Bloating • Burping • Nausea • Vomiting	
Bisacodyl	5–15 mg once daily	Oral	• Irritate smooth muscles of the intestine to increase peristalsis • Also increases intestinal fluid accumulation	30 mg	• Diarrhea • Nausea • Vomiting • Electrolyte and fluid imbalance	• Hypersensitivity • Obstruction of GI tract • Rectal bleeding • Symptoms of appendicitis or acute surgical abdomen

Contd...

Contd...

Name	Dosage	Route	Mechanism of action	Maximum dosage	Side effects	Contraindications
Loperamide	4 mg	Oral	Works by acting on mu-opioid receptors in the gut which in turn slows down contraction in the intestine	16 mg	• Stomach pain • Diarrhea • Bloating • Arrhythmia	• Ulcerative colitis • Bloody or tarry stool • Diarrhea with high fever
Diphenoxylate/atropine combination	Available as a 2.5 mg/0.025 fixed-dose tablet	Oral	GI propulsion is inhibited through direct action on the smooth muscle resulting in a peristaltic action	Maximum eight tablets	• Bloating • Constipation • Diarrhea • Difficulty swallowing • Drowsiness	• Known hypersensitivity • Pseudomembranous enterocolitis
Racecadotril	100 mg	Oral	Produces an antisecretory effect, and reduces the secretion of water and electrolytes from the intestine	300 mg	• Vomiting • Dizziness • Headache	• Diarrhea associated with purulent or bloody stools • Antibiotic-associated diarrhea
Bismuth subsalicylate	Two tablespoons every 0.5–1 hour	Oral	Causes reduction in prostaglandin formation as it inhibits cyclooxygenase	Not >16 tablespoons	• Darkening of stool • Vomiting • Diarrhea	• Allergy • G6PD deficiency
Cholestyramine (bile acid sequestrant)	4 mg	Oral	By removing excess bile, cholestyramine can help ease bile acid diarrhea	8–24 g	• Constipation • Diarrhea • Vomiting • Nausea • Stomach pain	• Allergic • Phenylketonuria
Ciprofloxacin	500 mg twice daily	Oral—intravenous	Being a bactericidal antibiotic, it inhibits DNA replication	1,000 mg once a day	• Nausea • Diarrhea • Prolonged QT interval • Hyperglycemia • Hypoglycemia	• Hypersensitivity • Myasthenia gravis

Contd...

Contd...

Name	Dosage	Route	Mechanism of action	Maximum dosage	Side effects	Contraindications
Ofloxacin	200 mg twice a day	Oral—intravenous	• Active against both gram-positive and gram-negative • Inhibits bacterial cell division	800 mg	• Diarrhea • Vomiting • Nausea	• Contraindication in pregnancy as animal studies have shown • Decreased fetal body weight and increased fetal mortality
Metronidazole	400 mg 8 hourly	Oral—intravenous	Used in the treatment of certain anaerobic bacterial and protozoal infections	4 g/day	• Nausea • Anorexia • Abdominal pain • Glossitis • QT prolongation • Hepatotoxicity	• Hypersensitivity • First trimester
Trimethoprim/sulfamethoxazole	160 mg/800 mg BD	Oral	The combination of these two agents creates a synergistic antifolate effect, hence acting in a bacteriostatic manner		• Loss of appetite • Nausea • Vomiting • Dyspepsia • Tinnitus • Rash	• Pregnancy • Liver parenchymal disease • Hematological disorder • Renal insufficiency
Rifaximin	400 mg	Oral	• Used to treat IBS-D • Broad-spectrum bactericidal activity against gram-positive and gram-negative aerobic and anaerobic bacteria	1,200 mg	• Loss of appetite • Stomach pain • Nausea • Headache	• Hypersensitivity • Severe hepatic impairment

(DNA: deoxyribonucleic acid; GI: gastrointestinal; G6PD: glucose-6-phosphate dehydrogenase; IBS-D: irritable bowel syndrome with diarrhea) should be advised to check frequently for fat-soluble vitamin deficiency and deranged clotting function.

Role of Antibiotics in Acute Infectious Diarrhea

Empiric antibiotics are routinely not advised in the management of acute diarrhea as symptoms are often mild, short-lived, and mostly of viral origin. Antibiotics should be advised in patients presenting with symptoms suggestive of invasive bacterial infection like bloody stools and, also in severe cases requiring hospitalization. Many antibiotics that are used to treat infectious diarrhea in the general nonpregnant population are contraindicated throughout or during specific gestation periods; these include metronidazole which is avoided in the first trimester as it has a potential risk of congenital disabilities in the fetus, tetracyclines in the last half of pregnancy as it is associated with risk of hepatotoxicity in the mother and potential for permanent teeth discoloration in the fetus and impairment of fetal long bone growth, and sulfa antibiotics which causes potential congenital malformations in the first-trimester use as well as jaundice and hemolytic anemia in the last month of pregnancy. In all these cases, antibiotics having a safer pregnancy profile, such as β-lactams including aminopenicillin (amoxicillin/ampicillin), cephalosporins, all erythromycins (except estolate), and metronidazole (after the first trimester) should be recommended.[2,9]

The American College of Obstetricians and Gynecologists (ACOG) recommends high-dose aminopenicillin (ampicillin intravenously 6–12 g/day or amoxicillin orally 100 mg/kg/day) for at least 14 days or until delivery for *Listeria monocytogenes*-induced diarrhea. The Infectious Diseases Society of America recommends vancomycin 125 mg four times daily or fidaxomicin 200 mg twice daily for 10 days to treat *C. difficile*-associated diarrhea. Both these antibiotics are safe to use in pregnancy.[12,13]

The safety profile of different antibiotics used for diarrhea during pregnancy is summarized in **Table 7**.

Role of Probiotics

Probiotics (nonpathogenic microorganisms) are usually not advised for acute diarrhea except in cases of postantibiotic-associated illness. In previous studies, the use of probiotics during pregnancy did not show any negative impact on childbirth, maternal, or infant outcomes.[9]

Chronic Diarrhea

In case of exacerbation of chronic functional diarrhea or irritable bowel syndrome (IBS-D), antidiarrheal agents (including bile acid sequestrants), 5-hydroxytryptamine type 3 (5-HT3) antagonists (ondansetron preferred over alosetron during pregnancy), and nonabsorbed oral antibiotic rifaximin (to be avoided in the first trimester) are prescribed.[2] Although, eluxadoline (a peripherally acting mixed kappa-opioid and mu-opioid receptor agonist/delta-opioid receptor antagonist) has been approved by the United States Food and Drug Administration (US FDA) in treating IBS-D in the general population, has no reports available of its use in human pregnancy at this time. Antispasmodics, selective serotonin reuptake inhibitors, and tricyclic antidepressants should only be used in severely symptomatic cases of IBS-D during pregnancy.[9] Managing cause-specific chronic diarrhea and fecal incontinence during pregnancy requires

TABLE 7: Medical management of diarrhea and irritable bowel syndrome (IBS-D).[2,3,9,12,13]

Medications		FDA classification	Comments
Antidiarrheal agents	Loperamide	C	• Weigh risk/benefit during pregnancy • *Human study:* Possible risk of teratogenicity • Contraindicated in bloody diarrhea
	Diphenoxylate with atropine	C	• To be avoided during pregnancy • Weigh risk/benefit during pregnancy if needed, especially in the third trimester • *Human studies:* Risk of fetal harm not expected, though the possible risk of neonatal respiratory depression and withdrawal seizures with near-term use
	Racecadotril	NA	• No specific clinical studies available • Should not be administered to pregnant women
	Bismuth subsalicylate	• C • D (in the third trimester)	• Weigh risk/benefit if <20 weeks gestation • *Human studies:* Avoid use starting at 20 weeks gestation (possible risk of fetal harm, including renal dysfunction and oligohydramnios, and premature fetal ductus arteriosus closure, starting at 30 weeks gestation)
	Bile acid sequestrant (cholestyramine)	C	• Weigh the risk/benefit during pregnancy, especially with prolonged use • Possible risk of fetal fat-soluble vitamin deficiency
Antibiotics	*Aminopenicillins:* Ampicillin/amoxicillin	B	Effective and safe (especially for Listeria)
	Cephalosporins	B	Effective and safe (third generations—for *Shigella* and *Salmonella*)
	Vancomycin	C	• May be used during pregnancy • Effective and low-risk (oral therapy for *Clostridium difficile*-associated diarrhea)
	Erythromycins (stearate) and azithromycin	B*	Effective and safe (especially for *Campylobacter jejuni*)
	Fidaxomicin	—	• Safe and may be used during pregnancy (for *C. difficile*-associated diarrhea) • *Human:* Insufficient data • *Animal:* Nontoxic

Contd...

Contd...

Medications		FDA classification	Comments
	Fluoroquinolones (ciprofloxacin and ofloxacin)	C	• Effective and low-risk (for *C. jejuni*, *Shigella*, and *Salmonella*) • Weigh risk/benefit during pregnancy • *Human data:* No known risk of teratogenicity, and possible risk of spontaneous abortion • *Animal data:* Risk of bone/cartilage damage
	Metronidazole	B	• May be used during pregnancy (used for giardiasis and amebiasis) (effective and low-risk in the second and third trimesters) • Avoided in the first trimester • *Human studies:* Possible risk of teratogenicity and the potential risk of spontaneous abortion
	Nitazoxanide	B	• Weigh risk/benefit during use in pregnancy (for cryptosporidiosis and giardiasis) • *Human:* Insufficient data • *Animal:* Nontoxic
	Trimethoprim/sulfamethoxazole (third trimester)	C	• Effective (for traveler's diarrhea and *Shigellosis*) and high-risk • Avoided in pregnancy • *Sulfamethoxazole:* Weigh risk/benefit during pregnancy, especially in the third trimester • *Human data:* Risk of kernicterus near-term • *Trimethoprim:* Consider risk/benefit during pregnancy, especially in the first trimester • *Human data:* Possible risk of abortion, possible risk of the congenital neural tube and cardiovascular defects
	Rifaximin	C	• Weigh risk/benefit during pregnancy [used in case of *Escherichia coli*-associated (ETEC and EAEC) traveler's diarrhea] • On the basis of the data available, there is no negative impact on the fetus as there is no or minimal systemic absorption • Though some animal data available showing risks of teratogenicity in the first trimester

Contd...

Contd...

Medications			FDA classification	Comments
IBS-D medications	Antispasmodics	Dicyclomine	B	• Can be prescribed during pregnancy • *Human data:* No known risk of fetal harm
		Hyoscyamine	C	Only used during pregnancy if needed
	Selective serotonin reuptake inhibitors	Fluoxetine	C	Adverse events in animal studies
		Paroxetine	D	Known fetal teratogenic effects
	Tricyclic antidepressants	Amitriptyline	C	• Weigh risk/benefit during pregnancy, especially in the third trimester • *Human data:* Risk of teratogenicity not expected
		Nortriptyline	D	• Weigh risk/benefit during pregnancy, especially in the third trimester • *Human data:* Possible risk of teratogenicity
		Desipramine	C	Generally, not recommended

*All except estolate—estolate should be avoided in pregnancy because of drug-related hepatotoxicity.

specialist intervention and assistance from an obstetrician, respectively.

Table 7 lists the drugs commonly used to treat diarrhea and IBS-D in pregnancy and their safety information.

Pregnancy causes several hormonal and/or anatomical changes that induce or exacerbate many GI problems in the pregnant population, including constipation and diarrhea. Most patients with these symptoms respond to oral rehydration, lifestyle, and dietary modifications. Whenever aggressive pharmacotherapy is needed, understanding the underlying pathophysiology is of utmost importance to guide treatment.

When selecting medications in pregnancy, the drug-related descriptive safety statement [Pregnancy and Lactation Labeling Rule (PLLR) system], which is based on animal and human studies accurately and effectively expressing the teratogenic and reproductive risks associated with drug exposure should be considered.

■ KEY POINTS

- Pregnancy causes several hormonal and/or anatomical changes that induce or exacerbate many gastrointestinal problems in the pregnant population, including constipation and diarrhea. Most patients with these symptoms respond to oral rehydration, lifestyle, and dietary modifications. Understanding the underlying pathophysiology is of utmost importance to guide treatment.

- After a thorough ongoing literature search, the most effective and safe therapeutic approach should be planned, considering maternal and fetal health and well-being when treating these symptoms in pregnancy. When selecting medications in pregnancy, the drug-related descriptive safety statement (PLLR system), based on animal and human studies accurately and effectively expressing the teratogenic and reproductive risks associated with drug exposure, is considered instead of the FDA pregnancy categories.

REFERENCES

1. Zielinski R, Searing K, Deibel M. Gastrointestinal distress in pregnancy: prevalence, assessment, and treatment of 5 common minor discomforts. J Perinat Neonatal Nurs. 2015;29(1):23-31.
2. Body C, Christie JA. Gastrointestinal Diseases in Pregnancy: Nausea, Vomiting, Hyperemesis Gravidarum, Gastroesophageal Reflux Disease, Constipation, and Diarrhea. Gastroenterol Clin North Am. 2016;45(2):267-83.
3. In: Feldman M, Friedman LS, and Brandt LJ (Eds). Sleisenger and Fordtran's Gastrointestinal and Liver Disease, 11th edition. Philadelphia: Saunders Elsevier; 2021.
4. Hestiantoro A, Baidah PA. The Prevalence and Risk Factors of Constipation in Pregnancy. Indones J Obstet Gynecol. 2018;6(2):84-8.
5. Fan W, Kang J, Xiao X, Li L, Yang X. Causes of constipation during pregnancy and health management. Int J Clin Exp Med. 2020;13(3):2022-6.
6. Cullen G, O'Donoghue D. Constipation and pregnancy. Best Pract Res Clin Gastroenterol. 2007;21(5):807-18.
7. Epocrates. Epocrates [online]. Available from: https://online.epocrates.com/drugs [Last accessed December, 2023].
8. Jessica C, Arif HL. Pregnancy Medications. Continuing Education Activities. In: Treasure Island (FL): StatPearls Publishing; 2023.
9. Menees SB, Lembo A, Charabaty A. Fecal Incontinence and Diarrhea During Pregnancy. Am J Gastroenterol. 2022; 117(10S):26-32.
10. Sharma JB, Karmakar D, Aggarwal S, Singhal S, Roy KK, Kumar S. Prevalence of gastro-intestinal symptoms during pregnancy: a questionnaire based study in a tertiary care center of South Asia. Int J Reprod Contracept Obstet Gynecol. 2014; 3(1):87-91.
11. Christie J, Rose S. Constipation, diarrhea, hemorrhoids, and fecal incontinence. In: Pregnancy in gastrointestinal disorders. Bethesda (MD): ACG Monograph American College of Physicians; 2007. pp. 4-9.
12. Play.google.com. Sanford Guide [Mobile application software]. [online] Available from: https://play.google.com/store/apps [Last accessed December, 2023].
13. Wald A. Constipation, diarrhea, and symptomatic hemorrhoids during pregnancy. Gastroenterol Clin North Am. 2003; 32(1):309-22,vii.

PART B: GYNECOLOGY

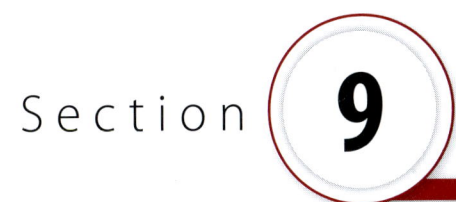

Section 9

Medical Management of Menstrual Disorders

- **Abnormal Uterine Bleeding**
  Latha Chaturvedula, Syed Habeebullah

- **Fibroids**
  Sumitra Yadav, Pooja Verma

- **Endometriosis**
  Archana Maurya, Vanshika Pundhir

Chapter 25

Abnormal Uterine Bleeding

Latha Chaturvedula, Syed Habeebullah

Abnormal uterine bleeding (AUB) refers to bleeding from uterine corpus that is abnormal in quantity, duration, and cyclicity—all these in the absence of pregnancy. It is of two types: (1) Chronic which is present for 6 months or more and (2) Acute which is sufficient enough to cause hemodynamic instability and warrants immediate treatment including hospitalization. As per the International Federation of Gynecology and Obstetrics (FIGO) (2018), the causes of AUB are either structural—polyp, adenomyosis, leiomyoma and malignancy (PALM), and hyperplasia or nonstructural—coagulopathy, ovulatory dysfunction, endometrial, iatrogenic and not otherwise classified (COEIN).[1]

Since the most common symptom of AUB is heavy menstrual bleeding (HMB), the drugs used are mainly to control HMB **(Box 1)**. The choice depends on the age, amount of bleeding, need for fertility, and associated pathology.

■ NONHORMONAL TREATMENT

Usually, they are the first-line drugs for AUB. But they are not very effective. The advantages of nonhormonal medications are:
- They need to be used only during menstruation thus reducing the cost and inconvenience.

BOX 1: Medications for abnormal uterine bleeding (AUB).
- The initial medications in the management of AUB can be nonhormonal or hormonal
- Mild excess bleeding with good hemoglobin levels treated with iron therapy
- Moderate/severe bleeding treated with nonhormonal/hormonal therapy
- Severe bleeding/severe anemia requires blood transfusion besides hormonal therapy
- Acute AUB is initially treated with hormones along with supportive measures
- Coagulopathy is treated with antifibrinolytic agents, combined oral contraceptives (COCs) and desmopressin

- They do not interfere with fertility.

The drugs commonly used are antifibrinolytic agents (tranexamic acid) and nonsteroidal anti-inflammatory drugs (NSAIDs).

Tranexamic acid acts by blocking the lysine binding sites on plasminogen resulting in reduced clot breakdown. It reduces flow by 40%.[2] It can be used in acute and chronic AUB. There is no increased risk of thrombosis with its usage.

Nonsteroidal anti-inflammatory drugs increase platelet aggregation and help in clot formation by blocking prostacyclin formation which is a vasodilator. They reduce blood loss by 25–50%.[3] They are used in patients with mild heavy bleeding with good Hb levels. They

TABLE 1: Commonly used nonhormonal agents in abdominal uterine bleeding (AUB).

Drug	Dosage	Side effects	Contraindications
Tranexamic acid	1 g TID orally	Nausea, vomiting, and headache	History of venous thromboembolism, impaired color vision
NSAIDs: • Mefenamic acid • Naproxen • Ibuprofen	All taken orally with food: • 500 mg TID with the onset of bleeding • 500 mg stat, 250–500 mg BD • 600 mg TID/QID	• Mostly common to all drugs in the group • Nausea, abdominal pain, and renal effects	• Renal dysfunction, coagulation disorders, inflammatory bowel disease, and asthma • Should be avoided in patients with coagulation disorders and platelet function abnormality
Ethamsylate	500 mg QID	Nausea, vomiting, skin rash, and headache	Asthma, porphyria, and breastfeeding
Desmopressin	0.3 µg/kg SC. If given IV diluted in 50–100 mL saline given over 30 minutes Rpt 12–24 hours	Flushing, headache, and tachycardia	Warmth and redness in face, fluid retention, hyponatremia

(NSAIDs: nonsteroidal anti-inflammatory drugs)

are less effective compared to tranexamic acid and levonorgestrel-releasing intrauterine system (LNG-IUS) but cheaper.[4] They should not be used if there is a coagulation disorder. They decrease cyclo-oxygenase enzyme and help in reducing inflammation and pain. Thus, they relieve dysmenorrhea too. When there is moderate to severe heavy menstrual bleeding with dysmenorrhea, a combination of tranexamic acid and mefenamic acid can be given. But the combination is expensive. Commonly used nonhormonal agents are described in **Table 1**.

Ethamsylate maintains capillary integrity has antihyaluronidase activity and inhibitory effect on PGs. Dosage is 500 mg QID starting 5 days before periods and continued for 10 days. It is expensive compared to NSAIDs and less effective than tranexamic acid in AUB.[5] It is not commonly used in practice.

Desmopressin is a vasopressin analog that helps in release of von Willebrand factor from its storage sites in endothelial cells and platelets. It is indicated for patients with mild-to-moderate classic von Willebrand's disease (Type I) with factor VIII levels >5%. The dosage is 300 µg given as puff in each nostril daily on days 2 and 3 of menstrual cycle.[6] To treat severe bleeding in von Willebrand disease, recombinant factor VIII and von Willebrand factor are used.

HORMONAL TREATMENT OF ABNORMAL UTERINE BLEEDING

Hormonal treatment is considered when there is no response to nonhormonal treatment in mild heavy bleeding and also in moderate/severe heavy bleeding. In acute AUB it is the first-line management. The commonly used hormones are given in **Box 2**.

PROGESTINS

In Heavy Menstrual Bleeding

Progestins are used to treat HMB and regularize the cycles in all age groups. They are used initially to stop the bleeding and then cyclically. They inhibit estrogen-receptor levels, convert estradiol to less potent estrone, and also make the endometrium atrophic when used for longer duration by inhibiting the mitotic activity of endometrial cells. The commonly used oral progestins are medroxy-progesterone acetate (MPA) and norethisterone acetate (NETA). The LNG-IUS contains 52 mg of the drug in its vertical arm and releases 20 μg of the drug daily. The systemic side effects are minimal and the efficacy is better than most of the other agents. Depot-medroxy-progesterone acetate (DMPA) 150 mg deep IM every 3 months has side effects similar to oral progestins. The dosages are shown in **Table 2**.

In Endometrial Hyperplasia without Atypia

The treatment of choice is LNG-IUS. If not willing, continuous administration of MPA 10–20 mg/day, or NET 10–15 mg/day. Cyclical usage is associated with less regression. Also, oral medications are less effective than LNG-IUS. This is continued for at least 6 months. Follow-up is with endometrial biopsy after 6 months. LNG-IUS can be retained for 5 years if needed. However, recent studies have shown that dienogest 2 mg given for 14 days cyclically was more effective than NETA 15 mg.[7]

In Endometrial Hyperplasia with Atypia

In these patients the usual treatment is total hysterectomy with bilateral salpingo-oophorectomy. However, in some pre-menopausal patients who are at low risk of developing ovarian cancer, ovaries can be retained with removal of uterus and fallopian

> **BOX 2:** Commonly used hormones.
>
> - Oral progestins
> - Levonorgestrel intrauterine system (LNG-IUS)
> - Injectable progestins
> - Combined oral contraceptive pills (COCs)
> - Estrogens
> - Estrogen receptor modulators, progesterone receptor modulators
> - Androgens (Danazol)
> - Gonadotropin-releasing hormone (GnRH) analogs

TABLE 2: Progestins and their dosages in heavy menstrual bleeding (HMB).

Preparation	Dosage to stop bleeding	Cyclical maintenance	Remarks
Medroxy-progesterone acetate (MPA)	10–20 mg TID/QID orally till bleeding stops (1–3 days); then 10 mg BD × 10–15 days	• *In anovulatory cycles:* 10 mg BD from day 16 × 10 days • *In ovulatory cycles:* 10 mg BD from D 5 × 21 days	
Norethisterone (NET)	5 mg TID oral till bleeding stops; then BD × 10–15 days	5 mg BD as above	
LNG-IUS	–	After insertion can be retained for 5 years	First-line choice for most of PALM-COEIN cases
Depot-Medroxy-progesterone acetate (DMPA)	–	Injection 150 mg deep IM every 3 months	Cheap. Provides contraception

(LNG-IUS: levonorgestrel intrauterine system)

tubes. In younger patients wanting to retain fertility, LNG-IUS or oral MPA/NET can be used in higher doses. They should be followed up with 3 monthly endometrial biopsies till two negative reports before they plan their pregnancies. Subsequently, annual follow-up is done.

Contraindications for progestins include history of thromboembolic disease, impaired liver function and breast cancer.

Side effects: Headache, dizziness, hair loss, fluid retention, insomnia, menstrual irregularity, low mood, and skin reactions.[8]

COMBINED ORAL CONTRACEPTIVES (BOX 3)

Estradiol valerate and dienogest-containing OCPs are shown to be effective in AUB with less thromboembolic and metabolic side effects.[9]

- Dienogest-containing OCPs are equally effective with less side effects in adenomyosis.[10,11]
- They can also be used continuously for a long period.

ESTROGEN RECEPTOR MODULATORS

Ormeloxifene (Centchroman)

It is a third-generation selective estrogen receptor modulator (SERM). It has both estrogenic and antiestrogenic activity. It is a nonsteroidal drug used originally for contraception; being also used to treat HMB for over 2 decades. The dosage is 60 mg twice weekly for 12 weeks followed by once weekly for next 12 weeks. Marked improvement was noted at 6 months in over 80% of perimenopausal women treated for acute HMB.[12] The side effects are minimal and include nausea, vomiting, weight gain, headache, and delayed menses.

> **BOX 3:** Combined oral contraceptives.
> - Useful to control acute bleeding in abnormal uterine bleeding (AUB)
> - Work well in AUB due to ovulatory dysfunction. Can be used to control bleeding in fibroids and adenomyosis
> - Reduce bleeding by 50%, relieve dysmenorrhea
> - Help in control of cycles and provide contraception
> - In the long term, they reduce the risk of ovarian and endometrial cancer
> - They are cheaper
> - Usually low-dose pills (estrogen 20–30 µg + progestin 0.5–0.75 mg) once daily are used except in acute bleeding where estrogen 50 µg is used two to three times daily till bleeding stops; then switched to low-dose pills once daily for at least 15 days. Then to be continued for three cycles
> - Contraindications include history of thromboembolic disorders, ischemic/valvular heart disease, liver dysfunction, migraine, current or past breast cancer and smokers over 35 years of age

PROGESTERONE RECEPTOR MODULATORS

Table 3 describes progesterone receptor modulators and their efficacy.

ANDROGENS

Danazol is a synthetic androgen, causes endometrial atrophy by inhibiting secretion of follicle-stimulating hormone (FSH) and luteinizing hormone (LH). At a dose of 200 mg daily orally, it is more effective than NSAIDs, COCs, and progestogens in HMB. But, the androgenic side effects (acne, reduced breast size, hirsutism, and deepening voice) that occur in the majority are unacceptable to most women.[16]

GONADOTROPHIC-RELEASING HORMONE AGONISTS

- They act by suppressing the release of FSH and LH thus producing pseudomenopause.

TABLE 3: Progesterone receptor modulators and efficacy.

Drug	Dosage	Efficacy	Side effects
Ulipristal acetate[13]	5–10 mg daily for 12 weeks. After 1 month another course of 12 weeks	Controls HMB in 90%, amenorrhea in 70%, fibroid size ↓ 45%	Hepatotoxicity. LFT done before tt and every month
Mifepristone[14]	10–25 mg daily × 12 weeks	• HMB control in 95% • Amenorrhea 84%	Headache, breast tenderness. Concern about endometrial hyperplasia
Asoprisnil[15]	10 mg daily	Highly effective in fibroid; ↓blood loss, size and amenorrhea	Mild ↑ endometrial thickness

(LFT: liver function test; HMB: heavy menstrual bleeding)

- They are effective in reducing blood loss in HMB associated with AUB-L.
- They take 1–2 weeks to stop bleeding; hence not useful in acute AUB.
- Though they reduce the size of fibroids, after stoppage of treatment, the fibroids start growing.
- They can be used 2–3 months prior to hysterectomy for AUB-L thus getting time to improve anemia and reduce operative blood loss.[17]
- The side effects include hot flushes, headaches, vaginal dryness, reduced libido, and reduced bone mineral density when used for prolonged periods.[18]
- The dosage of leuprolide acetate is 3.75 mg IM monthly for not >6 months.
  Other drugs in the group are nafarelin (200 µg intranasally twice daily) and goserelin (3.6 mg SC monthly). To reduce the side effects, add back therapy (estrogen + progestogen) is used.
- They are expensive.

GONADOTROPHIC-RELEASING HORMONE ANTAGONISTS

Gonadotropin-releasing hormone antagonists—elagolix, relugolix, and linzagolix used orally in fibroids reduce blood loss and size of fibroids. Elagolix 300 mg orally twice daily with low dose add back therapy was effective in control of HMB in fibroids with less significant side effects of hypogonadism mentioned above.[19] Linzagolix 100 mg once daily without add back therapy may also be useful in fibroids. But, these drugs are very expensive and hence have limited use.[20]

ESTROGENS

When bleeding is heavy, patient needs hospitalization for blood transfusion and if needed IV fluids. To arrest bleeding high-dose combined OCPs or progestins are given orally. Usually, bleeding stops in 2 days. Tranexamic acid orally also can be supplemented. When available injection conjugated equine estrogen 25 mg IV 4-6 hourly for 24 hours is used. This arrests the bleeding rapidly. Then OCPs/progestin are continued for 15 days. Contraindications for estrogens include risk of arterial/venous thromboembolism, breast cancer, and hepatic dysfunction.[21]

Table 4 summarizes the medical management of HMB in PALM COEIN conditions.

TABLE 4: Summary of medical management of HMB in PALM-COEIN conditions.[22]

Condition	First-line Mx	Second-line Mx	Remarks
Polyp	LNG-IUS (after hysteroscopic polypectomy)	GnRHa, progestins	Recurrence after stoppage high
Adenomyosis	LNG-IUS	GnRHa + add back. NSAIDs, COCs, oral progestins	Dienogest very promising
Leiomyoma	*Wanting fertility:* NSAIDs, COCs, Tranexamic acid	*Delay fertility:* LNG-IUS, ulipristal, mifepristone	LNG-IUS only when cavity regular
Malignancy/end hyperplasia	*Atypical hyperplasia, fertility sparing:* LNG-IUS	High-dose oral MPA/Megestrol acetate	Pregnancy after 3 monthly negative EBs twice
Coagulation abnormality	Tranexamic acid, COCs	LNG-IUS. *In von Willebrand disease:* Desmopressin, factor replacement	NSAIDs contraindicated
Ovulation dysfunction	*Not desiring fertility:* Low-dose of COCs, Oral progestins from D5 to 25	*Desiring fertility:* Oral progestins in second half of cycle	
Endometrial	Oral tranexamic acid + mefenamic acid	Low dose of OCPs, LNG-IUS	
Iatrogenic	*Poststerilization/IUCD HMB:* NSAIDs/Tranexamic acid	For break through bleeding with OCPs: Lasts 1–3 months, assurance	
Not otherwise classified	Tranexamic acid, NSAIDs	*If contraception needed:* OCPs, LNG-IUS	Rarely GnRHa

(COCs: combined oral contraceptive pills; GnRHa: gonadotrophin-releasing hormone agonists; HMB: heavy menstrual bleeding; IUCD: intrauterine contraceptive device; LNG-IUS: levonorgestrel intrauterine system; NSAIDs: nonsteroidal anti-inflammatory drugs; OCP: oral contraceptive pills)

■ KEY POINTS

- The first-line management of abdominal uterine bleeding is usually medical.
- Iron therapy alone is recommended in mild cases with good Hb.
- In acute/severe bleeding with severe anemia, blood transfusion is given.
- Nonsteroidal anti-inflammatory drugs are 40% effective in HMB, also relieve dysmenorrhea.
- Tranexamic acid is 50% effective. Can be combined with NSAIDs.
- Ethamsylate is less effective than tranexamic acid; not commonly used.
- Hormonal treatment is first line in acute AUB.
- Oral progestins can be used to arrest bleeding and regularize the cycles.
- Levonorgestrel intrauterine system provides long-term relief from AUB; can be used in AUB due to adenomyosis, some fibroids and endometrial hyperplasias.
- Combined oral contraceptive pills are effective in controlling bleeding besides giving relief from dysmenorrhea, regularizing the cycles, and provide contraception.
- Androgens (danazol) though effective are not used due to androgenic side effects.
- Selective estrogen receptor modulators (SERM) (ormeloxifene) can be used to control bleeding.

- Selective progesterone receptor modulators—ulipristal with some risk of liver toxicity and mifepristone with some risks of endometrial hyperplasia are being used in fibroid associated HMB; expensive.
- Gonadotropin-releasing hormone agonists and antagonists along with add back therapy can be used in HMB in fibroids. They are very expensive.

REFERENCES

1. Munro MG, Critchley HO, Fraser IS for the FIGO Menstrual Disorders Committee. The two FIGO systems for normal and abnormal uterine bleeding symptoms and classification of causes of abnormal uterine bleeding in the reproductive years: 2018 revisions. Int J Gynecol Obstet. 2018;143:393-408. Erratum in: Int J Gynecol Obstet. 2019;144(2):237.
2. Lukes AS, Moore KA, Muse KN, Gersten JK, Hecht BR, Edlund M, et al. Tranexamic acid treatment for heavy menstrual bleeding: a randomized controlled trial. Obstet Gynecol. 2010;116(4):865-75.
3. Cameron IT, Haining R, Lumsden MA, Thomas VR, Smith SK. The effects of mefenamic acid and norethisterone on measured menstrual blood loss. Obstet Gynecol. 1990;76(1),85-8.
4. Bofill Rodriguez M, Lethaby A, Farquhar C. Non-steroidal anti-inflammatory drugs for heavy menstrual bleeding. Cochrane Database Syst Rev. 2019.
5. Deeksha T, Ashok Kumar M, Suresh G. A Comparative Study of Tranexamic Acid and Ethamsylate in Dysfunctional Uterine Bleeding. Indian J Pharm Pract. 2021;14(3):205-10.
6. James AH. Heavy menstrual bleeding: work-up and management. Hematology Am Soc Hematol Educ Program. 2016; 2016(1):236-42.
7. Girbash EF, Sherif HE, Radwan AM, Abdeldayem HM. Dienogest versus norethisterone acetate in management of endometrial hyperplasia without atypia. Arch Gynecol Obstet. 2023;308(3):947-52.
8. Dhillon-Smith R, Latthe P. BritSPAG Guideline for the management of Heavy Menstrual Bleeding (HMB) in adolescents. Br Soc Paediatr Adoles Gynaecol. 2020.
9. Rafie S, Borgelt LM, Koepf ER, Temple ME, Lehman K. Novel oral contraceptive for heavy menstrual bleeding: Estradiol valerate and dienogest. Int J Women's Health. 2013;5(1):313-21.
10. Yang S, Liu Y, Wen J, Sun Y, Ren F. Clinical Efficacy of Dienogest versus Levonorgestrel-Releasing Intrauterine System for Adenomyosis. Evid-Based Complement Alternat Med. 2022;2022:1995472.
11. Ota I, Taniguchi F, Ota Y, Nagata H, Wada I, Nakaso T, et al. A controlled clinical trial comparing potent progestins, LNG-IUS and dienogest, for the treatment of women with adenomyosis. Reprod med biol. 2021;20(4):427-34.
12. Shrestha S, Thapa B, Baniya S, Pandey V. Ormeloxifene in acute heavy menstruation of menopause transition women. Asian J Med sciences. 2021;12(8):88-93.
13. Donnez J, Vazquez F, Tomaszewski J, Nouri K, Bouchard P, Fauser BC, et al. Long-term treatment of uterine fibroids with ulipristal acetate. Fertil Steril. 2014;101:1565-73. e1561-8.
14. Tristan M, Leonardo J, Orozco LJ, Steed A, Ramírez-Morera A, Stone P. Mifepristone for uterine fibroids. Cochrane Database Syst Rev. 2012;2012(8):CD007687.
15. Stewart EA, Diamond MP, Williams ARW, Carr BR, Myers ER, Feldman RA, et al. Safety and efficacy of the selective progesterone receptor modulator asoprisnil for heavy menstrual bleeding with uterine fibroids: pooled analysis of two 12-month, placebo-controlled, randomized trials. Hum Reprod. 2019;34(4):623-34.
16. Beaumont HH, Augood C, Duckitt K, Lethaby A. Danazol for heavy menstrual bleeding. Cochrane Database Syst Rev. 2007;3:CD001017.
17. Lethaby A, Vollenhoven B, Sowter M. Pre-operative GnRH analogue therapy before hysterectomy or myomectomy for uterine

fibroids. Cochrane Database Syst Rev. 2001;2:CD000547.
18. Telner DE. Approach to diagnosis and management of abnormal uterine bleeding. Can Fam Physician. 2007;53(1):58-64.
19. Archer DF, Stewart EA, Jain RI, Feldman RA, Lukes AS, North JD, et al. Elagolix for the management of heavy menstrual bleeding associated with uterine fibroids: results from a phase 2a proof-of-concept study. Fertil Steril. 2017;108(1):152-60.e4.
20. Donnez J, Taylor HS, Stewart EA, Bradley L, Marsh E, Archer D, et al. Linzagolix with and without hormonal add-back therapy for the treatment of symptomatic uterine fibroids: two randomised, placebo-controlled, phase 3 trials. Lancet. 2022;400(10356):896-907.
21. ACOG committee opinion no. 557: Management of acute abnormal uterine bleeding in nonpregnant reproductive-aged women. Obstet Gynecol. 2013;121(4):891-6.
22. Pajai S, Acharya N. Medical Management in Reproductive Age. In: Gandhi A, Shrikhande L (Eds). FOGSI focus: Abnormal Uterine Bleeding. New Delhi: CBS publishers and distributors Pvt Ltd; 2021. pp. 35-8.

Chapter 26

Fibroids

Sumitra Yadav, Pooja Verma

Expectant management can be carried in female with asymptomatic uterine fibroids regardless of the size and number, the status can be monitored over years using annual gynecological pelvic examination, aided by ultrasonography, and can be managed conservatively. Uterine fibroids are usually slow growing, a longitudinal USG-based study revealed that on an average a fibroid grows not >0.5 cm/year but some have shown a growth rate as fast as 3 cm/year.[1] In the past most common management consisted of surgical removal of fibroids but over the years watchful practices for management of asymptomatic fibroids have taken over. Medical therapy in symptomatic cases can be long term or short term as a preoperative therapy in order to decrease size of the fibroid thus reducing intraoperative blood loss and can also be used in perimenopausal women to alleviate symptoms till they attain menopause after which the fibroids are likely to regress.[1]

Note: Leiomyoma is a slow-growing benign tumor that grows at an average of 0.3–0.5 cm/year.

■ EXPECTANT MANAGEMENT

It is observing fibroid over years without any surgical or medical treatment, best suited for cases that are:
- Asymptomatic
- Size of the uterus is <12 weeks.
- Patient willing for follow-up visits.
- Diagnosis of fibroid is certain.

■ DEFINITIVE MANAGEMENT

In the form of medical or surgical resection is required in all symptomatic cases such as those presenting with:[2]
- Heavy menstrual bleeding
- Dysmenorrhea
- Pressure symptoms
- Infertility
- Recurrent pregnancy loss.

Definitive treatment comprises medical therapy and surgical resection that involves myomectomy and hysterectomy that can be performed abdominally, vaginally, or laparoscopically depending upon the size of uterus and expertise of the operating surgeon. Type of management will depend upon below-mentioned key points:
- Clinical presentation
- Size and number of myomas
- Site of fibroids
- Size of uterus
- Willingness to preserve fertility

Medical therapy is considered for women with small (<4 cm), asymptomatic or symptomatic fibroids who want to retain fertility. Usually, surgery is the mainstay for fibroids resulting in uterine size enlargement of >12 weeks. Medical treatments do not regress fibroids completely but are known to provide symptomatic relief and decrease size and volume of leiomyoma, so are used preoperatively to decrease operative morbidity and blood loss.

MANAGEMENT FOR LEIOMYOMA

- *Hormonal management:* Etiology of fibroid is multifactorial and is yet to be explored in depths, their seldom occurrence before menarche and regression after menopause signifies involvement of the two hormones; estrogen and progesterone.[3]
  - Antiprogestin **(Table 1)**
  - Gonadotropin-releasing hormone (GnRH) analogs **(Table 2)**

Add back therapy: Comprises low-dose estrogen prescribed to overcome the disadvantage of bone loss without inducing fibroid growth. It also induces menopause like vasomotor symptoms such as hot flashes, vaginal dryness. Usually, it is done by prescribing medroxyprogesterone acetate (MPA) 10 mg for day 16–25 and equine estrogen of 0.3–0.625 mg from day 1 to 25. Bone loss can also be prevented by adding selective estrogen receptor modulators (SERMs) such raloxifene and tibolone or bisphosphonates.[6]

Note: Salient features of GnRH analogs use:
- Reduces size of leiomyoma by 40–50% hence used preoperatively to decrease size of fibroid. The reversal of size occurs within 3 months after stopping treatment.
- Helps in treating anemia before surgery as it induces amenorrhea and prevents further blood loss.
  - Aromatase inhibitor **(Table 3)**
  - *Combined oral contraceptive pills:* They are used to treat heavy menstrual bleeding associated with myomas and reduce bleeding significantly primarily because of their suppressive effect on endometrium but have no effect in decreasing size or volume of fibroids.
  - *Levonorgestrel-releasing intrauterine system (LNG-IUS):* These are usually not recommended for cavity obliterating lesions such as intracavitary pedunculated leiomyomas and polyps, otherwise systemic reviews suggest their use to decrease menstrual blood loss and for increasing hematocrit for a period of time.[8]

NONHORMONAL THERAPY

- *Nonsteroidal anti-inflammatory drugs (NSAIDs):* It consists of nonsteroidal anti-inflammatory drugs which are used to treat dysmenorrhea related to fibroids by preventing prostaglandin release. Studies comparing their role in preventing bleeding are inadequate.
- *Antifibrinolytic drug:* Antifibrinolytics such as tranexamic acid is used to prevent blood loss in women with heavy menstrual bleeding which can be due to any underlying pathology. It blocks lysine-binding sites on plasminogen preventing its combination with fibrin and resulting in fibrinolysis. It can be administered orally 1 g thrice daily or can be injected 10 mg/kg/IV.

KEY POINTS

- Leiomyoma is a slow growing benign tumor that grows at an average of 0.3–0.5 cm/year.
- Type of management will depend upon below-mentioned key points: Clinical presentation, size, and number of myomas, site of fibroids, size of uterus, and willingness to preserve fertility.

TABLE 1: *Medical management of fibroids: Antiprogestin.*

Drug	Mechanism of action	Pharmacokinetics	Dosage	Side effects	Contraindications
Mifepristone (RU-486)	It is a 19-norgestin norethindrone derivative with potent antiprogestational and significant antiglucocorticoid and antiandrogenic action. It is a partial agonist and competitive antagonist at all progesterone receptor. It can bind to either progesterone receptor-A (PR-A) or progesterone receptor-B (PR-B), out of which PR-A receptors are present in higher concentration in leiomyoma compared to PR-B. Antiprogestin agents exert antagonistic effect by competitively binding to these receptors[4]	• Active orally • Bioavailability is 25% • Metabolized in liver by CYP3A4 • Half-life: 20–36 hours	2.5–10 mg for 3–6 months	• Headache • Nausea and vomiting • Abdominal pain • Endometrial hyperplasia • Vaginal bleeding	• Adrenal insufficiency • Allergy to the drug • Chronic systemic glucocorticoid use • Confirmed or suspected ectopic pregnancy • Inherited porphyria • Hemorrhagic disorders
Ulipristal acetate	It is a selective progesterone receptor modulator (SPRM). It exerts progestational effect in some tissue and antagonistic effect in others. It effectively decreases leiomyoma associated bleeding and decreases volume of leiomyoma, so commonly employed preoperatively[5]	• Active orally • Metabolized in liver by CYP3A4 • Half-life: 38 hours	5 mg and 10 mg prescribed for a duration of 13 weeks and 4 such courses should be given	• Headache • Breast tenderness • Vasomotor symptoms • Abdominal pain • SPRM-induced endometrial thickening	Pregnancy

SECTION 9: Medical Management of Menstrual Disorders

TABLE 2: *Medical management of fibroids: GnRH analogs.*

Drug	Mechanism of action	Pharmacokinetics	Dose	Side effects	Contraindications
GnRH analogs: Synthetic derivatives of GnRH decapeptide • Leuprolide acetate • Goserelin • Nafarelin	GnRH analogs activate pituitary gonadotrophs thus enhancing FSH and LH release, this phenomenon is called flare and lasts for a week after initiating therapy followed by downregulation of receptors resulting in decreased FSH and LH release thus reducing ovarian steroidogenesis and decreased estrogen and progesterone production ultimately in 1–2 weeks duration. They suppress leiomyoma cell proliferation and induce cellular apoptosis at around 4th week of initiating GnRH analogs therapy[6]	• Inactive when given orally • The duration of analogs used intramuscularly, subcutaneously, and intranasally is 3 hours	• FDA approved two depot formations: 3.75 mg given monthly and/or 11.25 mg for 3 months, both given intramuscularly • Two depot formation: 3.6 mg and 10.8 mg to be given once a month and 3 months respectively to be administered subcutaneously • 200 µg intranasally twice daily	• Hot flushes • Dyslipidemia • Osteopenia and osteoporosis if used for >6 months • Headache • Depression • Decreased libido • Fluid retention	• Pregnancy • Breastfeeding • Osteoporosis

(GnRH: gonadotropin-releasing hormone; FDA: Food and Drug Administration; FSH: follicle-stimulating hormone; LH: luteinizing hormone)

TABLE 3: Medical management of fibroids: Aromatase inhibitors (AIs).

Drug	Mechanism of action	Pharmacokinetics	Dose	Side effects	Contraindication
Letrozole	Aromatase is enzyme responsible for catalyzing the conversion of androgens to estrogen. As leiomyomas are sex-steroid hormones dependent tumors and these hormones mediate their effect by activating or inhibiting transcription and cellular growth factor production. Leiomyomas create a hyperestrogenic environment, which is mandatory for their growth and maintenance. When compared to normal myometrium, leiomyoma cells contain abundant estrogen receptors (ER), which result in larger estradiol binding. These tumors convert less estradiol to the weaker estrone. Another mechanism involves higher expression of cytochrome P450 aromatase in leiomyomas compared with normal myocytes[7]	• Bioavailability: 100% when given orally • Half-life: 40 hours	2.5 mg for a period of 12 weeks	• Headache • Visual symptoms • Nausea and vomiting • Antiestrogenic effects may result in hot flushes, vaginal dryness, and increase risk of osteoporosis and coronary artery diseases	• Hypersensitivity to AI use • Pregnancy • Lactation • Severe renal impairment

- Medical treatments do not regress fibroids completely but are known to provide symptomatic relief and decrease size and volume of leiomyoma, so are used preoperatively to decrease operative morbidity and blood loss.
- *progesterone receptor (PR):* A receptors are present in higher concentration in leiomyoma compared to PR-B receptors.
- Add back therapy with low-dose estrogen is advised to patients on GnRH therapy for a duration longer than 6 months to prevent bone loss and vasomotor symptoms.
- Levonorgestrel-releasing intrauterine system is not recommended for intracavitary pedunculated fibroids.
- *Gonadotrophic-releasing hormone agonists:* They suppress leiomyoma cell proliferation and induce cellular apoptosis at around 4th week of initiating GnRH analogs therapy.

REFERENCES

1. Williams book of gynaecology, Chapter 9, pelvic masses, p. 203.
2. Donnez J, Dolmans MM. Uterine fibroid management: from the present to the future. Hum Reprod Update. 2016;22(6):665-86.
3. De La Cruz MS, Buchanan EM. Uterine fibroids: Diagnosis and treatment. Am Fam Physician. 2017;95(2):100-7.
4. Strobl JS. chapter 61: Estrogens, Progestins, and SERMs. In: Craig CR, Stitzel RE (Eds). Modern Pharmacology with Clinical Application, 6th edition. 704. United States: Lippincott Williams & Wilkins; 2004.
5. NICE. (2018). NICE Guidelines 2018 on HMB—Heavy Menstrual Bleeding. [online] Available from: https://www.nice.org.uk/guidance/ng88/resources/heavy-menstrual-bleeding-assessment-and-management-pdf-1837701412549 [Last accessed December, 2023].
6. Hackenberg R, Gesenhues T, Deichert U, Duda V, Schmidt-Rhode P, Schulz KD. The response of uterine fibroids to GnRH-agonist treatment can be predicted in most cases after one month. Eur J Obstet Gynecol Reprod Biol. 1992;45(2):125-9.
7. Duhan N, Madaan S, Sen J. Role of the aromatase inhibitor letrozole in the management of uterine leiomyomas in premenopausal women. Eur J Obstet Gynecol Reprod Biol. 2013;171(2):329-32.
8. Stewart EA. (2019). Overview of treatment of uterine leiomyomas (fibroids). In: Barbieri RL, Eckler K (Eds). Waltham, MA: UpToDate. [online] Available from: https://www.uptodate.com/contents/overview-of-treatment-of-uterine-leiomyomas-fibroids [Last accessed December, 2023].

Chapter 27

Endometriosis

Archana Maurya, Vanshika Pundhir

Endometriosis is a chronic medical condition that affects around 6–10% of reproductive age women.[1]

Most common presenting symptoms are:
- Pelvic pain
- Dysmenorrhea
- Infertility

It is characterized by growth of the endometrial glands and stroma outside the endometrial cavity.

The diagnosis is made by histopathology of the endometriotic lesions.

Endometriosis has a classical triad of dysmenorrhea, dyschezia (pain during defecation), and dyspareunia (**Figs. 1 and 2**).

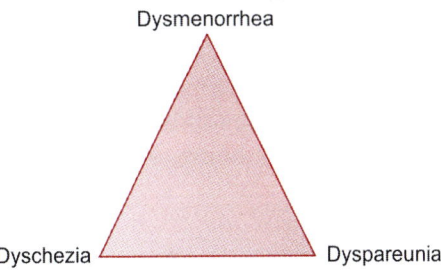

Fig. 1: Classic triad of endometriosis.

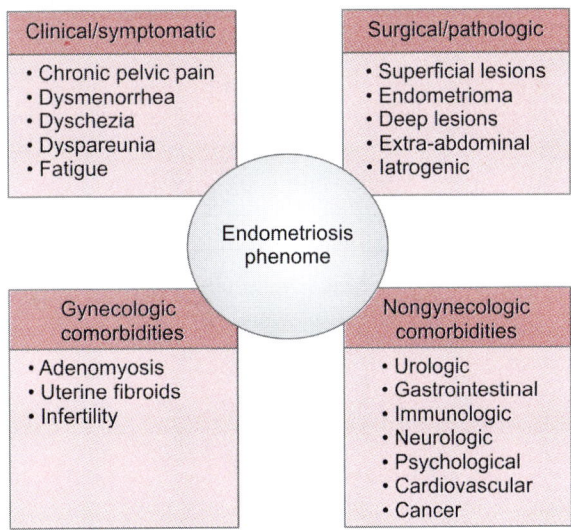

Fig. 2: Spectrum of endometriosis.

ETIOLOGY OF ENDOMETRIOSIS

Etiology of endometriosis can be described by the following theories:
- Sampson's theory
- Meyer's theory
- Halban's theory

SITES OF ENDOMETRIOSIS

- The most common site of endometriosis is the ovaries with spread to anterior and posterior cul-de-sac, broad ligament, fallopian tube, uterosacral ligaments, uterus, fallopian tubes, sigmoid colon, appendix, and round ligament.
- Other areas, which are less commonly involved, include the vagina, cervix, rectovaginal septum, cecum, ileum, inguinal canal, perineal scars, urinary bladder, ureter, and the umbilicus.
- Rare cases of endometriosis of gastrointestinal tract, bones, vertebra, central nervous system, and lungs have also been reported.
- Their appearance can range from red, brown, black, white, yellow, pink, and clear or red vesicle depending upon the degree of hemorrhage, fibrosis, inflammation, and duration of the lesions.

There are three types of endometriotic lesions:
1. Superficial peritoneal and ovarian implants
2. Endometriomas (ovarian cysts that are lined with endometrioid mucosa)
3. Deep infiltrating endometriosis (complex nodules comprised of endometriotic tissue, adipose tissue, and fibromuscular tissue)

The site and intensity of the symptoms seen in a patient of endometriosis can be attributed to the anatomical location and to the degree of the inflammatory response **(Table 1 and Fig. 3)**.

TABLE 1: Types of endometriotic lesions.

Ovarian endometriosis	Deep infiltrating endometriosis	Peritoneal endometriosis
Nodules implant in the lining of ovaries. When tissue around these areas hardens, it can develop and proliferate into the fallopian tubes and bowel	The nodules implant at least 5 mm below the peritoneum. Structures penetrated can include the uterosacral ligaments, bowel, bladder, and ureters	The peritoneum is the lining of the abdomen. Peritoneal endometriosis occurs when endometrial cells travel to and implant in the peritoneal wall

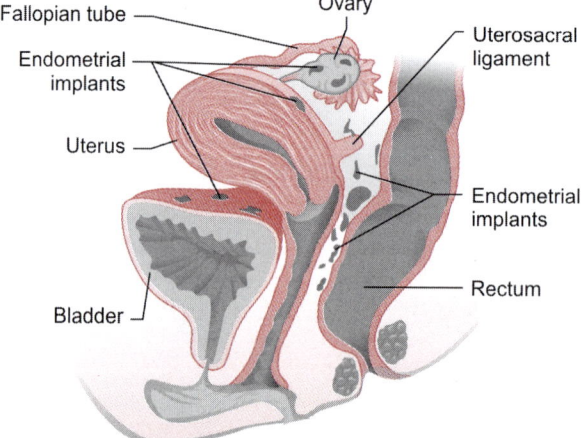

Fig. 3: Sites of endometriotic implants.

MEDICAL MANAGEMENT OF ENDOMETRIOSIS

Exaggerated inflammatory responses, along with excess production of estrogen, and progesterone resistance are the critical underlying mechanisms that lead to the symptoms of endometriosis. Endometriotic implants have impaired molecular and immunological functions. This leads to increased production of estrogen, pro-inflammatory cytokines, prostaglandins (PGs), and metalloproteinases and a failure of immune cells to suppress and clear the inflammatory response.

Constant supply of estrogen is crucial for the growth and persistence of the endometriotic implants, which comes from multiple sources.

- The endometrial implants have intrinsic aromatase activity, which leads to the conversion of cholesterol to estradiol.
- The endometrium is rich in PGE2 receptors and activation of the PG receptor subtype EP2 leads to activation of cyclic adenosine monophosphate (AMP), which increases the expression of key steroidogenic genes, and aromatase activity leading to increased estradiol production.
- Along with intrinsic aromatase activity estradiol produced from ovary and peripheral fat also reaches the sites of endometriosis. This continuous supply of estrogen is important for the continuous growth and survival of endometriotic implants.
- Pelvic pain in endometriosis is secondary to increased concentrations of PGs, especially of the subtype PGE2 and PGF2α. Cyclooxygenase (COX) catalyzes the conversion of arachidonic acid to PGH2 which is converted to PGE2 and F2α via the action of PG synthetase.
- COX-2 is expressed in higher concentrations in the endometrial implants as compared to the normal endometrial cells. Again, the increased concentration of PGE2 also provides a stimulus for estrogen production.
- Cytokines, especially interleukin 1β (IL-1β) and angiogenic factors like vascular endothelial growth factor (VEGF) in inducing COX-2 expression and increased PG production in endometriotic implants.
- Growing evidence also suggests a role of progesterone resistance in women with endometriosis. Studies have shown that the endometriotic lesions have a low progesterone receptor level. Progesterone is important for the activation of key enzyme 17-beta-hydroxysteroid dehydrogenase 2, which helps in converting estradiol to estrone, which is less biologically active. Thus, increased production of estradiol and decreased clearance leads to the growth of the endometriotic tissue.

TREATMENT DECISIONS

- *Pain:* Medical/surgical management
- *Infertility:* Surgery/medically assisted reproduction

Medications Used in Endometriosis

The medical management of endometriosis aims at controlling pain and suppression of the hormonally responsive endometriotic implants.

Empiric: [European Society of Human Reproduction and Embryology (ESHRE) 2022] NSAIDs (nonsteroidal anti-inflammatory drugs) for pain (*weak recommendations*).

Hormonal: (ESHRE 2022) **(Table 2)**
- Combined oral contraceptives (COCs) (*strong recommendations*)

TABLE 2: Hormonal treatment as an alternative to surgery for pain management.

	Recommendations (ESHRE 2022)
Presurgery	Not recommended to improve the pain outcome of the surgery
Postsurgery	COC/LNG-IUS for 18–24 months for secondary prevention of endometriomas if not seeking conception

(COC: combined oral contraceptive; ESHRE: European Society of Human Reproduction and Embryology; LNG-IUS: levonorgestrel-containing intrauterine system)

- Progestogens, dienogest, LNG-IUS (levonorgestrel-containing intrauterine system), danazol (strong recommendations)
- Gonadotropin-releasing hormone (GnRH) agonists (strong recommendations)
- GnRH antagonists (weak recommendations, second line)
- Aromatase inhibitors (strong recommendations); letrozole (pain refractory to above drugs) has hypoestrogenic effects after long-term use
- For antiprogestogens like gestrinone, ESHRE does not recommend.

Surgery for Pain Management

1. It is recommended to offer surgery as one of the option for pain management.
2. It is recommended to excise the lesions instead of ablation.
3. Laparoscopic excision (cystectomy) of the ovarian endometriomas is recommended to minimize the symptoms and recurrence of the endometriomas.
4. Addition of LUNA (laparoscopic uterosacral nerve ablation) to laparoscopic removal of the endometriomas does not improve the pain relief.
5. Presacral neurectomy (PSN) is beneficial for the treatment of the endometriosis-associated midline pain.
6. PSN requires high degree of skill.
7. PSN is associated with higher risk of intraoperative bleeding, postoperative constipation, and urinary urgency.

Preoperative Medical Management not Recommended (ESHRE 2022)

- Changes the appearance of the endometriomas
- Delay of the diagnosis
- Cost and side effects
- No difference for pain relief or infertility

Surgery or Medical Management (ESHRE 2022)

- No prognostic markers are currently available.
- Clinicians should take a shared decision-making approach, individual preferences, side effects, individual efficacy, costs, and availability considerations while choosing between hormonal and surgical treatment.

MEDICATIONS USED IN ENDOMETRIOSIS

Nonsteroidal Anti-inflammatory Drugs

These are the first-line agents in the management of endometriosis-related pain and dysmenorrhea.

These act by blocking the activity of the enzyme COX that plays the central role in the production of the inflammatory mediators.

Endometrial tissue have a higher concentration of COX-2 receptors.

The pain in endometriosis is secondary to elevated levels of PGs, interleukins, and cytokines.

Selective and nonselective COX inhibitors provide symptomatic relief.

Newer studies suggest that selective COX-2 inhibitors like rofecoxib can also inhibit the growth of the endometriotic implants.

Combined Hormonal Contraceptives

Combined oral contraceptives are the most commonly used first-line hormonal therapy. Estrogen and progesterone combinations or progesterone alone results in the decidualization of the endometriotic implants and slows down the progression of the disease.

Cost, ease of administration, and tolerability are some of the key features that have made their use popular.

As compared to cyclic administration, continuous therapy with COC has been shown to have better pain control.

Advantages
- Lower cost
- Ease of administration
- Easily tolerable

Limiting Factors (Fig. 4)
- Long-term administration
- Risk of thromboembolism
- High rates of recurrence after discontinuation
- Impaired fertility due to contraceptive action

Combinations with lower dose of ethinyl estradiol (20 µg) in comparison to higher dose have a lower risk of venous thromboembolism.

Gonadotropin-releasing Hormone Agonists

Gonadotropin-releasing hormone agonists act by blocking the ovarian estrogen

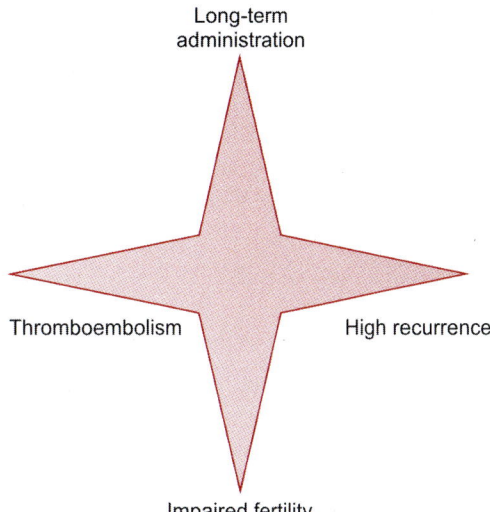

Fig. 4: Limiting factors of combined hormonal contraceptives.

production resulting in the retrogression of the endometriotic deposits.

During starting few days of GnRH agonists administration there is a flare effect due to the stimulation of the pituitary releasing follicle-stimulating hormone (FSH) and luteinizing hormone (LH).

However, upon continuous administration there is downregulation of pituitary GnRH receptors which eventually results in suppression of the hypothalamic–pituitary–ovarian axis, thereby causing anovulation.

This eventually results in hypoestrogenism, amenorrhea, and retrogression of the endometriotic deposits by cutting down the estrogen necessary for the proliferation of the implants.

Injection leuprolide acetate 3.75 mg monthly or 11.25 mg used three monthly, goserelin and nafarelin, are also the commonly used preparation.

Patients who are unable to tolerate oral contraceptive pills (OCPs) due to their medical conditions or who have not benefitted from the OCPs can be offered GnRH agonists.

The GnRH agonists are available in both nasal and injectable forms and offer high rates of pain relief and longer symptom-free period for up to 12 months.

Limitations of the GnRH Agonists (Fig. 5)

These are approved for continuous use for only up to 6 months due to side effects like:
- Bone loss
- Vaginal atrophy and dryness
- Hot flashes and abnormalities in lipid profile
- GnRH agonists suppress ovulation and cannot be used in women desiring fertility.

The addition of add-back therapy provides symptomatic relief and decreases the rate of bone loss.

Norethindrone acetate is the only Food and Drug Administration (FDA)-approved add-back therapy, but low-dose estrogen and a combination of estrogen and progesterone have also been used.

The combination of GnRH agonists and norethindrone acetate are only approved for use for duration of 12 months.

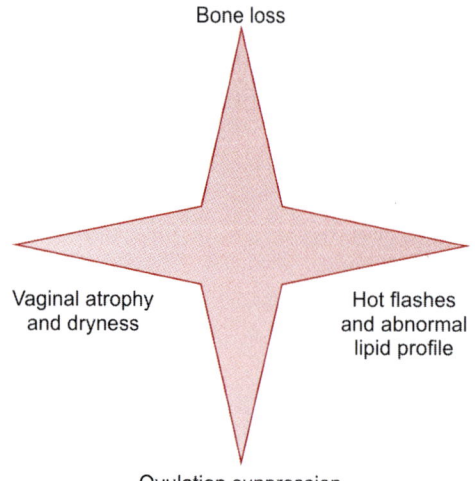

Fig. 5: Limitations of the gonadotropin-releasing hormone (GnRH) agonists.

Gonadotropin-releasing Hormone Antagonists

The GnRH antagonists do not cause the initial flare and have lower degree of hypoestrogenism. They are associated with lesser side effects and have a symptomatic improvement similar to GnRH agonists.

Progesterone-containing Contraceptives

Pathophysiologic basis of use of progesterone in endometriosis takes into accounts multiple mechanisms.
- It is responsible for the decidualization of the endometrium.
- It alters the estrogen receptors and hence inhibits the estrogen-induced mitosis.
- It inhibits the growth of the new vasculature (angiogenesis) and expression of matrix metalloproteinase needed for the growth of the endometriotic implants.

These can be administered by different routes oral, injectable, or intrauterine device and are a good alternative for women with contraindications to estrogens.

Cyproterone acetate, dienogest, dydrogesterone, gestrinone, lynesterole, medroxyprogesterone acetate, megesterol acetate, and norethindrone acetate are few of the progestins used in the patients of endometriosis.

Medroxyprogesterone is available as oral and injectable preparation and is administered 150 mg intramuscularly at 3 months' interval.

Oral medroxyprogesterone given in a dose ranging from 10 to 100 mg/day for 3–6 months have shown improvement in endometriosis.

Advantage of injectable progesterone lies in improved compliance and bypassing problems of gastrointestinal absorption.

Norethisterone acetate is a 19-nortestosterone derivative and is effective in control of dyspareunia, dysmenorrhea, pelvic pain, and dyschezia.

Dienogest is a 19-nortestosterone derivative. It has high specificity for progesterone receptors and less antiandrogenic side effects. Continuous administration results in decidualization and atrophy of the endometriotic implants. It also has anti-inflammatory, antiangiogenic and antiproliferative effects, thereby slowing down the progression of the disease process.

Dienogest is given in a dose of 2 or 4 mg/day. It is better tolerated and side effects like irregular bleeding eventually improves with time.

Levonorgestrel-containing Intrauterine Systems

The LNG-IUS is a T-shaped device that contains 52 mg of levonorgestrel, which releases 20 µg of hormone per day over a 5-year period.

The LNG-IUS delivers progesterone locally and avoids the systemic side effects.

A longer duration of activity further improves compliance.

The mechanism of action of LNG-IUS in endometriosis is progesterone induced:
- Decidualization and atrophy of the endometrium
- Hypomenorrhea and decreased retrograde menstruation
- Higher concentration of progesterone in the peritoneal cavity which suppresses the endometriotic implants by anti-inflammatory and immunomodulatory action

The LNG-IUS has a successful control endometriosis related pelvic pain and improve patient satisfactions.

They are also successfully used in patients with adenomyosis and deep rectovaginal endometriosis.

With its long-term use and better side effect profile LNG-IUS offers a great option in women who are do not desire to conceive.

Lesser side effects are seen with oral progesterons in comparison to combined hormonal contraceptives.

Etonogestrel Implant

It is inserted intradermally in the arm, it contains progestin etonogestrel and has contraceptive advantage of 3 years.

Medroxyprogesterone acetate and etonogestrel implants have similar pain relief and side effects.

Side effects include irregular menstrual bleeding, weight gain, nausea, headache, breast tenderness, and acne **(Fig. 6)**.

Etonogestrel implants and LNG-IUS are the options available to the women with symptoms of endometriosis where fertility is not an issue.

Selective Progesterone Receptor Modulators

Selective progesterone receptor modulators (SPRMs) have tissue action ranging from pure agonists to agonist/antagonist to antagonist. *Commonly used SPRM are:*
- *Mifepristone:* It acts as a progesterone antagonist and is commonly used for medical abortions.

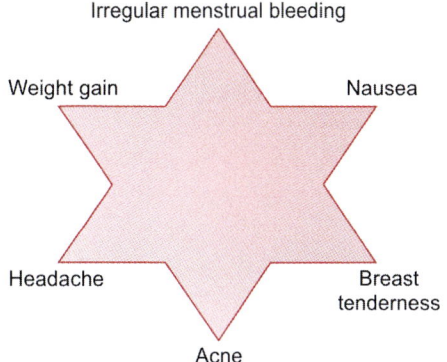

Fig. 6: Side effects of etonogestrel implant.

- *Ulipristal acetate:* It is commonly used for emergency contraception.

Advantage

They selectively inhibit the endometrial growth without the side effects of decreased estrogen, hence there is decreased menstrual bleeding.

Aromatase Inhibitors

Aromatase enzyme is responsible for the conversion of the steroid precursors into estrogen. It has been seen that there is no aromatase activity in normal endometrium while it is increased in the endometriotic implants; hence the increased estrogen production results in the proliferation of the endometriotic implants and sets up a vicious cycle of COX expression and increased PG production which furthermore increases the aromatase activity **(Fig. 7)**.

Mechanism of Action of Aromatase Inhibitor

Aromatase inhibitor allows blocking the action of aromatase enzyme in the ovary and adipose tissue (periphery), hence also benefitting the postmenopausal women where peripheral fat contributes the maximum estrogen.

- Anastrozole, letrozole, and exemestane are third-generation aromatase inhibitors that can be administered orally.
- They are reversible, more potent and have faster onset of action.
- Used in combination with COCs, GnRH agonists, and they markedly decrease the pain associated with endometriosis, hence improving the quality of life.

Side Effects

Long-term use is associated with ovarian follicular cyst and bone loss. Hence, they are used in combination with GnRH agonists and birth control pills.

Danazol

Danazol, a derivative of 17 alpha-ethinyltestosterone, inhibits LH surge and decreases ovarian steroidogenesis by direct inhibition of the ovarian enzymes.

It is successful in controlling pain associated with endometriosis but it is avoided due to androgenic side effects.

Dosage

It is administered in divided doses of 400–800 mg/day for 6 months.

Side Effects

These include acne, hirsutism, deepening of voice, weight gain, muscle cramps, liver dysfunction, and an abnormal lipid profile **(Fig. 8)**.

In studies by Selak et al. patients who were treated with danazol had improvement in the pain symptoms and also had improvement in the laparoscopic scores.

Also, danazol vaginal ring and intrauterine devices are associated with lesser side effects

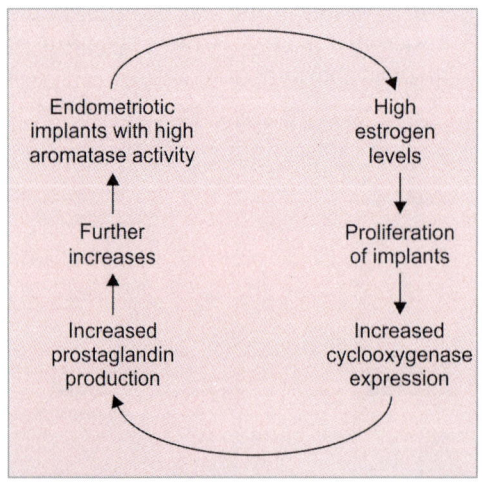

Fig. 7: Role of aromatase enzyme in endometriosis.

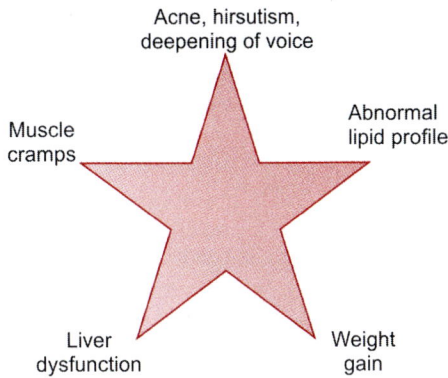

Fig. 8: Side effects of danazol.

hence better tolerability as compared to the oral administration.

NEWER TREATMENT OPTIONS STILL UNDER STUDY

Endometriosis affects women of reproductive age group. The treatment options that are available have a long-term side effects of hypoestrogenism and are associated with high rates of recurrence after the discontinuation of the therapy. The new therapies that are available are discussed in **Table 3**.

Antiangiogenesis Factors

The endometriotic implants secrete angiogenic factors like VEGF that are crucial for the formation of the network of capillaries crucial for the growth and survival of the implants. Hence by inhibiting the growth and survival of the implants it halts the progression of the disease.

Antiangiogenic agents that are under trial are as follows:
- TNP-470 (an analog of antibiotic fumagillin)
- Endostatin (a proteolytic fragment of collagen with endogenous antiangiogenic activity)
- Anginex (a synthetic peptide that stops the growth of blood vessels and induces apoptosis)
- Anti-VEGF antibody (Avastin)

But these drugs are still under trials and successful results have been seen in the animal models. *Dopamine receptor agonists, cabergoline and quinagolide*, act by dephosphorylation of VEGF2. They are being commonly used for the treatment of hyperprolactinemia and suppression of lactation. These agents have successfully shown the reduction the size of the implants. Treatment with ergot-derived dopamine agonist (cabergoline) and nonergot dopamine agonist (quinagolide) were effective in inhibiting angiogenesis and reducing the size of endometriotic lesions in the animal studies (mouse model).

In a study conducted by Gomez et al. it was seen that in women with endometriosis who underwent surgical resection of half of the endometriotic implant after receiving quinagolide for 18–20 weeks, there was significant reduction of the size of endometriotic lesions.

Statins

Statins are used in the treatment of hypercholesterolemia they act by blocking the conversion of 3-hydroxy-3-methylglutaryl coenzyme-A into mevalonate.

They have anti-inflammatory, anti-angiogenic, and antioxidant properties, hence their use in endometriosis is under study. They have been seen cause inhibition of the inflammatory [(PPAR-γ) peroxisome proliferator-activated receptor gamma, (LXRα) liver X receptor alpha, and (IGFBP-1) insulin-like growth factor binding protein 1] and angiogenic genes [COX-2, VEGF, RAGE (receptor for advanced glycation end-products), and (EN-RAGE)

TABLE 3: Drugs for medical management of endometriosis.

Drug	Dosage	Side effects	Mechanism of action
Oral contraceptives	Continuous/cyclical use	Nausea, headache, irregular bleeding	Decidualization of endometrial implants, ovarian suppression
Oral progestins: • Norethindrone acetate • Medroxyprogesterone acetate • Dienogest	*Continuous use:* • 5–20 mg daily • 30 mg daily, 150 mg monthly • 2 mg/day for 12–24 months	Weight gain, acne, breakthrough bleeding	• Suppression of ovarian steroidogenesis • Decidualization of the endometriotic implants • Decreases the activity of metalloproteinases and growth inhibitors • Dienogest inhibits angiogenesis and proliferation of stromal cells in endometrial implants
Levonorgestrel intrauterine device (IUD)	IUD releases 20 μg/day		Antiestrogenic action causes atrophy of endometriotic implants and amenorrhea
Antiprogestins: Gestrinone	1.25–2.5 mg twice a week	Nausea, muscle cramps, weight gains, acne, irreversible voice changes	Androgenic, antiestrogenic, and antigonadotropic action; hence causing degeneration of endometriotic implants
GnRH analogs: • Goserelin • Buserelin • Leuprolide acetate • Nafarelin • Triptorelin	All analogs are orally inactive: • Monthly/3 monthly injection • Nasal spray • Daily injection • Monthly/3 monthly nasal spray • Monthly/3 monthly	Hypoestrogenic side effects like hot flashes, vaginal dryness, reduced libido and reduced bone density	In the initial doses it causes flare reaction and later on receptor desensitization which causes pseudomenopause (reversible)
Danazol: Vaginal rings and intrauterine device	Divided doses of 400–800 mg/day for 6 months	*Androgenic side effect:* Acne, hirsutism, deepening of voice weight gain, muscle cramps, liver dysfunction and abnormal lipid profile	Acts by inhibiting LH surge and decreases ovarian steroidogenesis by suppression of the ovary
Aromatase inhibitor: • Anastrozole • Letrozole • Exemestane (third-generation aromatase inhibitors)	Orally: • 1 mg once daily • 2.5 mg once daily • 25 mg once daily	Long-term use is associated with follicular cyst and bone loss	Blocking the action of aromatase enzyme in the ovary and adipose tissue (periphery) decreasing the estrogen production

(GnRH: gonadotropin-releasing hormone; LH: luteinizing hormone)

extracellular newly identified RAGE]; also they decrease the matrix metalloproteinases, thereby decreasing the number and size of endometriotic implants.

Tumor Necrosis Factor Alpha Blockers

Tumor necrosis factor alpha (TNF-α) is a pro-inflammatory cytokine and its levels are increased in the peritoneal fluid of women with endometriosis.

Infliximab and etanercept are under study for the treatment of endometriosis.

Infliximab is a monoclonal antibody against TNF-α. Etanercept is a biologic fusion protein which blocks TNF-α.

The TNF-α blockers have shown good results in animal models, but same results are not seen in the humans.

Peroxisome Proliferator-activated Receptor Gamma Ligands

Peroxisome proliferator-activated receptors are ligand-activated nuclear receptors which have a role in inflammation and lipid and glucose metabolism. PPAR-γ ligands have anti-inflammatory properties and reduce estrogen synthesis by inhibiting aromatase enzyme. They inhibit cell proliferation, increase apoptosis, and inhibit the growth of the endometriotic lesions by an effect on the angiogenic factor VEGF.

Rosiglitazone and pioglitazone have been seen to reduce the size of the endometriotic lesions in the animal models but human studies are ongoing.

Pentoxifylline

Pentoxifylline has been studied in the treatment of endometriosis. It is currently being used in the treatment of intermittent claudication. It helps in improving the vascular supply in stenotic arteries by inhibiting the phosphodiesterase enzyme.

Pentoxifylline also has TNF-α blocking action, suppressing the release of inflammatory mediators. In animal studies pentoxifylline has shown successful results in improving fertility and reducing the size of the lesions. Human studies have shown limited results.

■ KEY POINTS

- Endometriosis is a chronic medical condition with pelvic pain, dysmenorrhea, and infertility the most common presenting symptoms.
- Etiology of endometriosis can be explained by Sampson's, Meyer's, and Halban's theories.
- Endometriosis has a complex pathophysiology involving the inflammatory mediators and exaggerated inflammatory response, excess production of estrogen, and progesterone resistance are the underlying mechanisms that lead to the symptoms of endometriosis.
- Endometriotic implants have impaired molecular and immunological functions.
- The medical management of endometriosis aims at controlling pain and suppression of the hormonally responsive endometriotic implants.
- *Treatment decisions*:
Pain: Medical/surgical management
Infertility: Surgery/medically assisted reproduction
- Drugs most commonly used for empiric treatment are NSAIDs.
- Hormonal drugs available are COCs, progestogens, dienogests, LNG-IUS, danazol, GnRH agonists, antagonists, and aromatase inhibitors.
- ESHRE guidelines 2022 for the pain management and recommendations
- Newer treatment options that are under evaluation are antiangiogenic factors, statins, TNF-α blockers, PPAR-γ ligands, and pentoxifylline.

■ REFERENCE

1. Rafique S, Decherney AH. Medical management of endometriosis. Clinical Obstetrics and Gynecology. 2017;60(3):485-96.

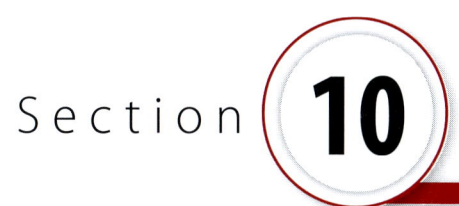

Medical Management of Endocrine Disorders

- **Polycystic Ovary Syndrome**
  Ruchika Garg, Mousumi Das Ghosh

- **Hirsutism**
  Ashima Taneja, Muskan Chaudhary

- **Primary Amenorrhea**
  Priyanka Dahiya

- **Secondary Amenorrhea**
  Ajit Kumar Nayak

Chapter 28

Polycystic Ovary Syndrome

Ruchika Garg, Mousumi Das Ghosh

Polycystic ovary syndrome (PCOS) is a widely prevalent endocrine disorder with an incidence of 8–13% in all reproductive age groups. PCOS is characterized by hypothalamic–pituitary–ovary axis dysfunction and anovulation. PCOS women typically have androgen excess, insulin resistance (IR), metabolic syndrome (MS), and low-grade chronic inflammation.

HORMONAL CONTRACEPTIVES—FIRST-LINE PHARMACOLOGIC THERAPY

Menstrual cycle abnormalities require management because oligo-ovulation, anovulation, and reduced progesterone exposure can all increase the risk of endometrial hyperplasia and malignancy.[1] Hormonal contraceptives are recommended for patients with irregular menstrual cycles and not keen to conceive.[2]

Apart from regulating menstrual cycle, combined oral contraceptive pills (OCPs) also improve features of hyperandrogenism and provide endometrial protection through withdrawal bleeding. These pills also improve menorrhagia and dysmenorrhea, and relieve premenstrual syndrome and pelvic pain related to endometriosis.[3] Long-term use protects against endometrial and ovarian cancer.

Selection of Oral Contraceptive

There is no optimal combined OCP in PCOS. Studies show almost similar efficacy among various oral contraceptives for regulating menstrual cycle or treating hyperandrogenism. The advantages of contraceptive pills outweigh the risks in most patients with PCOS and fertility is restored after discontinuing.[4]

Estrogen Component (Ethinyl Estradiol)[3,5,6]

Actions: This includes suppression of follicle-stimulating hormone (FSH), endometrial stabilization, potentiation of progestin action, suppression of dominant follicle formation, increase in sex hormone-binding globulin (SHBG) and decrease in free androgen.

Low-dose contraceptive pills (<50 µg) contain ethinyl estradiol (EE) in doses ranging from 15 to 35 µg.[7] World Health Organization (WHO) also recommends use of preparations with low dose and natural estrogens and low thromboembolic risk.[1]

Progestin Component

Mechanism of Action

It minimizes the frequency of gonadotropin-releasing hormone (GnRH) pulses, along with luteinizing hormone (LH) suppression, inhibition of LH surge, unreceptive endometrium, hostile cervical mucus, decrease in ovarian androgen and estrogen secretion, and increased SHBG concentration.

In menorrhagia, contraceptive pills with first- and second-generation progestin is preferred. After a few cycles when bleeding is controlled, we can switch over to third and fourth generation OCP.[3]

Newer OCPs contain fewer androgenic properties (such as norethindrone, desogestrel, and norgestimate). Progestins [cyproterone acetate (CPA) and drospirenone] function as androgen receptor antagonists.

Drospirenone is a spironolactone analog with mineralocorticoid activity; as a result, it has some diuretic property. However, it should not be prescribed to those predisposed to hyperkalemia.[8,9] Drospirenone and Dienogest are considered progestins with minimal androgenicity.

Side Effects

Most clinically important risk of oral contraceptive use is venous thromboembolism, especially in obese women. The new third-generation oral contraceptives have approximately twofold increased risk of venous thromboembolism compared with second-generation options. However, absolute risk of venous thrombosis is very small.

It takes a minimum time of 6 months for clinical improvement in acne and hirsutism. After a 6-month trial of oral contraceptive, an antiandrogen drug can be added in combination if there is suboptimal response.

If estrogen-containing pills are contraindicated then progestin-only pill (POP) should be prescribed in smokers and hypertensives.

Progesterone is used to induce withdrawal bleeding (medroxyprogesterone acetate 10 mg daily for 10–14 days, micronized progesterone 400 mg daily for 10–14 days).

Monitoring of Oral Contraceptive Effects

Measure blood pressure 3 months after start of oral contraceptives, then annually thereafter.

Measure glucose and lipid profile annually while oral contraceptives are used.

INSULIN-SENSITIZING MEDICATIONS

Metformin

Metformin increases insulin sensitivity in the liver to reduce gluconeogenesis and hyperinsulinemia. It leads to decreased androgen levels, increased rates of spontaneous ovulation, and enhanced ovulatory responses to clomiphene. It is used primarily to improve metabolic status in patients whose condition does not respond adequately to lifestyle measures.[10]

Metformin has some efficacy in normalizing ovulatory cyclicity but minimal impact on hirsutism. It does not provide endometrial protection unless normal ovulatory function is restored.

Metformin alone is less effective than clomiphene for ovulation induction, clinical pregnancy, and live birth.

Dose: Metformin hydrochloride oral tablet can be started 500 mg once in the evening, with a meal, for 1 week. Increase 500 mg a week if tolerates to goal of 1,500 mg or 2,000 mg/day.

Normal menstruation returns in 4–6 months. It also improves lipid profile. When added to clomiphene for infertility, ovulation and clinical pregnancy rates are markedly high compared to clomiphene alone. Weight loss and diet control is recommended to prevent metformin failure in severely obese patients.

Pharmacokinetics

Bioavailability: Under fasting conditions, the bioavailability of the metformin hydrochloride 500 mg tablet is 50–60%.

Food intake decreases and delays the absorption of metformin.

It takes 3 hours for effect after administration, half-life is about 20 hours.

Metformin is neither significantly metabolized in the liver nor exhibits substantial protein binding. Metformin is eliminated through the kidneys, mostly unchanged. Monitoring renal function is important.

Side Effects

Diarrhea, nausea, and vomiting are relatively common, affecting up to 30% of patients who take metformin. Gastrointestinal symptoms are dose-related and tend to resolve after several weeks.

Chest discomfort, headache, diaphoresis, hypoglycemia, weakness, and rhinitis are also included. Prolonged use of metformin can lead to decreased vitamin B_{12} levels.

A rare adverse effect of metformin therapy is *lactic acidosis,* which may occur in individuals with systemic and debilitating diseases. Lactic acidosis can be seen in 1 in 30,000 patients.

Therefore, metformin should not be prescribed to patients with renal, hepatic, or major cardiovascular disease.[2]

Monitoring of Metformin

Obtain serum creatinine level and estimated glomerular filtration rate (GFR) at least annually in all patients.

Thiazolidinediones—Rosiglitazone and Pioglitazone

This improves insulin sensitivity and also decreases androgen levels in women with PCOS. These insulin sensitizers act on intracellular metabolic pathways to enhance insulin action by regulating gene expression. Studies have shown resumption of ovulation following long-term treatment.

Administration

Taken orally once daily, with or without food. Monitoring of liver function test (LFT) levels is advocated along with check of rapid weight gain.

Side Effects

Use of thiazolidinedione causes dose-related fluid retention in 20% of patients. It is associated with weight gain and edema and there is evidence that both rosiglitazone and pioglitazone increase the risk of congestive heart failure (CHF). These drugs should be used with caution in patients with diastolic dysfunction or a history of CHF.

There is a risk of decreased bone density and fractures.

It should be avoided in patients with liver disease, heart failure, and those with increased risk of fractures.

As fetal safety is not well studied, these are contraindicated in pregnancy.[9]

TREATMENT OPTIONS FOR ACNE AND HIRSUTISM

This depends on patient's request and her degree of distress caused by hirsutism, rather than clinician's quantitative or qualitative assessments.

Hormonal contraceptives are first-line pharmacologic therapy. The Food and Drug Administration (FDA) approves EE/

norgestimate, EE/norethindrone, and EE/drospirenone for treatment of acne.[3] If these drugs are not effective, we can add antiandrogen drugs (e.g., spironolactone) after 6 months, preferably in combination with an oral contraceptive.

Antiandrogens

Primarily used to treat hirsutism (clinical hyperandrogenism), often in combination with an oral contraceptive.[11] With antiandrogens, concurrent contraception is crucial to limit risk of adverse pregnancy outcomes. This group of drugs can cross placenta and disrupt male sexual differentiation in a developing fetus resulting in genital ambiguity.[1,5]

Spironolactone (First-line Antiandrogen for Hirsutism and Acne)

Spironolactone is an aldosterone antagonist that, along with its major metabolite, canrenone, competes for T binding sites, thereby exerting a direct antiandrogenic effect at the pilosebaceous unit. In addition, spironolactone appears to interfere with cytochrome P450, thereby inhibiting steroid enzyme action and resultant androgen production.[2] Effective in decreasing degree of hirsutism and, to a lesser extent, acne.

Spironolactone oral tablet: 50–200 mg/day oral (PO) in one or two divided doses is prescribed.

It is a potassium-sparing diuretic. Serum potassium level has to be checked at 2 weeks after starting treatment. It has to be used cautiously if the patient is on any other medications or has a medical condition that may increase potassium.

Other side effects are breast tenderness, dehydration, and diarrhea.

Finasteride (Second-line Antiandrogen for Hirsutism)

Finasteride acts by inhibiting 5α-reductase. It decreases local dihydrotestosterone (DHT) levels in hair follicles with comparable effects to other antiandrogens. The effect of finasteride is dose-dependent.[5]

Dose: Finasteride oral tablet 2.5–5 mg PO once daily either alone or in combination with oral contraceptives has shown to reduce hirsutism in women with mild hirsutism. It has minimal adverse reaction compared to other antiandrogens. Daily use for 3 months or more is necessary before benefit is observed. Continued use is recommended to sustain benefit, which should be reevaluated periodically.

Cyproterone Acetate

The antiandrogen CPA is one of the most commonly used medications in the treatment of hirsutism, hyperandrogenism, and PCOS in women throughout the world.

Cyproterone acetate is a 17-hydroxyprogesterone acetate derivative with strong progestogenic properties. It is a competitive inhibitor at the androgen receptor.[12] It is available in combination with EE in the form of combined OCPs. Here, low-dose CPA in combination with EE is used to treat acne and has been found to result in overall improvement in 75–90% of women, with responses approaching 100%.

At a dose of 2 mg, its effect is equivalent to 50 mg of spironolactone. Orally administered CPA is rapidly and completely absorbed. Peak serum concentrations of 15 ng/mL are reached at about 1.6 hours after single ingestion. Bioavailability is about 88%. Discontinuation of CPA has been found to result in marked recurrence of symptoms in up to 70% of women.

It has a high risk of venous thromboembolism. It also causes fatigue, depression, weight gain and elevated liver enzymes.

Flutamide

Flutamide acts as a selective, competitive, silent antagonist of the androgen receptor. This competes for the androgen receptor and is effective for the treatment of hirsutism. Flutamide and its active form (hydroxyflutamide) stay in the body for a relatively short time, which makes it necessary to take flutamide multiple times per day. It has been used to treat hirsutism at dosages ranging from 62.5 to 750 mg/day.

Flutamide does not interact with the progesterone, estrogen, glucocorticoid, or mineralocorticoid receptor, and possesses no intrinsic progestogenic, estrogenic, glucocorticoid, or antigonadotrophic activity, hence, it does not cause menstrual irregularities in women.

The side effects are abdominal discomfort, and diarrhea, and methemoglobinemia in those who are susceptible to aniline toxicity or who are smokers. It is of limited value because of its dose-dependent hepatotoxicity.[4]

Monitoring of Antiandrogen Therapy

Monitoring response to treatment can be done objectively using Ferriman–Gallwey system, scoring at baseline and, if possible, at each visit.

Treatment can be continued as long as patient desires and should be discontinued if planning for pregnancy.

Monitoring testosterone levels after instituting pharmacologic therapy is generally unnecessary because hirsutism scores correlate poorly with serum androgen levels.

Other useful pharmacologic therapies can be advised based on symptoms related to hyperandrogenism like:

- Antibiotics, topical retinoids, or isotretinoin for acne
- Minoxidil topical solution to be applied on area of desired hair growth; maximum: 2 mL/day
- *Eflornithine for hirsutism:* Topical eflornithine slows growth of unwanted facial hair in 4–8 weeks. It inhibits hair growth (potentially by inhibiting ornithine decarboxylase)
- *Bicalutamide (≤50 mg daily)*

There is emerging data to support use with oral contraceptives in PCOS.[9]

Nonpharmacologic cosmetic therapies for hirsutism include shaving, depilating, hair bleaching, electrolysis, and laser hair removal.

TREATMENT OPTIONS FOR ANOVULATORY INFERTILITY

Preconception counseling for ideal body weight and blood sugar optimization is crucial. This improves ovulation and live birth rates.

Pharmacotherapy options include clomiphene, aromatase inhibitors, gonadotropins, and metformin. Ovulation induction can be done using either letrozole or clomiphene. Letrozole is superior to clomiphene for achieving pregnancy and live births. Clomiphene is also a first-line drug for ovulation induction because more safety data is available. The live birth rate following 6 months of clomiphene varies from 20 to 40%.[9] Letrozole may be preferred in overweight or obese patients.

Second-line pharmacologic option for infertility is usually ovarian stimulation using low-dose urinary or recombinant gonadotropins. Cumulative 1- and 2-year singleton live birth rates are approximately 50% and 70%, respectively. A low-dose, step-up protocol is generally favored aiming for mono-ovulation, with the ovary very sensitive to exogenous stimulation once a threshold dose has been reached.

For the purpose of treating infertility, metformin alone increases ovulation rate and use of metformin with clomiphene may offer better responses.

In vitro fertilization (IVF) for women with PCOS alone is recommended as third-line infertility therapy.[1]

Aromatase Inhibitors

Letrozole

Off-label letrozole is a first-line therapy used to achieve pregnancy with live birth for subfertile women with PCOS.[13] Letrozole diminishes hypothalamic estrogen negative feedback and transiently increases FSH release without depleting estrogen receptors (ERs).[10]

Letrozole oral tablet: 2.5, 5, or 7.5 mg PO once daily on days 3 through 7 of the menstrual cycle may be effective; alternatively, a 20-mg single dose on day 3 of the menstrual cycle has also been studied.

Generally, side effects include signs and symptoms of hypoestrogenism including fractures.

Anastrozole, which is a potent and highly selective aromatase inhibitor, is ineffective for ovulation induction.

Selective Estrogen Receptor Modulators

Clomiphene

Clomiphene citrate is a nonsteroidal, ovulation-inducing ER ligand with mixed agonist–antagonistic properties. It consists of a nonracemic mixture of zuclomiphene (~38%) and enclomiphene (~62%). Clomiphene acts as a selective estrogen receptor modulator (SERM). It blocks estrogen negative feedback and cause a prolonged increase in FSH secretion.[12]

Clomiphene is a prodrug most importantly of 4-hydroxyclomiphene and 4-hydroxy-N-desmethylclomiphene, which are the most active of its metabolites. The elimination half-life is about 4–7 days. Most clomiphene metabolism occurs in the liver, where it undergoes enterohepatic recirculation. Clomiphene and its metabolites are excreted primarily through feces (42%), and excretion can occur up to 6 weeks after discontinuation.

Clomiphene citrate oral tablet: Initially 50 mg PO once daily for 5 days. If ovulation does not occur with this dosing regimen, increase to 100 mg PO once daily for 5 days with the next cycle. The incidence rate of multiple pregnancy is 6–10%. If ovulation has not occurred after three courses of treatment, the patient needs reevaluation. If pregnancy does not occur within a total of six cycles, discontinue. Prolonged administration of the drug is not recommended.

Side effects: It may cause reversible ovarian enlargement. Other effects are visual symptoms (blurred vision, double vision, floaters, eye sensitivity to light, scotomata), headaches, vasomotor flushes (or hot flashes), light sensitivity and pupil constriction, abnormal uterine bleeding, and/or abdominal discomfort. Prolonged use may be associated with increased risk of ovarian cancer.

Gonadotropin Therapy

Typically used for ovulation induction after clomiphene or letrozole. Low-dose gonadotropin therapy aims to achieve a singleton live birth by creating a transient increase in FSH above a threshold dose for selecting a limited number of developing follicles, recognizing that PCOS women are prone to excessive follicle development.[2] Options include urinary gonadotropins or recombinant follicle-stimulating hormone.

DRUGS TO AID WEIGHT LOSS IN PCOS[14]

Orlistat

It assists in weight loss by inhibiting intestinal fat absorption (inhibits gastric and pancreatic lipases). There are various studies in PCOS obese patients with good results.

The person is advised to follow a low-fat diet that provides 30% of daily food energy as fat, distributed over three main meals a day. A weight loss goal is agreed upon and regularly reviewed, preferably after 12 weeks.

Bupropion/Naltrexone

It is a new antiobesity medication which suppresses appetite. Use and safety in PCOS needs further studies.

Glucagon-like Peptide-1 Receptor Agonists

This new group of medication which promotes weight loss in PCOS. Liraglutide has been shown to be superior to placebo as well as to metformin and orlistat in head-to-head comparisons. The efficacy of liraglutide in promoting weight loss in PCOS patients is proven.

Medical management may be needed for other associated problems in PCOS:[15]
- *Dyslipidemia:* Approximately 70% of patients with newly diagnosed disease have abnormal lipid levels, including increased total cholesterol level, high triglyceride levels, high low-density lipoprotein cholesterol (LDL-C) level, and decreased high-density lipoprotein cholesterol (HDL-C) level.
- *Hypertension:* Women with PCOS have risk of developing hypertension which if untreated may accelerate atherosclerotic cardiovascular disease.
- Nonalcoholic fatty liver disease is frequently seen in patients with PCOS, likely as a result of IR as well as obesity.
- *Depression and anxiety:* Increased incidence and prevalence over lifetime.

SPECIAL POPULATIONS

Adolescents

Diagnosis can be difficult in adolescents owing to overlap between normal pubertal development and characteristic features of PCOS. Suggested criteria include demonstration of chemical and/or biochemical hyperandrogenism and presence of persistent oligomenorrhea for at least 2 years after menarche.[16]

Hormonal Contraceptives

In early adolescence, using hormonal contraceptives is controversial. Ideal hormonal contraceptive regimen and appropriate duration of therapy for adolescents are uncertain. The standard practice is to wait for 2 years after menarche to prevent reduction in peak bone mass.[3]

Metformin Therapy

Small, short-term studies have found that metformin restores menstrual regularity and improves hyperandrogenemia, IR, and glucose intolerance in obese and nonobese adolescents with PCOS.

Postmenopausal Women

After menopause, two of the key diagnostic criteria of PCOS (irregular menses and polycystic ovaries on transvaginal ultrasonography) are no longer applicable.

Most women who had PCOS during their reproductive years continue to manifest both metabolic phenotype and unfavorable cardiovascular risk factors. Androgen levels are still higher than in postmenopausal women without history of PCOS.

It is advisable to maintain vigilance for monitoring lipid levels, blood pressure, and glycemia in accordance with standards of care in this population of women.

Polycystic ovary syndrome is a common condition affecting the reproductive, metabolic, and psychological health of a woman. First-line intervention is weight loss. OCPs form the first line of medical management, which is specially effective in restoring menstrual cycles and hirsutism. Insulin sensitizing agents, like metformin and thiazolidinediones, enhance metabolic response and fertility. Antiandrogens are used for hirsutism and acne along with contraceptive pills. For anovulatory infertility, ovulation induction with clomiphene or letrozole forms the mainstay of treatment. Drugs to aid in weight loss are also used in extreme obesity when lifestyle modification fails.

■ KEY POINTS

- Hormonal contraceptives are the first line pharmacologic therapy which regulates menstrual cycle and improves features of hyperandrogenism.
- Insulin sensitizing medications like Metformin is used to improve metabolic status, decrease androgen levels and increase rates of spontaneous ovulation.
- Treatment options for acne and hirsutism include hormonal contraceptives and antiandrogens.
- Anovulatory infertility is treated with clomiphene, aromatase inhibitors, gonadotropins, and metformin.
- Orlistat assists in weight loss.

■ REFERENCES

1. Joham AE, Norman RJ, Stener-Victorin E, Legro RS, Franks S, Moran LJ, et al. Review polycystic ovary syndrome. Lancet Diabetes Endocrinol. 2022;10:668-80.
2. Chang RJ, Dumesic DA. Polycystic ovary syndrome and hyperandrogenic states. In: Strauss JF III, Barbieri RL (Eds). Yen and Jaffs's Reproductive Endocrinology, 8th edition. Philadelphia: Elsevier; 2019. pp. 520-55.
3. Shah D, Patil M, On behalf of the National PCOS Working Group. Consensus statement on the use of oral contraceptive pills in polycystic ovarian syndrome women in India. J Hum Reprod Sci. 2018;11:96-118.
4. Bates GW Jr, Propst AM. Polycystic ovarian syndrome management options. Obstet Gynecol Clin North Am. 2012;39:495-506.
5. Sharma A, Welt CK. Practical approach to hyperandrogenism in women. Med Clin North Am. 2021;105:1099-116.
6. Nader S, Diamanti-Kandarakis E. Polycystic ovary syndrome, oral contraceptives and metabolic issues: New perspectives and a unifying hypothesis. Hum Reprod. 2007;22:317-22.
7. Shinkai K, Abudu B. Polycystic ovary syndrome. Treatment of Skin Disease. 6th edition. 2022;195;659-61.
8. Wu CQ, Grandi SM, Filion KB, Abenhaim HA, Joseph L, Eisenberg MJ, et al. Drospirenone-containing oral contraceptive pills and the risk of venous and arterial thrombosis: a systematic review. BJOG. 2013;120:801-10.
9. Badawy A, Elnashar A. Treatment options for polycystic ovary syndrome. Int J Womens Health. 2011;3:25-35.

10. Harborne L, Fleming R, Lyall H, Sattar N, Norman J. Metformin or antiandrogen in the treatment of hirsutism in polycystic ovary syndrome. J Clin Endocrinol Metab. 2003;88:4116-23.
11. Benjamins LJ, Barratt MS. Evaluation and management of polycystic ovary syndrome. J Pediatr Health Care. 2009;23:337-43.
12. Bulun S. Physiology and pathology of the female reproductive axis. In: Melmed S, Koenig R, Rosen CJ, Auchus RJ, Goldfine AB (Eds). Williams Textbook of Endocrinology, 14th edition. Netherlands: Elsevier; 2020. pp. 574-641.
13. Ali SS, Rehman R. Polycystic ovary syndrome and subfertility. In: Sheikh A, Rehman R (Eds). Subfertility: Recent Advances for Management and Prevention. Netherlands: Elsevier; 2021. pp. 115-34.
14. Markantes GK, Tsichlia G, Georgopoulos NA. Diet and exercise in the management of PCOS: Starting from the basics. In: Diamanti-Kandarakis E (Ed). Polycystic Ovary Syndrome: Challenging Issues in the Modern Era of Individualized Medicine. Netherlands: Elsevier; 2022. pp. 97-115.
15. Armeni E, Lambrinoudaki I. Long-term health in women of age more than 40 years with polycystic ovary syndrome. In: Diamanti-Kandarakis E (Ed). Polycystic Ovary Syndrome: Challenging Issues in the Modern Era of Individualized Medicine. Netherlands: Elsevier; 2022. pp. 245-85.
16. Makaya T, Basu S, Poole R. Symposium: Endocrinology. Management of teenagers with polycystic ovarian syndrome. Paediatr Child Health. 2019;29(7):303-8.

Chapter 29

Hirsutism

Ashima Taneja, Muskan Chaudhary

The management of hirsutism depends on the severity of the disease and reproductive status. The patient has to be counseled about the various modalities of treatment and the long duration of the treatment. A multimodal approach is preferred.[1]

Treatment of hirsutism includes:
- Lifestyle modification
- Pharmacological therapy
- Cosmetic methods

■ LIFESTYLE MODIFICATION

Lifestyle modification includes physical exercise, behavioral changes, and dietary changes.

Smoking cessation should be strongly discouraged because it aggravates the undesirable effects of many of the drugs available for hirsutism and related conditions.

Weight loss (5–10%) in obese patients with hyperandrogenemia decreases androgen excess, increases sex hormone binding globulin (SHBG), and reduces clinical hirsutism.[2]

A randomized control study by Wong et al. in 2016 documented that diet control for 6 months improved body mass index (BMI) levels, increased SHBG levels, and decreased lipid levels in polycystic ovary syndrome (PCOS) patients.[3] Cochrane study (2015) suggested no demonstrable benefits of weight loss in severe hirsutism.[4]

Pharmacological Treatment

The drugs used in the management of hirsutism include:
1. Combined oral contraceptives (COCs)
2. Antiandrogens
3. Insulin-sensitizing drugs
4. Glucocorticoids
5. Gonadotropin-releasing hormone (GnRH) agonists
6. Topical agents

Combined Oral Contraceptives

They contain combined oral estrogen and progestins.

Mechanism of Action of COCs

- *Estrogen* inhibits follicle-stimulating hormone (FSH) which prevents the growth of follicles.
- *Estrogen* also stimulates hepatic SHBG production. SHBG binds with the circulating androgens.
- Progestin inhibits luteinizing hormone (LH), which decreases ovarian androgens.
- Antiandrogenic progestins like cyproterone acetate (CPA) and drospirenone suppress adrenal androgen

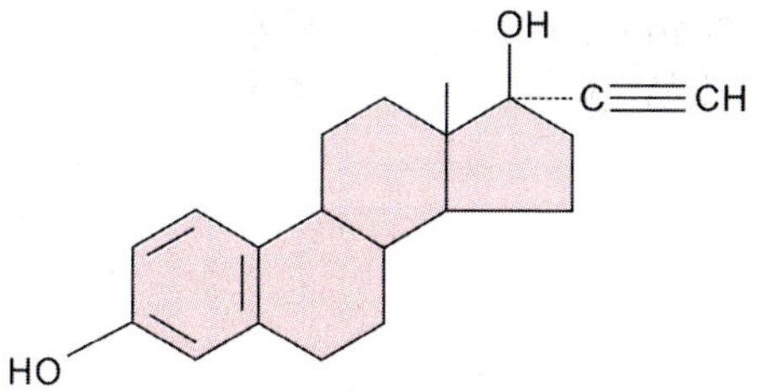

Fig. 1: Ethinylestradiol (EE) molecule.

TABLE 1: Different formulations of oral contraceptives available.

Estrogen	Progestin
Ethinylestradiol: • 20 µg • 20 µg	• Desogestrel (0.15 mg) • Drospirenone (3 mg)
Ethinylestradiol: • 30 µg • 30 µg • 30 µg	• Desogestrel (0.15 mg) • Levonorgestrel (0.15 mg) • Drospirenone (3 mg)
Ethinylestradiol: 35 µg	Cyproterone acetate (2 mg)
Ethinylestradiol: 50 µg	Norgestrel (0.5 mg)
Transdermal ethinylestradiol: 34 µg	Norelgestromin (200 µg)
Vaginal estrogen: 15 µg	Etonogestrel (0.12 mg)

secretion and increase the clearance of androgens.
- Androgenic progestins also increase the metabolic clearance of testosterone.
- Inhibition of 5α-reductase activity in the skin decreases the production of dihydrotestosterone (DHT) in hair follicles and sebaceous glands.[5]

Estrogen component of combination oral contraceptives: Ethinylestradiol (EE) is a very potent oral estrogen **(Fig. 1)**.

The dose of ethinylestradiol varies from 20 to 50 µg as given in **Table 1**.

The low-dose OCs (20–35 µg) have similar effectiveness for acne and hirsutism.

The transdermal contraceptive patch and the vaginal rings can also be used. The effect of transdermal contraceptive patches and oral contraceptives in suppressing serum androgen levels in hirsutism was found to be similar.[6]

Progestin component of combination oral contraceptives

Classification of progesterones:
- *First-generation progestins*—products containing estranes derived from testosterone such as norethindrone, norethynodrel, norethindrone acetate, and ethynodiol diacetate and pregnanes derived from 17-OH progesterone such as medroxyprogesterone acetate and chlormadinone acetate. They have medium androgenicity.
- *Second-generation progestins*—products containing gonanes derived from testosterone such as levonorgestrel and norgestrel. They have high androgenicity.
- *Third-generation progestins*—products containing desogestrel, gestodene, norgestimate/norelgestromin, and etonogestrel. They have low androgenicity.
- *Fourth-generation progestins*—products containing nonethylated estranes such as drospirenone and dienogest, or pregnanes (19-norprogesterones) such as nestorone, nomegestrol acetate, and trimegestone **(Box 1)**.

Progesterone alone or not recommended in hirsutism, as the suppression of androgens is not marked. It is recommended in patients where estrogen is contraindicated.

It is the first line of treatment in patients who are not seeking fertility (Endocrine Society Clinical Guideline) or patients with abnormal uterine bleeding or dysmenorrhea along with hirsutism.[7]

BOX 1: Classification of progestins.

- Combination of 19-nortestosterone derivatives (levonorgestrel and norethindrone) can worsen hirsutism.[8]
- *Levonorgestrel (LNG) is not preferred for the treatment of hirsutism but the risk of thromboembolism with LNG is less as compared to other progestins.*[9]
- *Drospirenone* is a newer progestin with antiandrogenic properties but has higher risk of thromboembolism.
- *Cyproterone acetate (CPA)* (2 mg) has superiority over other progestins after 12 months of use but has a risk of thromboembolism.
- Progesterones alone regimens include medroxyprogesterone acetate (MPA) 10–20 mg daily and injection depot medroxyprogesterone acetate (DMPA) 150 mg intramuscular every 3 months.

TABLE 2: Antiandrogens used for the treatment of hirsutism.

Antiandrogens	Dosing
Cyproterone acetate	- 50–100 mg/day on menstrual days 5–15 in combination with ethinylestradiol - 20–35 mg on days 5–25
Spironolactone	100–200 mg/day given in divided doses twice daily
Finasteride	2.5–5 mg/day
Flutamide	- 250–500 mg/day (high dose) - 62.5 to <250 mg/day (low dose)

Side effects of oral contraceptive pill: These newer oral contraceptive pill (OCP) formulations might cause:

- Mild increase in blood pressure
- May have deleterious effects on coagulation
- Increase the risk of nonfatal venous thromboembolism compared with second-generation OCPs.[10]

The choice of an OCP for the treatment of hirsutism must balance carefully the greater efficacy of third-generation pills against the safer coagulation profile of second-generation OCP, especially in adolescents, hypertensive women, and smokers.

Antiandrogens

Various antiandrogen drugs are described in **Table 2**.

Mechanism of action: It inhibits testosterones and androgens at the level of the pilosebaceous gland.[11]

Indications for Antiandrogens in Hirsutism (Table 3)

- Patients with contraindications to combined oral contraceptives
- Inadequate response to combined oral contraceptives.

Cyproterone acetate blocks the action of dihydrotestosterone and testosterone. It should be administered along with ethinylestradiol to prevent menstrual irregularities and ovulation. It is available as a combined estrogen–progestin oral contraceptive (2 mg cyproterone acetate and 35 µg ethinylestradiol) available as *Diane-35*.

Improvement of hirsutism is observed after 3-6 months of therapy.

- *Mechanism of action:*
  - It decreases androgen by competing with androgen receptors
  - It inhibits 5α-reductase enzyme activity
- The dose is 50–100 mg/day on menstrual cycle days 5–15 for 3–6 months with ethinylestradiol 20–35 mg on days 5–25 for 3–6 months.
- *Side effects:* Nausea, weight gain, loss of libido, and breast pain.

TABLE 3: Medications commonly used for treatment of hirsutism.

Medication	Dosage	Side effects	Remarks
Oral contraceptives	One tablet daily	Gastrointestinal upset, headaches	Recommended first-line agents
Metformin	500–2,500 mg daily in divided doses	Gastrointestinal upset	Useful in the treatment of PCOS
Cyproterone acetate	50–100 mg/day	Nausea, weight gain, loss of libido, and breast pain	Administered along with ethinylestradiol to prevent menstrual irregularities
Spironolactone	100–200 mg daily	Hyperkalemia, irregular menses	Risk of pseudohermaphroditism in males
Finasteride	5 mg daily	Hepatotoxicity, decreased libido, mastalgia, dry skin	–
Glucocorticoids	5–10 mg daily	Weight gain, osteoporosis, adrenal suppression	Congenital adrenal hyperplasia
GnRH (leuprolide)	3.75 mg weekly, 11.25 mg 3 monthly intramuscular	Hot flushes, osteoporosis, atrophic vaginitis	Consider adding add-back therapy
Ketoconazole	200 mg daily	Dry skin, headache, hepatotoxicity	Used after failure of other drugs
Eflornithine	13.9% topical	Acne, erythema, burning, itching, dry skin	Consider as a combination therapy
Flutamide	250 mg daily	Hepatotoxicity	

(GnRH: gonadotropin-releasing hormone; PCOS: polycystic ovary syndrome)

Spironolactone is an aldosterone antagonist. It works as a competitive inhibitor of the androgen receptor and 5α-reductase inhibitor.

- *Mechanism of action:*
  - It is a competitive inhibitor of the androgen receptor.
  - It inhibits 5α-reductase enzyme activity
- *Dose:* 50–100 mg twice daily.
- *Side effects* include menstrual irregularities (dose-dependent), fatigue, hyperkalemia, and feminization of the male fetus
- *Caution:* Not to be used with oral contraceptives containing drospirenone.

Flutamide: It is as effective as spironolactone. A minimum of 3 months of therapy is required to observe the results.

- *Mechanism of action:*
  - It blocks androgen receptors
  - It decreases testosterone synthesis
- *Doses:*
  - 250–500 mg/day (high dose)
  - 250 mg/day (low dose)
- *Side effects:* The major side effect is hepatotoxicity (flutamide is not recommended due to hepatotoxicity). Others include nausea, dry skin, and headache. It is also not cost-effective.

Finasteride: It acts by inhibiting 5α-reductase activity. Finasteride is effective in the treatment of hirsutism in women.

- The required daily dose is 5 mg/day.

- Adverse effects include libido reduction, mastalgia, and dry skin.
- *Caution:* It should be used with an effective method of contraception.

Ketoconazole: Ketoconazole is an orally active antimycotic agent and a potent inhibitor of gonadal and adrenal steroidogenesis.

The dose is 200 mg/day.

Insulin-sensitizing Drugs

The most common cause of hirsutism is PCOS. It is associated with insulin resistance and is the most commonly used drugs for hirsutism.
- *Mechanism of action:*
  - Decrease androgen levels
  - Decrease circulating androgens
- *Drugs used:*
  - Metformin
  - Thiazolidinediones (rosiglitazone)

Although these drugs decrease levels of circulating insulin and androgens, however, it is concluded from various systematic reviews and meta-analyses that they are not recommended for the treatment of hirsutism.[12]

Glucocorticoids

Corticosteroids are less effective in the treatment of hirsutism as compared to COC.
- *Uses:* To suppress endogenous adrenocorticotropic hormone (ACTH) secretion and to suppress adrenal androgen levels in cases with congenital adrenal hyperplasia.
- *Adverse effects:* Obesity, hypertension, weight gain, Cushing syndrome, and osteoporosis.

Gonadotropin-releasing Hormone Agonists

- *Mechanism of action:*
  - Decreases LH
  - Decreases androgen levels
- *Indications:*
  - Severe hyperandrogenism
  - Women who do not respond to a combination of COC and antiandrogens.
- *Drugs:*
  - Leuprolide
  - Nafarelin
  - Goserelin
- *Disadvantage:*
  - Costly therapy
  - Causes osteoporosis and decreased bone mineral density
  - Menopausal symptoms
- *Efficacy:* The efficacy of GnRH agonists is similar to COCs.

Topical Agents (Eflornithine Hydrochloride)

It is a topical antiandrogen cream.

Preparation: 13.9% of *eflornithine hydrochloride*
- *Mechanism of action:*
  - Irreversible inhibiting ornithine decarboxylase catalyzes the rate-limiting step for follicular polyamine synthesis
  - It reduces the growth and appearance of facial hair
- *Results:* Take 6–8 weeks and after discontinuation of treatment, reappearance of facial hair to pretreatment levels after 8 weeks of stopping the treatment.
- *Indication:* Mild hirsutism.
- *Efficacy:* When used in conjunction with laser hair removal, eflornithine produces a more rapid response than laser treatment alone.[13]
- *Side effects:* Itching and dry skin.

■ COSMETIC METHODS

Cosmetic methods of hair removal are depicted in **Flowchart 1**.

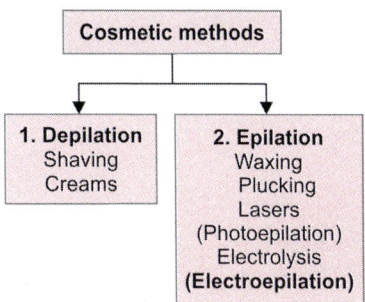

Flowchart 1: Cosmetic methods of treatment for hirsutism.

TABLE 4: Comparison of photoepilation and electrolysis.

Photoepilation	Electrolysis
• Works on dark hair • Rapidly cover large areas • High chances of paradoxical hair growth • Shorter treatment duration	• Works on any hair type • Covers small areas • Less paradoxical hair growth • Longer treatment time

- *Depilation:* It is the removal of the hair shaft and includes shaving and chemical depilatory (creams and gels)
- *Epilation:* It removes the hair shaft, follicle, and bulb. It includes threading, lasers, waxing, and plucking.
  - Side effects of creams include hyperpigmentation, irritation, itchy skin, and possible skin discoloration
    * *Side effects of shaving:* Short-lived, lasts for 1–3 days
    * Side effects of plucking or waxing include scarring and folliculitis
  - Lasers and light-based technology for hair removal have become the fastest-growing procedures. It causes selective hair damage and is less time-consuming.
    * It has longer hair food in the world and fewer side effects
    * Photoepilation uses a long pulse-duration light source such as Nd: YAG or diode laser (FDA approved). Topical treatment or electrolysis is preferred over photoepilation in such patients.
    * Topical eflornithine cream is added with this treatment for rapid response.
- Complete or nearly complete alopecia occurs for 4–6 weeks after each photoepilation treatment.[14]

- *Side effects:*
  * Thermal injury
  * Hhyperpigmentation
  * Multiple treatments are required.

The difference between photoepilation and electrolysis is elaborated in **Table 4**.

- *Duration of photoepilation:*
  - 4–6 cycles 4–6 weeks apart
  - Maintenance treatments every 6–12 months
- The success rate is 10–40% with single cycle and 90% with repeated cycles.[15]

Electrolysis damages hair follicles through an electric current. This treatment is safe and effective. Side effects include pain.

■ FOLLOW-UP

Before starting any method, the outcomes of treatment should be discussed with the patient. Patients are to be reassessed at routine intervals (every 3–6 months).

The minimum duration of treatment required is 6 months.

A summary of the management of hirsutism is depicted in **Flowchart 2**.

■ KEY POINTS

- *First line of treatment* for hirsutism is low-dose combined oral contraceptive pills.
- In case of contraindication to oral contraceptives, antiandrogens can be used.

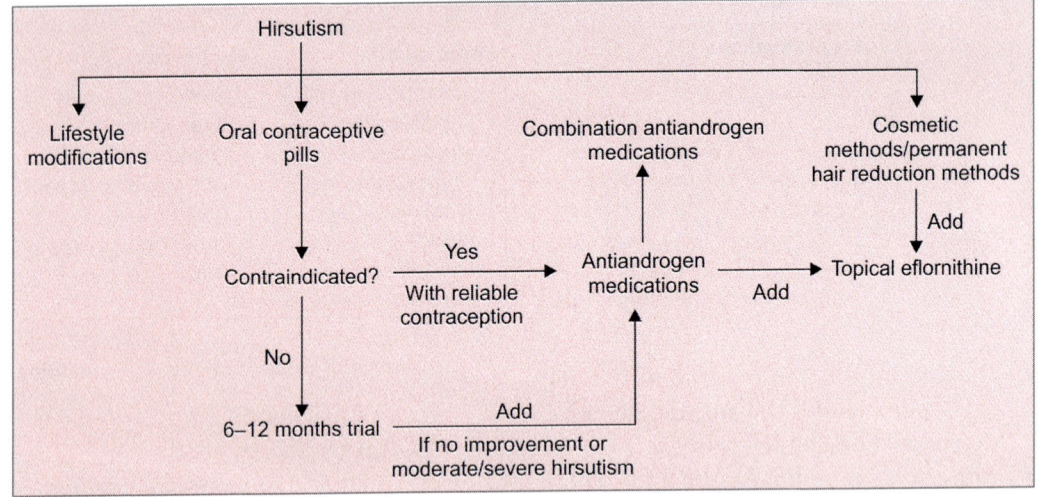

Flowchart 2: Management of hirsutism.

- Inadequate response to treatment with COCs, combine an antiandrogen agent.
- GnRH agonist therapy should be considered in management severe hyperandrogenism.
- Cosmetic methods to be used in combination with pharmacological therapy.
- Eflornithine cream can be added to pharmacological therapy for faster response.

REFERENCES

1. Screening and Management of the Hyperandrogenic Adolescent: ACOG Committee Opinion, Number 789. Obstet Gynecol. 2019; 134(4):e106-e114.
2. NHS. (2019). Dietary Advice for Polycystic Ovary Syndrome (PCOS). [online] Available from: https://www.swft.nhs.uk/application/files/8015/6586/5352/Dietary_Advice_for_Polycystic_Ovary_Syndrome_A4_2019.pdf [Last accessed December, 2023].
3. Wong JM, Gallagher M, Gooding H, Feldman HA, Gordon CM, Ludwig DS, et al. A randomized pilot study of dietary treatments for polycystic ovary syndrome in adolescents. Pediatr Obes. 2016;11(3):210-20.
4. Lim SS, Hutchison SK, Van Ryswyk E, Norman RJ, Teede HJ, Moran LJ. Lifestyle changes in women with polycystic ovary syndrome. Cochrane Database Syst Rev. 2019;3(3):CD007506.
5. Taylor HS, Pal L, Seli E, Fritz MA. Speroff's Clinical Gynecologic Endocrinology and Infertility. Philadelphia: Lippincott Williams & Wilkins; 2019.
6. White T, Jain JK, Stanczyk FZ. Effect of oral versus transdermal steroidal contraceptives on androgenic markers. Am J Obstet Gynecol. 2005;192(6):2055-9.
7. Endocrine Society. (2018). Hirsutism Guideline Resources. [online] Available from: https://www.endocrine.org/clinical-practice-guidelines/hirsutism#1 [Last accessed December, 2023].
8. Parkin L, Sharples K, Hernandez RK, Jick SS. Risk of venous thromboembolism in users of oral contraceptives containing drospirenone or levonorgestrel: nested case-control study based on UK General Practice Research Database. BMJ. 2011; 342:d2139.
9. Moubasher AEA, Abdel Basset HA, Khalil AAM, Youssef EMK. Levonorgestrel vs combined oral contraceptive pills in the treatment of female acne and hirsutism. Dermatol Ther. 2020;33(6):e13700.
10. Escobar-Morreale HF, Carmina E, Dewailly D, Gambineri A, Kelestimur F, Moghetti P, et al.

Epidemiology, diagnosis, and management of hirsutism: a consensus statement by the Androgen Excess and Polycystic Ovary Syndrome Society. Hum Reprod Update. 2012;18(2):146-70.
11. Martin KA, Anderson RR, Chang RJ, Ehrmann DA, Lobo RA, Murad MH, et al. Evaluation and treatment of hirsutism in premenopausal women: An Endocrine Society Clinical Practice Guideline. J Clin Endocrinol Metab. 2018;103(4):1233-57.
12. Cosma M, Swiglo BA, Flynn DN, Kurtz DM, Labella ML, Mullan RJ, et al. Clinical review: Insulin sensitizers for the treatment of hirsutism: a systematic review and metaanalyses of randomized controlled trials. J Clin Endocrinol Metab. 2008;93(4): 1135-42.
13. Shehzad T, Iqbal F, Iqbal N. A randomized study of eflornithine cream combined with intense pulsed light versus intense pulsed light treatment alone for hirsutism in women. J Pakistan Assoc Dermatol. 2018;28(4):482484.
14. Avci P, Gupta GK, Clark J, Wikonkal N, Hamblin MR. Low-level laser (light) therapy (LLLT) for treatment of hair loss. Lasers Surg Med. 2014;46(2):144-51.
15. Lepselter J, Elman M. Biological and clinical aspects in laser hair removal. J Dermatolog Treat. 2004;15(2):72-83.

Chapter 30

Primary Amenorrhea

Priyanka Dahiya

Absence of menstruation by 15 years of age with normal development of secondary sexual characteristics (or pubertal development) or by 13 years of age along with absence of development of secondary sexual characteristics.[1] It has been classified in various ways: according to presence or absence of secondary sexual characters, by gonadotropin [follicle-stimulating hormone (FSH)] levels or according to the level of compartmental defect.

Table 1 highlights the important points of consideration while recording history, examination, and investigating a case of primary amenorrhea. For simplified understanding and approach toward

TABLE 1: Important points of considerations while recording history, examination, and investigating a case of primary amenorrhea.

History	Examination	Investigations
• *Sexual history:* Rule out pregnancy • Cyclical lower abdominal pain • Stress, weight loss, lifestyle, any chronic systemic illness • Family history of late menarche, genetic abnormalities • Headaches, visual disturbance • Galactorrhea • *Medications:* Antipsychotics, illicit drug abuse, chemo/radiotherapy	• BMI and height • Secondary sexual characteristics (Tanner staging) • Signs of thyroid or other endocrine disorder • Galactorrhea • Hirsutism, virilization, clitoromegaly • Turner's syndrome and androgen insensitivity body habitus • *Neurological:* Visual fields, smell, fundus • *Abdominal:* Mass arising from pelvis, inguinal area—gonads, hernia • Pelvic examination (imperforate hymen, transverse vaginal septum, blind vagina) • Digital rectal examination	• Karyotyping • *Hormonal assay:* FSH, LH, prolactin, thyroid profile, androgen levels (testosterone, androstenedione, 17α-hydroxyprogesterone) • *Pelvic ultrasound:* Uterus and ovaries • CT/MRI head

(BMI: body mass index; CT: computed tomography; FSH: follicle-stimulating hormone; LH: luteinizing hormone; MRI: magnetic resonance imaging)

managing such a case, it may be broadly categorized as amenorrhea with presence or absence of secondary sexual characters. **Flowcharts 1 and 2** depict management algorithm for primary amenorrhea with normal secondary sexual characters and that with either absence or underdeveloped secondary sexual characters respectively.

HYPERGONADOTROPIC PRIMARY AMENORRHEA

- This is the most common cause of primary amenorrhea (40%).
- It includes:
  - *Gonadal dysgenesis:* Turner's syndrome (TS) (45,X), mixed gonadal dysgenesis (45,X/46,XY), pure gonadal dysgenesis (46,XX), Swyer syndrome (46,XY)

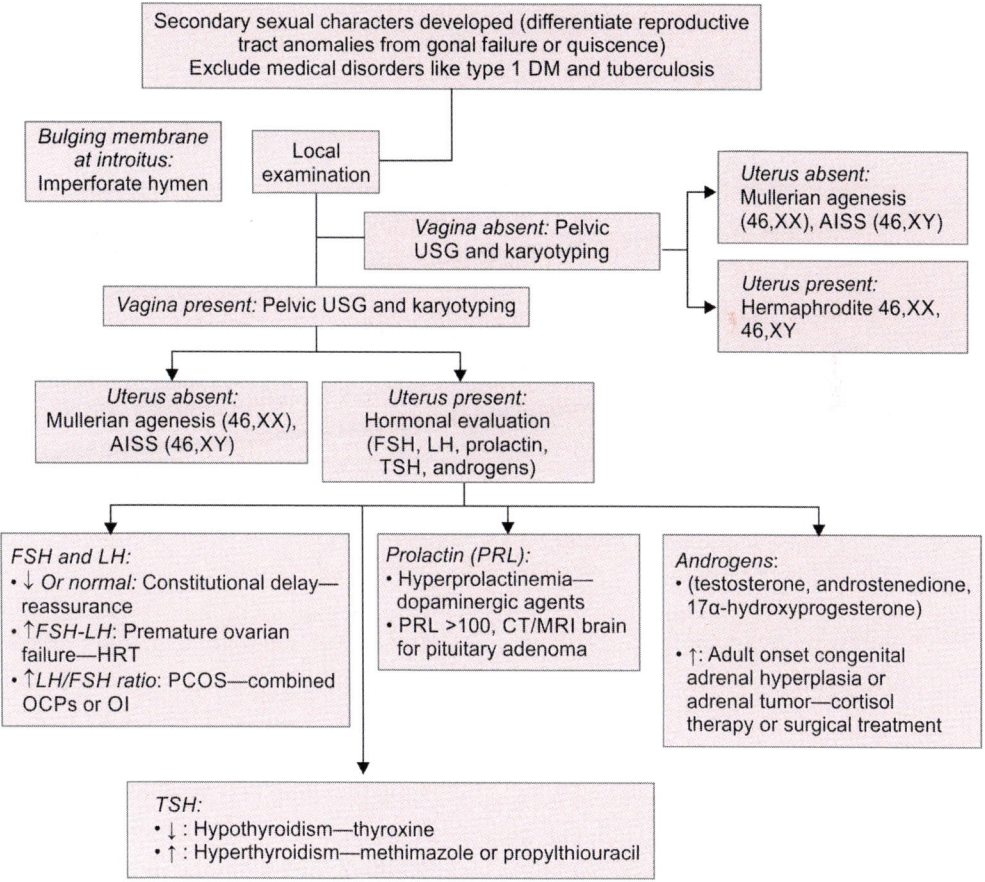

Flowchart 1: Depicts management algorithm for primary amenorrhea with normal secondary sexual characters.

(AISS: androgen in sensitivity syndrome; CT: computed tomography; DM: diabetes mellitus; FSH: follicle-stimulating hormone; HRT: hormone replacement therapy; MRI: magnetic resonance imaging; LH: luteinizing hormone; OCPs: oral contraceptive pills; OI: ovulation induction; PCOS: polycystic ovary syndrome; TSH: thyroid-stimulating hormone; USG: ultrasonography)

Flowchart 2: Management algorithm for primary amenorrhea with absent or underdeveloped secondary sexual characters.

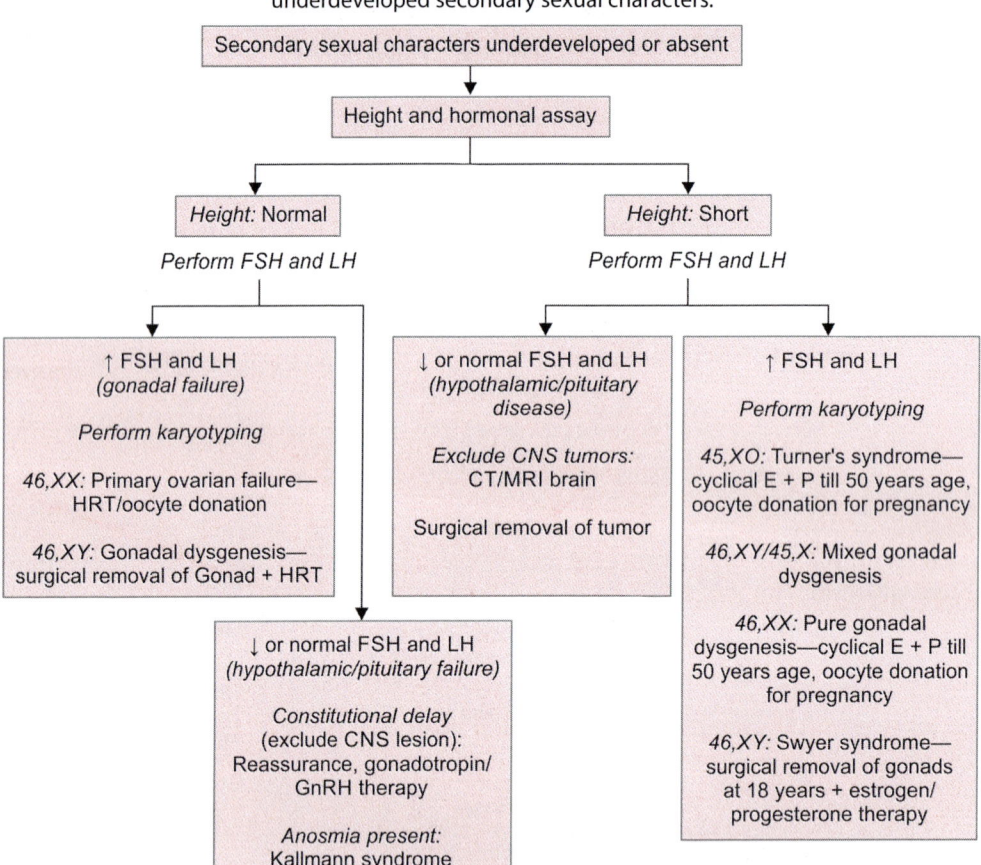

(CNS: central nervous system; CT: computed tomography; FSH: follicle-stimulating hormone; GnRH: gonadotropin-releasing hormone; HRT: hormone replacement therapy; LH: luteinizing hormone; MRI: magnetic resonance imaging)

- Premature ovarian failure (POF), resistant ovary syndrome

Turner's Syndrome

- Streak gonads with external female genitalia, absent secondary sexual characters
- Short stature, webbed neck, widely spaced nipples, wide carrying angle, cardiac anomalies (coarctation of aorta), renal anomalies
- *Associated medical disorders:* Hypertension, thyroiditis, sensorineural deafness, learning disabilities
- In Turner's mosaic (45,X/46,XX), physical findings may be absent, they may menstruate and conceive.
- **Tables 2 and 3** depict various estrogen and progesterone replacement therapy options available for treatment of Turner's syndrome.

TABLE 2: Estrogen therapy in Turner's syndrome.

Mechanism of action: Bind to specific nuclear receptors in target cells (ER) → regulate protein synthesis; estrogen agonists bind to EREs of target genes → promote or repress the gene transcription

Metabolism: Aromatic hydroxylation at either the C2 or C4 position, in liver by microsomal cytochrome P450

S/E: Epiphysis fusion resulting in stunted growth, ↓libido, gynecomastia, ↑incidence of gall stones, benign hepatomas, migraine, worsening of epilepsy

Low-dose estrogen treatment options available for use:

Preparation	Dose	Considerations for use
Transdermal patch		
Estraderm (matrix)	50/100 μg patch twice weekly, increment after every 6 months to adult dose by 50–100 μg twice weekly	• Applied to non-hairy skin below waist, replace and change site every 3–4 days • Not small enough to initiate puberty
Menostar (Bayer) (matrix)	14 μg patch, weekly	Easiest way to give low dose; once-a-week dosing
Vivelle-Dot (Novartis) (matrix)	25/50/75/100 μg patch twice weekly	To initiate puberty one patch per month, can be incremented by 25–100 μg twice weekly; designed for twice-weekly dosing, but can give once per week to increase dose more slowly
Oral route		
Premarin (Pfizer) (conjugated equine estrogen)	• 0.3, 0.625 mg/day, one-half pill daily • Increment by 0.625–1.25 mg/day after 6 months till adult dose	
17-beta-E2 (Estrace)	0.5, 1, 2, 4 mg/day, pill daily	Cheapest option, brands vary by country
EE	Started at 2 μg/day, increment by 10–20 μg/day	Not available in many countries
Depot		
Depot E2 (E2 cypionate)	5 mg/mL, started at 0.2 mg/mL	

(E2: estradiol; EE: ethinyl estradiol; ER: estrogen receptor; ERE: estrogen response element; S/E: side effect)

- **Table 4** enlists guidelines for hormone replacement therapy (HRT) in treating TS.

The investigations in a case with Turner's syndrome are shown in **Box 1**.

Box 2 shows the treatment in a case with Turner's syndrome.

Points of Consideration

- *Goal of estrogen replacement:* To mimic normal physical and social development and progression of puberty; best when started between 11 and 12 years of age and increasing over 2–3 years; neurocognitive benefits are inconclusive.

TABLE 3: Progesterone and combined E + P HRT for Turner's syndrome.

Mechanism of action: Progesterone agents can bind to the progesterone receptor (PR) as well as the androgen, glucocorticoid, and mineralocorticoid receptors according to their class.

The 19-norprogesterone derivatives are associated with androgenic action, medroxyprogesterone acetate with glucocorticoid-agonistic action, and drospirenone with antiandrogenic and antimineralocorticoid action.

Progesterone binds to PR → dimerization → attaches to PRE of target genes → regulates transcription through coactivators.

Metabolism: Mainly hepatic, excretion: Renal

S/E: Headache, breast engorgement, edema, mood swings, irregular bleeding when given continuously.

Regimens of estrogen + progestin are either combined sequentially with an estrogen for 21–25 days and the progestin for only 10–14 days, or combined continuously.

Progestin and estrogen/progestin combination treatment options available for use after pubertal induction:

Preparation	Dose	Considerations for use
Oral		
Medroxyprogesterone acetate	10 mg/day for 10 day	Give with TD E2 or alone for 10 day
Micronized progesterone	100 mg/day	Give continuously with TD E2, ↓ risk of breast cancer over long-term usage
Combined E2/progestin sequential patch (TD)		
Climara pro (Bayer)	E2 0.045 mg and levonorgestrel 0.015 mg/ 24 hours	Not used to initiate puberty One patch weekly
Combipatch (Noven)	E2 0.045 mg and norethindrone 0.14 or 0.25 mg/24 hours	Not used to initiate puberty One patch weekly
Combined E2/progestin sequential pills		
Combined OCPs		Not used to initiate puberty
Divina plus	Estradiol valerate 2 mg and medroxyprogesterone acetate 10 mg; 1 pill/day	Not used to initiate puberty, not available in India
Trisequens (Novo Nordisk)	E2 2 mg and norethisterone acetate 1 mg; 1 pill/day	Not used to initiate puberty Not available in India

(E2: estradiol; HRT: hormone replacement therapy; OCPs: oral contraceptive pills; PRE: progesterone response element; S/E: side effect; TD: transdermal)

- The transdermal (TD) patches may be split into halves and quarters, allowing for a steady increase in dosage.
- The likelihood of achieving uterine size normalization is positively correlated with both the length and dosage of estrogen replacement therapy. This outcome has significance only in the context of individuals considering pregnancy as a viable option.

TABLE 4: Guidelines for hormone replacement therapy in Turner's syndrome.[6]

Age	Proposed treatment
Childhood	• Consider GH treatment when linear growth velocity declines • Begin to monitor for autoimmune thyroid disease
8–10 years	• Anticipatory guidance regarding induction of puberty • Obtain family history regarding disorders associated with thrombophilia
9–11 years	• Obtain LH and FSH concentrations to assess for ovarian failure • Consider obtaining AMH and inhibin B concentrations • Obtain bone age X-ray to assure that bone age is >8 years of age (to accurately interpret LH and FSH concentrations)
12–14 years	• Begin low-dose estrogen monotherapy preferably using transdermal route • Begin the discussion regarding fertility and reproductive options • Encourage parents to initiate and continue this discussion at home
Next 1–2 years	Gradually increase estrogen dose
13–16 years	Add progestogen therapy
17–50 years	• Continue cyclic hormone replacement therapy • Monitor glycemic status (earlier if clinically indicated)
50 years	Consider continuation of hormone replacement therapy with consideration of risk factors (similar to normal women undergoing menopause)

(AMH: anti-Mullerian hormone; FSH: follicle-stimulating hormone; GH: growth hormone; LH: luteinizing hormone)

BOX 1: Investigations in a case with Turner's syndrome.

- ↑ FSH (>40 mIU/mL)
- ↓ Estradiol (<25 pg/mL)
- ↓ Inhibin B
- ↓ AMH
- PCT is negative

(AMH: anti-Mullerian hormone; FSH: follicle-stimulating hormone; PCT: post coital test)

- In the context of oocyte donation, it is sometimes required to administer dosages that exceed the standard amount. For instance, oral doses of up to 8 mg have been employed for a duration of up to 2 years in order to attain optimum uterine development.[7]
- The recommended method of administering low-dose estradiol (E2) is through a systemic route, as supported by research that demonstrates its efficacy and theoretical advantages. In situations when TD E2 is unavailable or poses compliance challenges, the utilization of oral micronized E2 or depot E2 preparations is supported by empirical data.
- The administration of progestin is recommended with the onset of vaginal bleeding or following a 2-year course of estrogen therapy. During that period, several women revealed a preference for the convenience associated with the utilization of an oral combination of estrogen and progestin.
- The monitoring of treatment involves the assessment of patient satisfaction as well as the evaluation of growth and development indicators.

> **BOX 2:** Treatment in a case with Turner's syndrome.
>
> - *Estrogen replacement (ER) therapy:* To promote feminization, prevent osteoporosis, neurocognitive benefits, lipid metabolism
>   - Starting at age 11 and continuing until age 50, with dose increments spaced out over a couple of years
>   - Starting pubertal estrogen replacement with low-dose transdermal (TD) estrogen is recommended (benefits include avoiding procoagulation effects, first-pass metabolism, and increased stroke risk), as reported in the literature.[2-4]
>   - Side effects (S/E): Breast tenderness, nausea, vomiting, bloating, stomach cramps, headaches, weight gain, darkening of the skin, hair loss, vaginal itching, abnormal uterine bleeding
> - *Growth hormone (GH) therapy:*
>   - In order to optimize growth potential, it is advisable to consider initiating GH therapy prior to commencing low-dose estrogen therapy.
>   - This approach results in an annual net height gain of 1 cm.
>   - IGF-1 levels can be monitored to facilitate dosage changes.
>   - S/E: The individual presents with a combination of medical conditions including benign intracranial hypertension, scoliosis, slipping capital femoral epiphysis (SCFE), and aberrant glucose metabolism. Symptoms reported include headache and vomiting.[5]
> - *Progestins:*
>   - The administration of progestins should be initiated either with the onset of breakthrough bleeding or after a duration of 2 years of estradiol (E2) therapy.
>   - This effectively reduces the potential dangers associated with endometrial hyperplasia, such as irregular bleeding and the development of endometrial cancer resulting from extended exposure to unopposed estrogen.

- Individuals with TS have an elevated risk of developing both type 1 and type 2 diabetes mellitus (DM). However, studies have shown that the method of estrogen delivery does not have a significant impact on glucose and lipid metabolism in these individuals.[8]
- GH:
  - Oxandrolone has anabolic properties that facilitate the promotion of linear development in females who are diagnosed with Turner syndrome.
  - The potential adverse effects linked to the use of this medication include virilization and a lack of therapeutic effectiveness.
- A comprehensive approach including an eclectic group of medical professionals, including pediatric endocrinologists, reproductive endocrinologists, cardiologists, geneticists, otolaryngologists, mental health specialists, and social workers, is considered to be the most effective strategy.

Swyer Syndrome (46,XY)

- This is also known as acquired male pseudohermaphrodite with pure XY gonadal dysgenesis.
- *Etiology:* Genetic mutation of *SRY* gene
- Failure of development of internal and external male genitalia
- *Absence of MIF (Mullerian inhibiting factor):* Phenotypically female with absent secondary sexual characters
- *Treatment:*
  - Surgical removal of gonads (risk of malignancy)
  - Cyclical E + P (estrogen + progesterone) therapy (to induce menstruation)

- Pregnancy possible with donor egg/in vitro fertilization (IVF)

Premature Ovarian Insufficiency/Failure

- Loss of ovarian activity before the age of 40 years and characterized by menstrual disturbance (amenorrhea or oligomenorrhea) with raised gonadotropins and low E2
- Causes:
  - *Primary* (FSH receptor gene polymorphism, autosomal, inhibin B mutation, enzymatic defects, autoimmune disorders)
  - *Secondary* (chemo/radiotherapy, oophorectomy, uterine artery embolization, infections like mumps, herpes, and HIV)
- *Diagnosis* **(Table 5)**
- *Increased risk of:* Infertility, fractures, progression to cardiovascular disease, type 2 DM, cognition decline, concurrent autoimmune diseases.
- Indications for HRT in premature ovarian insufficiency (POI) **(Table 6)**
- Risks of HRT **(Table 7)**
- *Recommendations:*
  - Gonadectomy for all women with detectable Y chromosomal material
  - Fragile X premutation testing is indicated in POI women.
  - Autosomal genetic testing is not at present indicated in women with POI,

TABLE 5: Important points for establishing clinical diagnosis of a premature ovarian insufficiency (POI) case.

Presentation	Exclusion criteria	Diagnostic criteria	Investigations
• Less than 40 years with amenorrhea of ≥4 months • *Hypoestrogenic symptoms*: Night sweats, hot flushes, irritability, insomnia, reduced libido, vulvovaginal atrophy • Accelerated cognitive impairment	• Chromosomal abnormalities • Iatrogenic factors • RT/CT • Ovarian surgery • Autoimmune factors • Autoimmune thyroid, Addison's disease, SLE, rheumatoid arthritis, antinuclear antibodies • Inborn errors of metabolism (galactosemia) • *R/O*: Hyperprolactinemia, eating disorder/low BMI, PCOS, pregnancy	• Oligo/amenorrhea ≥4 months • FSH >25 IU/L* (on two separate occasions >4 weeks apart)	• hCG • FSH • TSH • Serum prolactin • *R/O associated autoimmune disorders*: TPO antibodies, anti-21 hydroxylase antibody • *Others*: – AMH – DEXA scan – Vitamin D levels – USG pelvis (ovarian volume, AFC) – Karyotype, FMR permutation analysis

* European Society for Human Reproduction and Embryology (ESHRE) Guideline Group on POI; Webber L, Davies M, Anderson R, Bartlett J, Braat D, Cartwright B, et al. ESHRE guideline: Management of women with premature ovarian insufficiency. Hum Reprod. 2016;31(5):926-37.

(AFC: antral follicle count; AMH: anti-Mullerian hormone; BMI: body mass index; CT: chemo therapy; DEXA: dual-energy X-ray absorptiometry; FSH: follicle-stimulating hormone; hCG: human chorionic gonadotropin; PCOS: polycystic ovary syndrome; RT: radiotherapy; SLE: systemic lupus erythematosus; TPO: thyroid peroxidase; TSH: thyroid-stimulating hormone; USG: ultrasonography)

TABLE 6: Indications for commencing HRT in POI cases.

S. no.	Indication	Comments
1.	Vasomotor symptoms	Indication to start HRT
2.	Bone health	Recommended to maintain bone health and prevent osteoporosis
3.	Genitourinary symptoms	Both systemic and local estrogens are effective
4.	Cardiovascular health	Early initiation is strongly recommended to control future risk of cardiovascular disease; and it should be continued at least until the average age of natural menopause
5.	Sexual function	Local estrogen may be required to treat dyspareunia
6.	Quality of life	Indirect benefit
7.	Neurological function	Indirect benefit
8.	Life expectancy	Indirect benefit

(HRT: hormone replacement therapy; POI: premature ovarian insufficiency)

TABLE 7: Risks associated with hormone replacement therapy (HRT).

S. no.	Risk	Comments
1.	Breast cancer	Found to increase the risk of breast cancer before the age of natural menopause
2.	Endometrial hyperplasia and cancer	Progestogen should be given in combination with estrogen therapy to protect the endometrium in women with an intact uterus
3.	Thromboembolic events and stroke	No evidence on increased risk

unless there is evidence suggesting a specific mutation [e.g., (BPES) blepharophimosis syndrome].

- *If cause is unknown or an immune disorder is suspected:* Screen for 21OH-Ab [adrenocortical antibodies (ACA) and thyroid peroxidase (TPO) antibodies]. In patients with a positive TPO-Ab test, thyroid-stimulating hormone (TSH) should be measured every year.
- Dietary supplementation (calcium + vitamin D) and estrogen replacement are recommended to maintain bone health and prevent osteoporosis.
- It is recommended that treatment for women diagnosed with primary ovarian insufficiency should be maintained until they reach the average age of natural menopause, which typically occurs around 50–51 years of age.
- Estrogen-only therapy is often indicated for women who have undergone a hysterectomy. For women who desire monthly withdrawal bleeds, cyclical progestin combined with estrogen is advised. Alternatively, continuous combined therapy may be suitable for patients who choose not to have monthly withdrawal bleeds **(Table 8)**.
- Women who have a higher risk of liver illness, migraines, or venous

TABLE 8: Hormone replacement therapy (HRT) for premature ovarian insufficiency (POI) cases.

	Recommended HRT for POI	
	Progestogen	
Estrogen	*Continuous*	*Sequential*
1–2 mg micronized 17β-estradiol (oral)	2.5–5 medroxyprogesterone acetate (MDPA) (oral)	10 mg MDPA, 12 days each month
100 μg 17β-estradiol (transdermal)	100 mg micronized progesterone (oral)	200 mg micronized progesterone (oral), 12 days each month
0.625–1.25 mg conjugated equine estrogen (oral)		

Source: American College of Obstetricians and Gynecologists. (2017). Hormone Therapy in Primary Ovarian Insufficiency. [online] Available from: https://www.acog.org/clinical/clinical-guidance/committee-opinion/articles/2017/05/hormone-therapy-in-primary-ovarian-insufficiency [Last accessed December, 2023].

thromboembolism should use TD estrogen (*see* **Table 8**).
- For the purpose of optimizing bone health, HRT may be better than combined oral contraceptive pill (COCP), however, the necessity of contraception must be considered.
- Specialist referral is necessary for patients who have primary amenorrhea and need pubertal induction but have contraindications to HRT due to hormone-sensitive tumors, or have a medical history of thrombophilia or endometriosis.
- Hormone treatment is recommended as a means of mitigating the risk of osteoporosis, cardiovascular disease, and urogenital atrophy, while also enhancing the overall quality of life for women diagnosed with primary ovarian insufficiency.
- Screen for osteoporosis with DEXA (dual-energy X-ray absorptiometry) scan, vitamin D supplementation, lifestyle changes, weight bearing exercises, include dairy products in diet (more than three servings).
- In contrast to the conventional approach of using bisphosphonates as the major therapeutic intervention for postmenopausal osteopenia or osteoporosis, the optimal management strategy for addressing low-bone density in women with primary ovarian insufficiency primarily involves the utilization of hormonal therapy.
- Oocyte donation option for fertility in women with POI.

EUGONADOTROPIC PRIMARY AMENORRHEA

- This is the second most common cause of primary amenorrhea (30%).
- It includes:
  - Absence of Mullerian development [(MRKH) Mayer–Rokitansky–Küster–Hauser syndrome, androgen insensitivity syndrome (AISS)]
  - Normal Mullerian development [imperforate hymen, transverse vaginal septum, polycystic ovary syndrome (PCOS) (7%), adult-onset congenital adrenal hyperplasia (CAH)

(1%), Cushing's disease (1%), thyroid disease (1%)].

Mullerian Agenesis/Mayer–Rokitansky–Küster–Hauser

- Normal height and hair growth
- Normal external genitalia, secondary sex characteristics
- Short blind-ending vagina (0–3 cm) with no cervix at the apex
- *Ultrasonography (USG) (transvaginal/perineal):* Absent uterus/vaginal canal, ovaries normal
- *Pelvic magnetic resonance imaging (MRI):* Determines the presence of rudimentary uterine buds/complete uterovaginal agenesis
- Renal abnormalities are found in approximately 30% of patients
- *Biochemical:* Gonadotropins, androgens, E2—normal
- *Chromosomal analysis:* 46,XX
- *Treatment:* Surgical
  The treatment modality entails a vaginoplasty, which aims to create a functioning neovagina.
- The *McIndoe vaginoplasty* procedure involves the utilization of a split-skin graft to cover a mold that is positioned into the dissected pouch located between the rectum and bladder.
- The *Baldwin vaginoplasty*, focuses on the utilization of a bowel transplant.
- The *Davydov vaginoplasty* procedure, employs a peritoneal graft for the creation of a neovagina.
- *William's vulva vaginoplasty* (labia majora flaps)
- *Cultured autologous vulvar tissue*/tissue-engineered biomaterial
- The *laparoscopic Vecchietti vaginoplasty* procedure involves the placement of a surgical traction device on the anterior abdominal wall, with subperitoneal threads connected to a mold positioned inside the vagina.

Androgen Insensitivity Syndrome

- Karyotype 46,XY
- *Gonads:* Present in inguinal canal—produce testosterone and MIF
- Deficiency of androgen receptors at target organs/or lack of 5α reductase enzyme (resulting in undermasculinization)
- *There are three overarching phenotypes that may be identified:*
  1. Complete androgen insensitivity syndrome (CAIS) is characterized by the presence of normal female external genitalia.
  2. Partial androgen insensitivity syndrome (PAIS) is characterized by varying degrees of insensitivity to androgens, resulting in individuals presenting with mainly female, mostly masculine, or ambiguous external genitalia.
  3. The individual presents with mild androgen insensitivity syndrome (MAIS), characterized by the presence of normal male external genitalia.
- *Treatment:*
  • *CAIS:* Gonadectomy can be performed after puberty when feminization has fully occurred, or it can be done during the prepubertal stage along with estrogen replacement therapy (see **Table 2**). Vaginal dilatation may be employed as a preventive measure against dyspareunia.
  • *PAIS:* Individuals who are assigned male at birth can undergo urologic surgical interventions, such as orchiopexy and hypospadias correction. Individuals assigned female at birth who have gonadectomy after puberty, with the

aim of preventing the development of clitoromegaly, may require combined estrogen and androgen replacement treatment.
- MAIS: For gynecomastia, MAIS patients may need a mammoplasty. Prenatal virilization may be enhanced by androgen medication **(Box 3 and Table 9)**.
- For the skeletal system's optimization: Weight-bearing workouts, together with the addition of calcium

BOX 3: Side effects and contraindications of androgen pharmacotherapy.

Side effects of androgen replacement therapy:
- Generally reversible with cessation of therapy
- High doses pose hepatic adverse effects
- Virilization in children/women (deepening of voice, terminal body hair, stunting of height)
- Intolerable increase in libido and erection frequency
- Seborrhea, acne
- *With high dosages:* Salt retention, edema, cholestatic jaundice

Contraindication: Prostate or breast cancer, congestive heart failure (CHF)

TABLE 9: Androgen replacement therapy.

Goal: To maintain stable, physiologic testosterone levels for prolonged periods using convenient depot testosterone formulations and avoid excessive fluctuation of androgen levels; plasma $t^{1/2}$ is only 10–20 minutes.

Mechanism of action: Testosterone is converted to dihydrotestosterone → binds to cytoplasmic androgen receptors (ARs) → ↑/↓DNA transcription: tissue specific → modified protein synthesis

Testosterone implants[9]	• Subdermal implants (200-mg pellets) at lateral abdominal or hip • Absorbed from reservoir into extracellular fluid	S/E: Bleeding or infection at implant site (<1%), extrusion
Transdermal testosterone[10] (andractim: dihydrotestosterone 25 mg/g gel)	• Transdermal patches, topical gels, creams • Gradual release diffusion down a concentration gradient into the blood stream	• *Benefits:* Uniform blood levels, circumvent the first pass metabolism • *S/E:* Skin reaction (20%), risk for an intimate partner in case of direct skin contact
Testosterone microspheres[11]	• Biodegradable microspheres injection, consisting of polyglycolide–lactide matrix • Every 2–3 months IM	Limitations of microsphere technology such as loading capacity, large injection volumes, and batch variability
Oral testosterone[12]	200–400 mg	Low oral bioavailability requiring high daily doses (200–400 mg) to maintain physiologic testosterone levels; not commercially available
Buccal/sublingual testosterone[13]		Sublingual cyclodextrin formulation/ buccal lozenge
Steroidal androgen[14] nandrolone (19-nortestosterone) 7α-methyl 19-nortestosterone (MENT)[15]	MENT is being developed as a depot androgen for androgen replacement and male contraception in an androgen-progestin combination regimen	• *Minimal aromatizability:* Suitable for treatment of osteoporosis in women in whom estrogen therapy is C/I due to hormone sensitive cancers (breast, uterus) • *S/E:* Virilization

(C/I: contraindication; IM: intramuscular; S/E: side effect)

and vitamin D supplements, are recommended for optimal bone health. Patients who reveal signs of reduced bone mineral density and/or multiple fractures should get bisphosphonate medication.

Imperforate Hymen (Cryptomenorrhea)

- Cyclical abdominal pain
- Palpable abdominopelvic mass (hematocolpos)
- Bluish bulging membrane at introitus
- *Treatment:* Surgical (cruciate incision and drainage)

Transverse Vaginal Septum

- Cyclical abdominal pain
- Palpable abdominopelvic mass (hematocolpos, hematometra)
- *Treatment:* Surgical (Septum excision and vaginoplasty)

Polycystic Ovary Syndrome

- Clinical features of hyperandrogenism (hirsutism, male pattern alopecia, acne)
- Normal menstrual cycles or chronic anovulation [oligomenorrhea, primary or secondary amenorrhea, dysfunctional uterine bleeding (DUB) or infertility]
- *Investigations:*
  - ↑LH (luteinizing hormone)/FSH
  - ↑AMH (anti-Mullerian hormone)
  - Normal/↑serum testosterone (≤150 ng/dL)
  - Normal/↑DHEA-S (dehydroepiandrosterone-sulfate) (<800 µg/dL)
  - Mild ↑serum prolactin (5–30%)
  - USG
- *Management:*
  - Lifestyle modification and weight loss
  - OCPs (oral contraceptive pills)
  - Antiandrogens
  - Insulin sensitizers
  - Ovulation induction

The details have been covered in Chapter 31.

Adult Onset Congenital Adrenal Hyperplasia

- Deficiency of 17-α-hydroxylase enzyme
- ↑ACTH (adrenocorticotropic hormone), ↓Cortisol
- *Clinical features:* Hypertension, hypernatremia, hypokalemia, amenorrhea
- *Treatment:* Cortisol therapy (refer to endocrinologist).

HYPOGONADOTROPIC PRIMARY AMENORRHEA

- Hypothalamic disorders (constitutional delay, Kallmann syndrome, Eating disorders, weight loss, malnutrition, stress)
- Pituitary disorders (Pituitary tumors, pituitary hypoplasia, empty sella syndrome).

Delayed Puberty (Constitutional Delay)

- History of delayed puberty may be present in mother or sister
- *On investigation:* No neurological or anatomical abnormalities are found.
- Further investigation is needed if puberty is delayed beyond 18 years of age.

Kallmann Syndrome

- Congenital form of hypogonadotropic hypogonadism (deletions/point mutations in the *KISS1R/KAL-1* gene)
- Manifests with hypo- or anosmia and lack of sexual maturation
- *Signs and symptoms:* Anosmia, reduced libido, cleft palate/lip, hypodontia, cleft hand or foot, unilateral (U/L) renal

agenesis, hearing impairment, mirror movements of the hands (synkinesis), ataxia, color blindness and ocular window defects; lack of testicular development in males, primary amenorrhea in women, poorly defined secondary sexual characteristics (sparse pubic hair and underdeveloped mammary glands or micropenis).
- *Evaluation* **(Box 4)**
- At risk of developing osteoporosis due to decreased sex hormones production
- *Treatment:* Lifelong HRT
  - Sex hormone replacement (testosterone or estrogen/progesterone) (*see* **Tables 2, 3 and 9**)
  - Fertility enhancement: Gonadotropin-releasing hormone (GnRH) injections (to induce ovulation), human chorionic gonadotropin (hCG) injections (to increase sperm count in males)
  - GnRH pulsatile therapy
  - *Monitoring HRT:* In males, measurement of serum testosterone, inhibin B, hematocrit and prostate-specific antigen (PSA)
  - In females, measurement of estrogen, FSH, LH, inhibin B and AMH
- Vitamin D supplementation and bisphosphonates are required.

Anorexia Nervosa

- Weight loss, body mass index (BMI) <10th percentile, ↓FSH, LH, E2.
- Appetite stimulant, antidepressant, dietary supplement, psychiatric consultation

Pituitary (Prolactinoma/Microadenoma)

- *Moderate:* High levels of serum prolactin (>50 µg/L)
- *Computed tomography (CT)/MRI:* Micro/macroadenoma
- *Treatment:* Medical (dopamine agonist)/surgical **(Table 10)**

BOX 4: Evaluation of Kallmann syndrome.

Clinical:
- Growth evaluation using standard height charts
- Tanner staging of sexual development
- Males: Look for undescended testis, testicular volume
- Females: Breast development, menarche
- Checking sense of smell using odorant panel
- Check hearing impairment, neurodevelopmental delay, synkinesis

Investigations:
- FSH, LH, testosterone, estrogen, prolactin
- GnRH and/or hCG stimulation test
- LFT, KFT
- inflammation marker testing
- Karyotype to check for chromosomal abnormalities
- MRI brain
- DEXA scan
- Renal USG

(DEXA: dual-energy X-ray absorptiometry; FSH: follicle-stimulating hormone; GnRH: gonadotropin-releasing hormone; hCG: human chorionic gonadotropin; KFT: kidney function test; LFT: liver function test; LH: luteinizing hormone; MRI: magnetic resonance imaging; USG: ultrasonography)

TABLE 10: Management of hyperprolactinemia.[16]

Dopamine agonists	Dose	Medical Mechanism of action	Common S/E
Bromocriptine (Criptal/ B-Crip/Brom/Bromogen)	• 2.5–15 mg daily • Start with low dose and increment after 4–6 weeks	Partial agonist at central and peripheral D2 receptors; decreases prolactin release from pituitary by activating dopaminergic receptors on lactotrope cells	GI (nausea, vomiting), CVS (postural hypotension, dizziness), CVS (headache, drowsiness), cardiac valvulopathy with high doses
Cabergoline (Caberlin/ Cabergoline/Cabliz)	• 0.25–1 mg twice weekly • Or 0.5–2 mg once weekly	Long-acting, D2 selective receptor agonist	S/E are less severe, short lasting with cabergoline

Surgical: Transsphenoidal resection of adenoma

(CVS: cyclic vomiting syndrome; GI: gastrointestinal; S/E: side effect)

KEY POINTS

- Role of HRT is to mimic the normal physical, social development, and progression of puberty.
- Estrogen replacement is best started between 11 and 12 years of age and increased slowly over 2–3 years.
- Progestin should be added once vaginal bleeding occurs or after 2 years of estrogen treatment.
- Dietary supplementation (calcium + vitamin D) and estrogen replacement is recommended to maintain bone health and prevent osteoporosis. Bisphosphonate therapy for those with evidence of decreased bone mineral density and/or multiple fractures.
- Treatment for all women with primary ovarian insufficiency should continue until the average age of natural menopause is reached (age 50–51 years).
- Lifelong HRT is needed for Kallmann syndrome with sex hormone replacement and GnRH therapy.
- Pituitary disorders can largely be managed medically with dopamine agonists.

REFERENCES

1. ACOG Committee Opinion No. 651: Menstruation in girls and adolescents: using the menstrual cycle as a vital sign. Obstet Gynecol. 2015;126:e143-6.
2. Torres-Santiago L, Mericq V, Taboada M, Unanue N, Klein KO, Singh R, et al. Metabolic effects of oral versus transdermal 17β-estradiol (E_2): a randomized clinical trial in girls with Turner syndrome. J Clin Endocrinol Metab. 2013;98(7):2716-24.
3. Mohammed K, Abu Dabrh AM, Benkhadra K, Al Nofal A, Carranza Leon BG, Prokop LJ, et al. Oral vs Transdermal Estrogen Therapy and Vascular Events: A Systematic Review and Meta-Analysis. J Clin Endocrinol Metab. 2015;100(11):4012-20.
4. Canonico M, Carcaillon L, Plu-Bureau G, Oger E, Singh-Manoux A, Tubert-Bitter P, et al. Postmenopausal Hormone Therapy and Risk of Stroke: Impact of the Route of Estrogen Administration and Type of Progestogen. Stroke. 2016;47(7):1734-41.
5. Ross JL, Quigley CA, Cao D, Feuillan P, Kowal K, Chipman JJ, et al. Growth hormone plus childhood low-dose estrogen in Turner's syndrome. N Engl J Med. 2011;364(13):1230-42.
6. Gonzalez L, Witchel SF. The patient with Turner syndrome: puberty and medical management concerns. Fertil Steril. 2012;98(4):780-6.
7. Foudila T, Söderström-Anttila V, Hovatta O. Turner's syndrome and pregnancies after

oocyte donation. Hum Reprod. 1999;14(2): 532-5.
8. Klein KO, Rosenfield RL, Santen RJ, Gawlik AM, Backeljauw PF, Gravholt CH, et al. Estrogen Replacement in Turner Syndrome: Literature Review and Practical Considerations. J Clin Endocrinol Metab. 2018;103(5):1790-803.
9. McCullough AR, Khera M, Goldstein I, Hellstrom WJ, Morgentaler A, Levine LA. A multi-institutional observational study of testosterone levels after testosterone pellet (Testopel(®)) insertion. J Sex Med. 2012;9:594-601.
10. Meikle AW, Mazer NA, Moellmer JF, Stringham JD, Tolman KG, Sanders SW, et al. Enhanced transdermal delivery of testosterone across nonscrotal skin produces physiological concentrations of testosterone and its metabolites in hypogonadal men. J Clin Endocrinol Metab. 1992;74:623-8.
11. Amory JK, Anawalt BD, Blaskovich PD, Gilchriest J, Nuwayser ES, Matsumoto AM. Testosterone release from a subcutaneous, biodegradable microcapsule formulation (Viatrel) in hypogonadal men. J Androl. 2002;23:84-91.
12. Amory JK, Page ST, Bremner WJ. Oral testosterone in oil: pharmacokinetic effects of 5alpha reduction by finasteride or dutasteride and food intake in men. J Androl. 2006;27:72-8.
13. Salehian B, Wang C, Alexander G, Davidson T, McDonald V, Berman N, et al. Pharmacokinetics, bioefficacy, and safety of sublingual testosterone cyclodextrin in hypogonadal men: comparison to testosterone enanthate—a clinical research center study. J Clin Endocrinol Metab. 1995;80:3567-75.
14. Frisoli A Jr, Chaves PH, Pinheiro MM, Szejnfeld VL. The effect of nandrolone decanoate on bone mineral density, muscle mass, and hemoglobin levels in elderly women with osteoporosis: a double-blind, randomized, placebo-controlled clinical trial. J Gerontol A Biol Sci Med Sci. 2005;60:648-53.
15. Sundaram K, Kumar N, Bardin CW. 7a-Methyl-nortestosterone (MENT): the optimal androgen for male contraception. Ann Med. 1993;25:199-205.
16. Webster J, Piscitelli G, Polli A, Ferrari CI, Ismail I, Scanlon MF. Cabergoline Comparative Study Group A comparison of cabergoline and bromocriptine in the treatment of hyperprolactinemic amenorrhea. N Engl J Med. 1994;331:904-9.

Chapter 31

Secondary Amenorrhea

Ajit Kumar Nayak

Management according to the underlying cause of secondary amenorrhea is described in the following text.

Causes of secondary amenorrhea:
- *Physiological:* Pregnancy, lactation
- *Pathological:*
  - *Genital tract:* Acquired cervical atresia, cervical stenosis, vaginal atresia, Asherman syndrome, and vesicovaginal fistula (VVF)
  - *Ovarian causes:* Surgical extirpation, radiotherapy, autoimmune disease (thyroid, diabetes), polycystic ovarian syndrome (PCOS), resistant ovarian syndrome, infection, masculinizing ovarian tumors, and premature ovarian failure
  - *Pituitary causes:* Simmond disease, Sheehan syndrome, hyperprolactinemia, pituitary adenomas, Cushing's disease, and empty sella syndrome
  - *Hypothalamic causes:* Gonadotropin-releasing hormone (GnRH) deficiency, vigorous exercise, stress, obesity, pseudocyesis, and eating disorders
  - *Thyroid disorder:* Both hypothyroidism and hyperthyroidism
  - *Suprarenal cause:* Addison disease, adrenogenital syndrome, and suprarenal tumor.

■ INVESTIGATION

Investigation for secondary amenorrhea is mentioned in **Flowchart 1**.[1]

Progesterone Challenge Test

Tablet medroxyprogesterone acetate (MPA) 10 mg daily for 5–10 days or injection progesterone 100–200 mg intramuscularly single dose or cap. oral micronized progesterone 200–300 mg daily for 10 days is prescribed.

If withdrawal bleeding occurs within 2 weeks progesterone challenge test (PCT) is positive.

Positive test indicates amenorrhea secondary to anovulation. Most common causes include PCOS, thyroid disorder, hyperprolactinemia, obesity, and hypothalamic causes.

Negative test suggests hypothalamic hypoestrogenism, compromised outflow tract (Asherman syndrome, cervical stenosis), and premature ovarian failure.

Estrogen–Progesterone Challenge Test

Tablet conjugated estrogen 1.25–2.5 mg one daily or tab. estradiol valerate 2 mg BID for 25 days and tab. MPA 10 mg one daily for 10 days from 16th to 25th day.

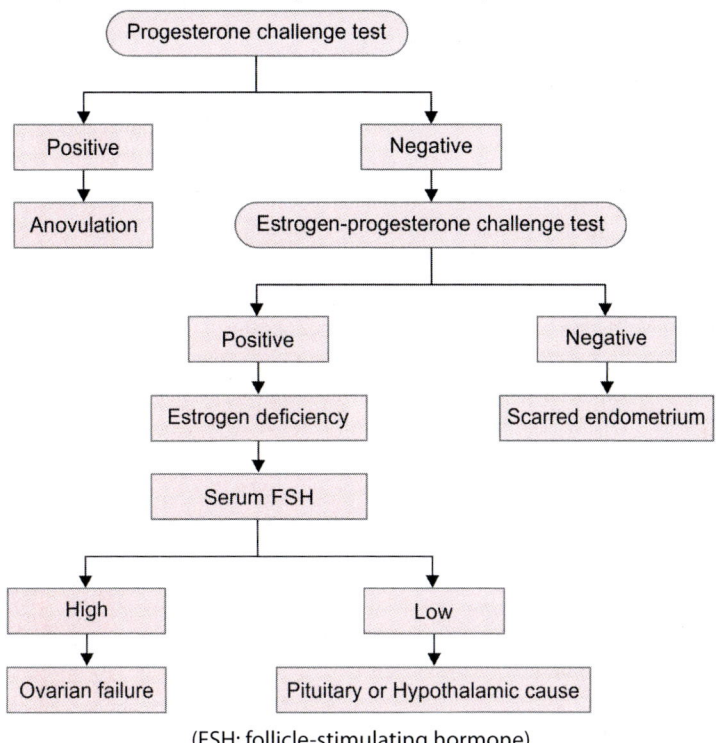

Flowchart 1: Investigation for secondary amenorrhea.

(FSH: follicle-stimulating hormone)

If bleeding occurs, amenorrhea due to hypoestrogenism (hypothalamic amenorrhea or premature ovarian failure).

If bleeding does not occur, then most likely it is an outflow tract obstruction (Asherman syndrome, cervical stenosis).

HYPERPROLACTINEMIA

Treatment with dopamine agonist restores ovulatory function and menses within several weeks. Bromocriptine and cabergoline are commonly used. Treatment should begin with a low-dose regimen and should gradually be adjusted in increments to achieve normal prolactin levels **(Table 1)**.[2]

Given the concerns relating to long-term use of dopaminergic drugs, a trial discontinuation of treatment should be attempted if prolactin levels have been normal for 2 or more years.

Treatment should be focused on patient and not the prolactin levels as hyperprolactinemia itself poses no particular health risk. In women with no risk of unwanted pregnancy, cyclic progestin therapy will prevent the clinical consequences of chronic unopposed estrogen. For those who are frankly hypogonadal, combined estrogen–progesterone treatment in physiological dose should be used. In women who need contraception, low-dose oral contraceptive pills can be used. The same are useful in the management of drug-induced hyperprolactinemia when drugs cannot be discontinued.

POLYCYSTIC OVARIAN SYNDROME

Weight reduction and lifestyle modification is the mainstay of treatment.[3]

TABLE 1: Drug therapy.			
Drugs	**Bromocriptine**	**Cabergoline**	**Pergolide**
Class	Dopamine agonist (DA) and antiparkinsonian	Long-acting selective dopamine receptor agonist, with high affinity for D2 receptors	• Antiparkinsonian and long-acting DA • Ergot derivative and a D1 and D2 receptor agonist
Mechanism of action	Activates postsynaptic DA receptors to inhibit prolactin secretion	Stimulating D2 receptors of the pituitary lactotrophs	Highly potent long-acting inhibitor of prolactin secretion
Adverse effects	Postural hypotension, constipation, nausea, vomiting, dizziness, headache and fatigue, behavioral alteration	Nausea is less common, cardiac valvulopathy reported with high dose (>4 mg daily)	Increased risk of newly diagnosed cardiac valve regurgitation
Contraindication	• Cardiovascular disease • Uncontrolled hypertension	Uncontrolled hypertension	• Uncontrolled hypertension • Cardiovascular disease
Dosing	2.5–15 mg daily oral (PO) in 2–3 divided doses; therapy started with low dose (0.625–1.25) at bedtime	0.25–1 mg PO twice weekly	0.025–0.6 mg PO once daily

- *Combined oral contraceptive pills (COCP):* In women who do not wish to conceive, COCP given cyclically will confer regular monthly withdrawal bleeds. Estrogen suppresses androgens and adrenal hormones. It raises the secretion of sex hormone-binding globulin (SHBG) in the liver which binds with testosterone, thus reducing free testosterone. It also suppresses luteinizing hormone (LH). It is best given as lose-dose pills having progestogens with lesser androgenic effect. Fourth generation of combined pills which contains 30 μg of E2 and 2-3 mg drospirenone (progestin with antiandrogenic and antimineralocorticoid effect) are best for PCOS. It helps to reduce acne, prevents water retention, reduces weight, and maintains a lipid profile.

Adverse effects: These include intermenstrual spotting, headache, dizziness, breast tenderness, cervical mucorrhea, chloasma, vaginitis and vulvovaginitis, weight gain, mood changes, venous thrombosis, myocardial infarction, stroke, gallbladder disease, hypertension, and to a lesser degree breast cancer.

Specific types or doses of COCP cannot currently be recommended in adults and adolescents with PCOS and practice should be informed by general population guidelines.

Preparations:
COCP – 30 μg of ethinyl estradiol (EE) + 3mg drospirenone (21 days)
COCP – 20 μg of EE + 3mg drospirenone (24 days)
COCP – 30 μg of EE + 3mg drospirenone (28 days)
COCP – 20 μg of EE + 3mg drospirenone (28 days, 24 active, 4 placebos)
COCP – 35 μg of EE + cyproterone acetate 2 mg (21 days) (should not be

considered as first line in PCOS due to adverse effects including venous thromboembolic risks) the COCP alone should be recommended in adults with PCOS, adolescents with a clear diagnosis of POCS, and who deemed at risk but not yet diagnosed for management of hyperandrogenism and/or irregular menstrual cycles.

- *COCP plus metformin:* Metformin is oral biguanide (insulin sensitizer) approved for treatment of type 2 diabetes mellitus.

   This combination drug is considered in women with PCOS for management of metabolic features where COCP and lifestyle changes do not achieve desired goals. This could be considered in adolescent with PCOS with body mass index (BMI) >25 kg/m². This is most beneficial in high metabolic risk groups including those with diabetes risk factors, impaired glucose tolerance, or high-risk ethnic group.

   Mechanism of action are reduction of hepatic gluconeogenesis and increase in peripheral glucose uptake by liver, skeletal muscle, and adipose tissue. It stimulates glycolysis in liver.

   Dosage of metformin: 500–850 mg three times per day

   Adverse effects: Dose-dependent nausea/vomiting, bloating, cramps, diarrhea, flatulence, lactic acidosis, vitamin B_{12} deficiency

- *Progestin:* Another alternative to treat menstrual irregularity is to take progestin (Tab. MPA 10 mg one daily) for 10–14 days every 1–3 months. This will induce period in almost all women with PCOS but it does not help with the cosmetic concerns and does not prevent pregnancy. Another option is to consider progesterone secreting intrauterine device, i.e., LNG IUS (levonorgestrel-releasing intrauterine system).

- *Inositol [myoinositol (MI) or d-chiro-inositol (DCI)]:* Administration of MI or DCI in the physiological plasma ratio ensures better clinical results. MI acts at the ovary by reducing hyperandrogenemia, regularizes cycle with spontaneous ovulation, improves ovarian response, and improves oocyte quality. DCI acts at the periphery and reduces insulin resistance, improves glucose metabolism, and improves lipid profile. Inositol in any form should currently be considered an experimental therapy in PCOS.

   Dose: 2–4 g/day

- *Other adjuvant drugs:*
  - *N-acetyl cysteine:* Decreases serum insulin, total cholesterol, low-density lipoprotein (LDL) and homocysteine levels, increase ovulation rate and pregnancy rates and high-density lipoprotein (HDL) levels; prescribed as an adjuvant to clomiphene citrate in the dose 600 mg twice a day for 6 weeks
  - *Vitamin D:* Has beneficial effects on insulin resistance, hyperandrogenism, follicular maturation, menstrual regularity. and ovulation; given orally at a dose 400–2,000 IU/day or 50,000 IU/week
  - *L-Methylfolate:* It is the active form of folic acid that helps in DNA synthesis and reduces homocysteine levels and thereby improves endothelial function.
  - *Antioxidants:* Like omega-3 fatty acids, melatonin, soy and phytoestrogens, chromium and zinc

- Combinations of metformin, inositol, and other adjuvants

THYROID DISORDER

Both hypothyroidism and hyperthyroidism result in chronic anovulation and amenorrhea. Any abnormal thyroid-stimulating hormone (TSH) value should be confirmed by repeat testing that includes measurement of serum thyroxine (T4) levels to better define the nature and extent of thyroid disorder.

Hypothyroidism

Hypothyroidism can lead to disturbance in both cycle length and amount of bleeding. Menstrual disturbances in hypothyroidism is three times more common than that of normal population. Most common presentation is oligomenorrhea. The plasma-binding activity of SHBG is decreased, which in turn leads to decreased plasma concentration of total testosterone and estrogen and free fractions of these hormones are increased. Also there is decreased rate of metabolic clearance of estrone and androstenedione along with increased peripheral aromatization. Serum prolactin concentration is often increased and this in turn is due to hypothalamic thyrotropin-releasing hormone (TRH), which not only increases TSH, but also prolactin levels. All of the above factors lead to anovulation.[4]

In clinical hypothyroidism, serum TSH is raised and serum T4 and triiodothyronine (T3) are low whereas in subclinical hypothyroidism only serum TSH is raised. American thyroid association defines it as TSH value greater than upper limit of normal range (4.5–5.0 mIU/L) with normal free T4 level. European Thyroid Association defines it as mild with TSH levels 4–10 and severe with TSH level >10 with normal free T4 levels.

Management: Levothyroxine replacement remains the gold standard treatment. It is very effective when administered orally and has a long half-life permitting once-a-dose dosage. The aim is to reach normal TSH levels (0.3–2.5 mIU/L). When possible, levothyroxine should be administered separately from other interfering medications and supplements such as calcium carbonate and ferrous sulfate. A 4-hour difference in administration is desirable. Starting replacement therapy should be decided based on factors such as patient weight (1.6–1.8 µg/kg), BMI, pregnancy status, history of infertility, etiology of hypothyroidism, and age. The dose for replacement should be with an initial full replacement or alternatively partial replacement with gradual increase in the dose titrated upward or downward using serum TSH levels.

Preparations: Synthetic levothyroxine sodium.

Hyperthyroidism

Menstrual irregularities are 2.3-fold higher in thyrotoxic women than in general population. Common manifestation being amenorrhea, oligomenorrhea, hypomenorrhea, and anovulation. Hyperthyroidism leads to increase in concentration of SHBG. Plasma levels of testosterone, androstenedione, and estradiol are higher in all phases of menstrual cycle.

Management: Treatment of clinical hyperthyroidism may include antithyroid drugs, radioactive iodine, or surgery.

Thionamides: Mechanism of action: They bind to thyroid peroxidase and prevent oxidation of iodine and iodotyrosyl residues, thereby inhibiting iodination of tyrosine residues in thyroglobulin and inhibiting coupling of iodotyrosine residues to form T3 and T4. The important drugs used are propylthiouracil, carbimazole, and methimazole **(Table 2)**.

TABLE 2: Mechanism of action of propylthiouracil and carbimazole.

Propylthiouracil	Carbimazole
Less potent	Five times more potent
High plasma protein-bound	Less plasma protein-bound
Less transferred across placenta	Large amounts cross placenta
t½ 1–2 hours	t½ 6–10 hours
No active metabolite	Produced active metabolite—methimazole
Multiple daily dose needed	Single dose
Inhibits peripheral conversion of T4 To T3	No such action

(T3: triiodothyronine; T4: thyroxine)

Adverse effects: Hypothyroidism occurs due to overtreatment, gastrointestinal (GI) intolerance, skin rashes, and joint pain, hepatitis in propylthiouracil, loss of hair, and loss of taste. A rare but serious adverse effect is agranulocytosis.

Preparation and dose: Propylthiourcil: 50–150 mg TDS followed by 25–50 mg BD–TDS for maintenance.

Carbimazole: 5–15 mg TDS initially, maintenance dose 2.5–10 mg daily in 1–2 divided doses.

Methimazole: 5–10 mg TDS initially, maintenance dose 5–15 mg daily in 1–2 divided dose.

PREMATURE OVARIAN INSUFFICIENCY

It is defined as hypergonadotropic hypogonadism and amenorrhea arising before age of 40 years. Causes include numerical and structural chromosomal abnormalities, fragile X premutation, autoimmune disorder, galactosemia, radiation therapy, and chemotherapy. The basic pathophysiology involves accelerated follicular atresia.[5]

Management

Effective management of premature ovarian insufficiency (POI) requires careful counseling and emotional support. Attention should focus on excluding those causes having important potential health consequences for the patient or other members of her family.

The short-term as well as long-term management of women with POI centers on hypogonadism and its sequelae. They are at real risk of skeletal fragility and low bone mass, increased risk of coronary heart disease, and vasomotor and genitourinary symptoms that can be debilitating.

Hormone therapy with estrogen and progesterone is the treatment of choice. This treatment should continue up to at least the age of 50 years.

- *Estrogen:* Estrogen lowers total cholesterol and LDL, increases HDL, has antiatherogenic effect on arterial wall, causes augmentation of vasodilators like nitric oxide and prostacyclin, reduces levels of renin and angiotensin converting enzyme, decreases insulin resistance and inhibits oxidation of LDL.

  Preparations: Oral, transdermal (patch, gel, spray), vaginal (creams, rings, tablets) implants, and injectable.

  Products name: 17beta-estradiol, conjugated estrogen.

- *Progesterone:* Addition of progesterone is mandatory in woman with intact uterus to counter endometrial hyperplasia and cancer due to unopposed estrogen cyclic treatment.

Cap. micronized progesterone 200 mg daily or Tab. MPA 10 mg daily for 12–14 days each month.

Preparation: Oral, intramuscular, implants, IUS, vaginal tablets and rings, skin patches.

Adverse effects of hormone therapy: Major: Venous thromboembolism, stroke, coronary artery disease, pulmonary embolism, increased risk of breast cancer, endometrial cancer when estrogen is used alone, increased incidence of Alzheimer's disease, and gallbladder disease.

Minor: Nausea, bloating, leg cramps, breast tenderness, break through bleeding, vaginal discharge, mood swings, etc.

Contraindications of hormone therapy are undiagnosed genital tract bleeding, hormone-dependent neoplasia in the body, suspected pregnancy, history of venous thromboembolism, severe active liver disease, and strong family history of breast cancer.

ASHERMAN SYNDROME

Intrauterine adhesions are a consequence of trauma to the endometrium, producing partial or complete obliteration in the uterine cavity and cervical canal. It presents as menstrual abnormality in about 68% as amenorrhea or hypomenorrhea.[6]

The gold standard for the treatment is hysteroscopic-guided adhesion lysis. It is safe and effective procedure for restoring the normal menstrual pattern and fertility. Prevention of recurrent adhesion is essential for a successful treatment.

Methods include second and third look hysteroscopic adhesiolysis; barrier methods like seprafilm, hyaluronic acid gel, amnion graft; mechanical methods like IUD, Lippes loop, Foley balloon; hormone treatments like estrogen–progesterone, GnRH analogs, and danazole; and pharmacological agents like antibiotics, nonsteroidal anti-inflammatory drugs (NSAIDs), antihistamines.

MEDICAL MANAGEMENT FOR PREVENTION OF RECURRENT ADHESIONS

Barrier methods:
- Seprafilm is a bioresorbable membrane of chemically modified hyaluronic acid and carboxymethylcellulose, shown to be effective in reducing adhesion formation
- Autocross-linked hyaluronic acid gel.
- Fresh amnion graft draped over an inflated Foley catheter balloon.

Hormone treatment: Estrogen–progestin therapy significantly increases endometrial thickness and volume, but there is no objective evidence based on randomized controlled trials to confirm the efficacy of hormone treatment on the reduction of reformation of intrauterine adhesions.

Preparations: Tab. conjugated estrogen 2.5 mg one daily or Tab. estradiol valerate 2 mg BID for 25 days and Tab. MPA 10 mg one daily for 10 days from 16th to 25th day.

Genital tuberculosis: Antitubercular drugs: The endometrium is affected in 50–80% (average 70%) patients through hematogenous, lymphatic, or contagious route. Destruction of the endometrium may occur with Asherman's syndrome manifesting as secondary amenorrhea and infertility.
- *Intensive phase daily (2 months):*
  - Drug (mg) if weight <45 kg: 2HRZE: Isoniazid (INH) 300, rifampicine 450, pyrazinamide 1,250, and ethambutol 800

- *Drug (mg) if weight >45 kg: 2HRZE:* INH300, rifampicine 600, pyrazinamide 1,750, and ethambutol 1,200.
- Continuation phase daily (4 months):
  - *Drug (mg) if weight <45 kg: 4HRZE:* INH300, rifampicine 450, and ethambutol 800.
  - *Drug (mg) if weight >45 kg: 4HRZE:* INH300, rifampicine 600, and ethambutol 1,200.

Anorexia or bulimia nervosa: No medications, antidepressant can be tried to deal with anxiety and depression associated with it. Nasogastric feeding or IV fluid is recommended.[7]

Obesity:
- Lifestyle and behavioral changes
- *Drugs:* Orlistat 120 mg, liraglutide, naltrexone, bupropion, phentermine.[8]

Malnutrition: Iron, calcium, vitamin A, vitamin D, B-complex supplementation.

Stress or depression: Healthy diet, 7–8 hours of sleep per night, regular exercise, minimize caffeine, alcohol, stay socially connected, make time for rest and relaxation, deep breathing, anti-anxiety and antidepressant drugs.

Extreme weight loss: Try to avoid excess weight loss, nutritional supplementation.

Exercising too much: Reduce vigorous exercise.

Central nervous system tumor: For prolactinoma tablet cabergoline 0.5 mg twice a week for 3–12 months.

Chronic illness:
- Chronic liver disease
- Chronic renal insufficiency
- Diabetes
- Immunodeficiency state
- Inflammatory bowel disease
- Thyroid disease
- Severe depression or psychosocial stressors.

Treatment: Treat the underlying cause.

Hypothalamic or pituitary destruction:
- *Kallmann syndrome:* Steroid replacement therapy such as testosterone or estrogen–progestin supplementation.
- *Sheehan syndrome:* Hormone replacement, i.e., ovarian, thyroid, and adrenocortical hormones (ACTH).

Amenorrhea associated with depot MPA: Counseling and reassurance.[9]

Post-pill amenorrhea:
- Bromocriptine
- Clomiphene
- Reassurance
- Periodic follow-up
- Progesterone withdrawal bleeding.

KEY POINTS

- In any patient with secondary amenorrhea pregnancy has to be ruled out first.
- Progesterone challenge test to be done as initial line of management.
- Serum TSH, prolactin and FSH estimation to be done along with pelvic ultrasound.
- Weight reduction and lifestyle modification to be tried first in PCOD cases before giving any drugs.
- Full course of antitubercular drugs to be given for genital tuberculosis cases with amenorrhea.
- Synechiolysis with adhesion preventive measures to be taken for Asherman syndrome.
- Cabergoline should be given for hyperprolactinemia and L-thyroxin for hypothyroidism.

REFERENCES

1. Klein DA, Paradise SL, Reeder RM. Amenorrhea: a systematic approach to diagnosis and management. Am Fam Physician. 2019;100(1):39-48.
2. Goswami B, Patel S, Chatterjee M, Koner BC, Saxena A. Correlation of prolactin and thyroid hormone concentration with menstrual patterns in infertile women. J Reprod Infertil. 2009:10:207-12.
3. Balen AH, Morley LC, Misso M, Franks S, Legro RS, Wijeyaratne CN. et al. The management of anovulatory infertility in women with polycystic ovary syndrome: an analysis of the evidence to support the development of global WHO guidance. Hum Reprod Update. 2016;22:687-708.
4. Koutras DA. Disturbances of menstruation in thyroid disease. Ann N Y Acad Sci. 1997; 816:280-4.
5. Starup J, Sele V. Premature ovarian failure. Acta Obstet Gynecol Scand. 1973;52:259-68.
6. Dreisler E, Kjer JJ. Asherman's syndrome: current perspectives on diagnosis and management. Int J Womens Health. 2019; 11:191-8.
7. Gordon CM, Ackerman KE, Berga SL, Kaplan JR, Mastorakos G, Misra M, et al. Functional Hypothalamic Amenorrhea: An Endocrine Society Clinical Practice Guideline. J Clin Endocrinol Metab. 2017; 102(5):1413-39.
8. Wood PL, Bauman D. Gynaecological issues affecting the obese adolescent. Best Pract Res Clin Obstet Gynaecol. 2015;29(4): 453-65.
9. Ingerslev M, Jeppesen T, Ramsing EM. Secondary amenorrhoea and oral contraceptives. Acta Obstet Gynecol Scand. 1976; 55(3):233-8.

Section 11

Medical Management of Anovulation

▲ **Ovulation Induction in Intrauterine Insemination**
Reeta Bansiwal, Anshika Agarwal

▲ **Ovulation Induction in IVF-ET**
Renu Tanwar, Renu Singh

Chapter 32

Ovulation Induction in Intrauterine Insemination

Reeta Bansiwal, Anshika Agarwal

Ovulation induction (OI) is often the first treatment for infertility with or without intrauterine insemination (IUI). OI is a pharmacological treatment of women with anovulation or oligo-ovulation with the intention of inducing normal ovulatory cycles, whereas, ovulation stimulation (OS) is a pharmacological treatment with the intention of inducing the development of ovarian follicles. OS can be used for two purposes—(1) for timed intercourse or insemination and (2) in in vitro fertilization (IVF), to obtain multiple oocytes at follicular aspiration.[1] Drugs used for inducing ovulation in anovulatory women are called ovulogens. Once limited to clomiphene citrate (CC) and urinary gonadotropins in 1961, but lot more added since then in the armamentarium. This chapter aims to overview the developments, structure, mode of action, and side effects of drugs used for OI in IUI cycles.

Various drugs used for OI:
- *Selective estrogen receptor modulator:*
  - Clomiphene citrate
  - Tamoxifen
- *Aromatase inhibitor:*
  - Letrozole
  - Anastrozole
- *Insulin sensitizing agent:* Metformin
- *Gonadotropins:* Human menopausal gonadotropin/follicle-stimulating hormone (hMG/FSH)
- *Clomiphene/letrozole with gonadotropins.*

NATURAL OVULATION PHYSIOLOGY

Every month from the primordial follicles pool of ovary, few follicles are recruited under the effect FSH derived from pituitary. It requires a certain amount of FSH known as FSH threshold and for a certain period of time called FSH window to cause follicular recruitment. When follicles grow, they secrete estrogen and estrogen concentration increases which causes negative feedback on hypothalamus and pituitary, thereby reducing the FSH level. Only that follicle which has more FSH receptors and maintains high estrogen microenvironment even in low FSH, survives while rest get atretic, leading to selection of dominant follicle. Estrogen at high doses causes positive effect on pituitary to secrete more luteinizing hormone (LH), causing LH surge, and enabling ovulation.[2] Ovulogens work on the principle of increasing FSH to recruit follicles and selection of dominant follicle.

SELECTIVE ESTROGEN RECEPTOR MODULATOR

Clomiphene Citrate

Clomiphene citrate was first synthesized in 1956 and got approved for infertility treatment by the US Food and Drug Administration (US FDA) in 1967.

Structure

It is a nonsteroidal triphenylethylene derivative having both estrogen agonist and antagonist properties. It is a racemic mixture of two different isomers—enclomiphene (62%) and zuclomiphene (38%) **(Fig. 1)**. Enclomiphene is more potent isomer and the one responsible for its OI action. Enclomiphene is short-acting but zuclomiphene is cleared slowly and can be deducted for weeks after the single dose.[3]

Mechanism of Action

Principle: It mainly acts centrally at hypothalamus and pituitary. Due to its structurally similarity to estrogen, it competes with endogenous estrogen *(competitive antagonist)* for nuclear estrogen receptors (ER) and causes a reduction in the negative feedback of endogenous estrogens due to prolonged depletion of hypothalamic and pituitary ERs.[3] This in turn leads to an increase in the release of gonadotropin-releasing hormone (GnRH) from the hypothalamus into the hypothalamic–pituitary portal circulation, instigating an increase in the release of pituitary gonadotropins which lead to follicle formation in the ovary. It does not have progestational, corticotropic, and androgenic effects.

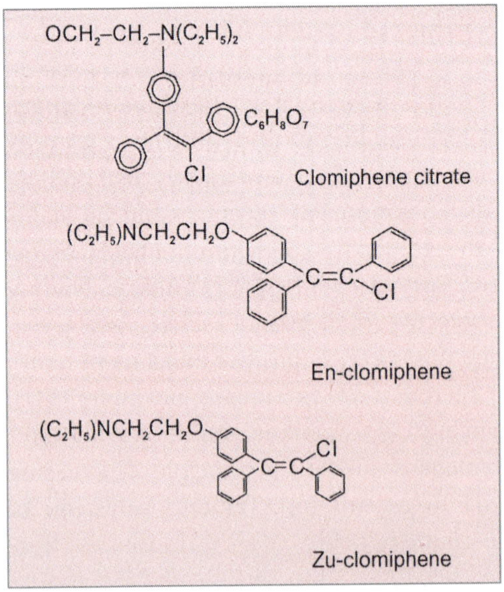

Pharmacokinetics

- *Oral bioavailability:* >90%
- *Half-life:* 7 days (its metabolites may be found in feces up to 30 days)
- *Metabolism:* Liver
- *Excretion:* Mainly through feces and some in urine
- *Dosage:* 50–150 mg/day
- *Standard regime:* Starting of minimum dose 50 mg/day from day 2 to 5 of menstrual cycle for 5 days. Dose is increased by 50 mg in next cycle if ovulation is not achieved till maximum 150 mg dose.

CC Success and Efficacy

The ovulation rate ranges between 70 and 92%, but the pregnancy rate is much lower. The discrepancy between the high ovulation rates and relatively low pregnancy rates may be due to the following factors—(1) antiestrogen effects on the endometrium, (2) antiestrogen effects on the cervical mucus, (3) decrease in uterine blood flow, (4) impaired placental protein 14 synthesis, (5) subclinical pregnancy loss, (6) effect on tubal transport, and (7) detrimental effects on the oocytes.[4] Evidence suggests majority

Fig. 1: Structure of clomiphene and its isomers.

of IUI pregnancies occur in the first three to four cycles of IUI. 88% of all successful IUIs happen within three cycles and 95% within four.[5] Long-term (>12 months) CC therapy is associated with a slight increase in future risk of ovarian cancer [relative risk (RR) = 1.5–2.5].[6]

Side Effects

Hot flushes (10%), abdominal discomfort, bloating (5%), breast discomfort (2%), nausea and vomiting (2%), visual symptoms (floaters, flashes, and abnormal perception), and headache (1.5%). These symptoms are temporary and usually goes after stopping drug. The multiple pregnancy rate is approximately 5% and almost exclusively due to twins. There is no evidence of increased overall risk of congenital anomalies or of any one anomaly in particular.[7] No causal relationship has been found between CC use and ovarian, breast, or endometrial cancer as per Cochrane database.

Contraindications

- Preexisting ovarian cysts
- Suspected malignancy
- Liver disease

Clomiphene resistance: Failure to ovulate after receiving 150 mg of CC daily for 5 days per cycle, for at least three cycles. It occurs in approximately 15–40% in women with polycystic ovary syndrome (PCOS),[8] whereas, clomiphene failure is defined as failure to conceive despite successful CC- induced ovulation.

Management of Clomiphene Resistance in Polycystic Ovarian Syndrome

The major factors involved in clomiphene resistance are insulin resistance (IR), hyperandrogenism, and obesity.

Different therapy evaluated are as follows:
- Insulin-sensitizing agents:
  - About 50–70% of PCOS women present with IR, more in obese than lean PCOS.[9] IR with compensatory hyperinsulinemia causes increase in ovarian androgen production leading to oligo/anovulation.
  - Several insulin-sensitizing drugs have been proposed to treat IR, such as metformin, pioglitazone, troglitazone, and myoinositols in order to reduce serum androgens and improve ovulation alongside making lifestyle changes.[10]
    - *Metformin:* It is a biguanide, commonly used in noninsulin-dependent diabetes mellitus, has been recommended along with clomiphene in CC resistance cases in women with body mass index (BMI) >30 kg/m^2 in a dose (1,500–2,000 mg/day).[11]
    - *Myoinositol:* It takes part in many signal pathways, such as the pathways of insulin and gonadotropins. It acts as second messenger of FSH and LH, hence helps in glucose uptake, follicle maturation and reducing hyperinsulinemia and thereby improving ovulation in infertile PCOS patients.[12] Dose recommended is 4 g/day.
- *Clomiphene citrate with glucocorticoids:* Glucocorticoids are used when serum dehydroepiandrosterone-sulfate (DHEA-S) concentration is >200 µg/dL. It reduces the adrenal androgens and thereby improves ovarian hormonal milieu and induces ovulation in infertile PCOS patients. Dose—0.5–2 mg from day 2 of menstrual cycle for 10 days.[13]

- *Clomiphene with gonadotropins:* Gonadotropins act by inducing ovulation, maintaining, and provoking optimal follicle growth via controlled administration of FSH. Risk of ovarian hyperstimulation syndrome (OHSS) and multiple pregnancies is the main drawback.
- *Extended CC regime:* The duration of clomiphene is extended beyond 5 days. Dose—100 mg (day 2–day 9) resulted in modest ovulation, pregnancy rate with no side effects and offers safety, efficacy, and economic advantage.[14]
- *Stair step protocol (SSP):* CC 50 mg/day is started from day 2 of menstrual cycle for 5 days and in nonresponsive patients, the dosage was increased to 100 mg/day for 5 days in the same cycle. Maximum dose of 150 mg was given until the dominant follicle was generated. USG after the dose increment is done 2 days after the last dose. SSP helps in effective treatment in significantly shorter time period without any detrimental effect on the ovulation and pregnancy rates.[15]
- *CC with bromocriptine/cabergoline:* It is used in women with hyperprolactinemia and ovulatory dysfunction. Both are ergot alkaloids that mimic the actions of dopamine via their binding to dopamine receptors. Serum concentrations peak 1–3 hours after an oral dose of bromocriptine, and very little remains in the circulation 14 hours after administration; an oral dose of 2.5 mg generally lowers prolactin concentrations for up to 12 hours. It can be administered orally/rectally. Cabergoline is a longer-acting dopamine agonist with high affinity for the dopamine receptor. A single dose of cabergoline effectively inhibits prolactin secretion for 7 days or longer. They act through lowering the prolactin levels and thereby allowing the hypothalamic-pituitary-ovarian axis to escape from the suppressive influence that hyperprolactinemia has on pulsatile GnRH secretion and restoring normal ovulatory function.

Tamoxifen

Tamoxifen is US FDA approved for the treatment of both early and advanced ER-positive (or ER+) breast cancer in pre- and postmenopausal women. It has also the OI property and used off-label for the same.

Pharmacokinetics

- *Oral bioavailability:* 100%
- *Protein bound:* >99% (albumin)
- *Half-life:* 5–7 days
- *Metabolism:* Liver
- *Excretion:* Feces 65% and urine 6%.

Dosage

- 20 mg daily for 5 days starting from day 3 to 5 of menstrual cycle
- *Maximum dose:* 80 mg/day.

Efficacy

It is similar to clomiphene and relatively safe and can be a good alternative to CC. Unlike clomiphene, tamoxifen acts as an agonist on the ERs of the vaginal mucosa and endometrium but studies on the effects of tamoxifen on cervical mucus have been inconclusive.[16]

Side Effects

- Endometrial polyp and hyperplasia
- Endometrial cancer
- Liver toxicity
- Deep vein thrombosis
- Pulmonary embolism
- Stroke

AROMATASE INHIBITORS

Aromatase is a cytochrome P450-dependent enzyme that acts as the ultimate step in the synthesis of estrogen. It catalyzes the conversion of androgens to estrogens. Aromatase inhibitor is a competitive inhibitor of the aromatase enzyme system, and inhibits the conversion of androgens to estrogens. The conversion of androgens to estrogens also occurs at peripheral sites, such as in muscle, fat, and the liver.

Aromatase inhibitors are classified into first, second, and third generations as per their chronologic development and type I (steroid analogs of androstenedione) and type II (nonsteroidal) **(Table 1)**. Anastrozole (1 mg daily) has been used for a 5-day interval. When early on, a phase II randomized controlled trial comparing a single-dose therapy with anastrozole and 5-day course of clomiphene reported significantly lower ovulation rates with anastrozole and the sponsoring company stopped the development of the drug.[17] Thus, letrozole is the most studied and the most commonly used aromatase inhibitor in OI.

Only third-generation aromatase inhibitors are safe and with oral bioavailability. Letrozole is mainly used for suppressing estrogen production in postmenopausal women with breast cancer. Its use in infertility is "off label" for OI. It is now the first drug of choice for OI.[11]

Mechanism of Action

It competitively binds to heme of the aromatase-cytochrome P450 subunit of enzyme which results in reduction of estrogen biosynthesis. It effectively lowers serum estrone, estradiol, and estrone sulfate but has no effect on corticosteroid synthesis, aldosterone or thyroid synthesis.

Pharmacokinetics

- *Oral bioavailability:* >95%
- *Half-life:* 48 hours
- *Protein binding:* 60% mainly to albumin
- *Metabolism:* Liver
- *Excretion:* Biliary (85%) and urinary (11%)
- *Dosage:* 2.5–7.5 mg/day from day 2–5 of cycle for 5 days
- *Regime:* The starting dose for letrozole is 2.5 mg a day for 5 days. If 2.5 mg/day fails to induce ovulation, the dosage can be increased by 2.5 mg increments up to a maximum of 7.5 mg/day for 5 days. Dose increments can be done in the same cycle without inducing bleeding, like the stair-step protocol with clomiphene.

Side Effects, Safety, and Efficacy

Side effects are hot flushes (18%), bone pain (20%), back pain (17%), nausea (15%), and dyspnea (44%). These are usually after long-term use. October 12, 2011, letrozole was banned from sale and distribution in India due to a report (abstract only) of an increase in cardiac and bone malformations in letrozole-treated pregnancies.[18] After the report, the manufacturer of letrozole, novartis stated to clinicians that letrozole was not safe for use in women who were either desiring pregnancy or pregnant. After this many reports came stating the safety of letrozole.[19,20]

TABLE 1: Classification of aromatase inhibitors.

Generations	Type 1 steroidal analog	Type 2 nonsteroidal analog
First	None	Aminogluthethimide
Second	Formestane	• Fadrozole • Rogletimide
Third	Exemestane	• Anastrazole • Letrozole • Vorozole

On March 1st, 2017, ban on letrozole was revoked in India. Letrozole has no antiestrogenic effect on endometrium and cervical mucous and has been proven to be more effective than clomiphene (RR: 1.148, 95% CI: 1.077–1.223, 3,017 women, 19 trials, I²: 47.7%, low-quality evidence). It has ovulation rate of 75%, pregnancy rate of 25%, and multiple pregnancy rate of <4%.[21]

METFORMIN

It is a dimethylbiguanide, an oral antihyperglycemic agent widely used in the management of noninsulin-dependent diabetes mellitus. It is an insulin sensitizer that reduces IR and insulin secretion. For last few years, it has gained popularity in increasing ovulation frequency, mainly in women with PCOS. Cochrane systematic review concluded metformin as an effective treatment for anovulation in women with PCOS and recommended as first-line treatment.[22] However, ovulation rates were higher when combined with clomiphene rather than alone (76% vs. 46%). It is to be used as an adjuvant to general lifestyle improvements and not as a replacement for increased exercise and improved diet.

Pharmacokinetics

- *Oral bioavailability:* 50–60%, food interferes with absorption
- *Protein bound:* None
- *Excretion:* Renal
- *Half-life:* 4–8.7 hours
- *Dose:* 1,500–2,000 mg/day in divided doses.

Side Effects and Safety

- Diarrhea (53%)
- Nausea/vomiting (25.5%)
- Flatulence (12.1%)
- Asthenia (9.2%)
- Indigestion (7.1%)
- Abdominal discomfort (6.4%)
- Headache (5.7%)

Overall, metformin use in women of reproductive age has an assured safety record.[23]

GONADOTROPINS

It is a second line of treatment for OI, first being letrozole. Though it was discovered way back in 1927 that pituitary hormone controls ovarian function,[24] it was only in 1950 when first urinary extract of gonadotropin containing both FSH and LH called "pergonal" was approved for selling by Italy. Initially, hMG was highly impure with lots of proteins and many isoforms of FSH and LH. It leads to allergic reactions and pain at injection site and also discrepancies in patient response. Purification of hMG leads to introduction of "Metrodin" in mid-1980 and further purification led to development of highly purified urinary FSH (>95% purity) in 1993. Then, with the help of recombinant technology, the world's first r-hFSH (follitropin-α) preparation for clinical use was produced by Serono Laboratories in 1988, and was licensed for marketing in the European Union as GONAL-f in 1995. In 1996, Organon Laboratories brought r-hFSH (follitropin-β; Puregon). Recently, follitropin-δ (Rekovelle, Ferring Pharmaceuticals, UK) has been granted for marketing in 2016. Similarly, the genes for the other gonadotropins have also been transfected into mammalian cell lines and led to the development of recombinant human LH (r-hLH) and recombinant human chorionic gonadotropin (r-hCG). They are now commercially available (r-hLH as Luveris, Merck, Germany; r-hCG as Ovidrel/Ovitrelle, Merck; and r-hFSH and r-hLH in a 2:1 ratio, Pergoveris, Merck).

Human Menopausal Gonadotropin

It is extracted from the urine of post-menopausal women as levels of FSH and LH are high in them. It was successfully introduced into clinical use by Bruno Lunenfeld in 1961. It contains FSH and LH in the ratio of 1:1. The early preparations were originally only about 5% pure and contained varying amounts of FSH, LH, and hCG. Improvements in purification techniques resulted in standardization of the FSH and LH activity to 75 IU for each type of gonadotropin, although extraneous urinary proteins still existed.[25] Human urinary-derived menotropin preparations are exposed to the theoretical risk of infection from menopausal donors of urine. Therefore, highly purified preparations came which can be given as subcutaneous (SC) administration and intramuscular (IM) administration.

- *Generic name:* Menotropin
- *Half-life:* Elimination half-life of 11–13 hours
- *Brand:* Menopur (5 mL vial contain 75 IU FSH and 75 IU LH), Humog, Pergonal, Repronex, etc.
- *Route of administration:* IM or SC
- *Side effects:*
  - Mild bloating
  - Pain swelling, rash, or irritation at injection site
  - Stomach pain/pelvic pain.

Follicle-stimulating Hormone

It is of broadly of two types:
1. Urinary derived
2. Recombinant

Urinary derived: Extracted from the urine of postmenopausal women. It is then purified to remove various proteins and other substances. Depending upon the degree of purification, it comes as purified FSH or in highly purified form.

Purified Urinary Follicle-stimulating Hormone

It was formed by removing LH from urinary extracts using immunoaffinity columns containing polyclonal anti-hCG antibodies. It contains 75 IU FSH and ≤1 IU of LH but considerable amount of other urinary proteins and required intramuscular route of administration.[25]

Generic name: Urofollitropin, purified.

Brand names: Bravelle, Metrodin, Fertinorm, etc.

Highly Purified Urinary Follicle-stimulating Hormone

It was formed by using monoclonal antibodies specific for FSH. It contains 75 IU of FSH and <0.1 IU of LH and <5% of unidentified proteins. The even more highly purified preparations are available containing <0.001 IU of LH and very low levels of urinary proteins. They can be administered by SC route.[25]

Generic name: Urofollitropin, highly purified.

Brand names: Fertinex.

Recombinant Follicle-stimulating Hormone

They are manufactured by inserting the genes encoding for the alpha and beta subunits of FSH into expression vectors that are transfected into Chinese hamster ovary cell lines, which then synthesizes and secretes a glycosylated bioactive dimeric FSH that is purified by immunochromatography using a specific anti-FSH monoclonal antibody (follitropin-α and follitropin-β).

Recombinant FSH preparations contain less acidic FSH isoforms that have a shorter half-life of 24 hours than those derived from human urine but stimulate estrogen secretion as or even more efficiently.[26] Recently follitropin-δ has been developed using a cell line of human fetal retinal origin. The amino acid sequences of the α- and β-subunits of are identical to that of natural human FSH, but the sialic acid content of the FSH molecule is higher, which gives it a longer elimination half-life of 30 hours.[26]

Corifollitropin Alfa

It has been formed by recombinant technology where FSH β-subunits are combined to the C-terminal peptide of the hCG β-subunit (containing additional glycosylation sites). It has a longer half-life of 7 days and sustains follicular growth for 1 week. So, daily seven injections can be replaced by its one injection, which makes it patient friendly. It is designed for multifollicular growth so not feasible for OI, where aim is unifollicular growth. Its approval for marketing was given to Merck pharmaceuticals on February 15, 2010.

Side effects of FSH preparation:
- Local irritation at the injection site
- Feeling of fullness, bloating, and tenderness in the abdomen
- Mood swings
- Fatigue
- Risk of OHSS if higher doses are used
- Multiple pregnancy 15%.

Regime

1. *Low step-up dose protocol:* Starting dose is 75 IU (low daily dose) for 7 days and step-up by 37.5 IU after 7 days or more if no follicle is >10 mm, cycle monitoring is done transvaginally every 1–2 days. Step-up gonadotropins in small increments every 7 days till dominant follicle appear. Trigger for oocyte maturation is given once dominant follicle >18 mm. It can be started at a lower dose of 37.5 IU in PCOS patients.

2. *Low slow step-up protocol:* It is a chronic low dose step-up protocol. Low starting dose—37.5–75 IU. Smaller increments are done over longer duration. It is suited for PCOS women who are sensitive to low-dose stimulation and avoids OHSS, multiple pregnancy, and overall reduction in cycle cancellation but the overall cost of cycle may increase.

3. *Sequential treatment (CC/letrozole with gonadotropins):* Standard dose of CC/letrozole from D2 to D6, followed by addition of low dose hMG on last day of CC/letrozole or the next day. Cycle monitoring and gonadotropin dose adjusted as per step-up protocol.

4. *Step-down protocol:* Mimics physiology and more suitable for hypogonadotropic hypogonadism anovulation (WHO type 1). Starting dose—150 IU, it is continued till dominant follicle >10 mm seen in transvaginal scan. Gradually, gonadotropin dose is reduced and promotes the development of most sensitive follicle. Trigger of ovulation done once dominant follicle >18 mm.

HUMAN CHORIONIC GONADOTROPIN

Human chorionic gonadotropin belongs to the same glycoprotein family as FSH, LH and thyroid-stimulating hormone (TSH). All members of this family share the same alfa subunit, but have different β-subunits.

There is 80% homology between hCG and LH, hence both are capable of stimulating the same hormone receptor.[27] Therefore, hCG is used as a surrogate LH surge.

Mechanism of Action

Due to molecular homology with LH, it binds to the LH receptor and initiates the resumption of meiosis and the maturation of the oocyte from the immature "metaphase I" stage to the mature "metaphase II" stage of development. Although hCG activates the LH receptor, it does not do so in an identical manner to LH. In a natural LH surge, it consists of three phases—(1) abrupt onset (14 hours), (2) LH peak/plateau (14 hours), and (3) gradual descent to baseline (20 hours), lasting a mean duration of 48 hours. Whereas, hCG has fivefold more affinity and much longer action.[27] It not only causes oocyte maturation but also supports the early pregnancy due to its extended action and thereby a threat for OHSS as well.

Human chorionic gonadotropin available in two forms:
1. Urinary hCG
2. Recombinant hCG

Pharmacokinetics

Urinary hCG

- *Dose:* 5,000–10,000 IU
- *Route:* HP form can be given SC
- *Action:* Ovarian LH receptors
- *Half-life:* 33.5 hours

Recombinant hCG

- *Dose:* 250–500 µg
- *Route:* SC injection
- *Half-life:* 28–29 hours
- *Action:* Ovarian LH receptors

Side Effects

- Acne
- Changes in emotions or mood
- Headache
- Pain, irritation, or inflammation at the injection site
- Allergic reactions such as skin rash, itching or hives, swelling of the face, lips, or tongue
- Breathing difficulty
- Breast enlargement
- Ovarian hyperstimulation syndrome
- Nausea, vomiting
- Pelvic pain and bloating

Other Uses

- Male hypogonadotropic hypogonadism
- Prepubertal cryptorchidism

Commercial Brands

Urinary hCG: Pregnyl, Profasi, Coriosurge XP, etc.

Recombinant hCG: Ovidrell

Drugs used for OI in IUI cycles are mentioned in **Table 2**.

■ KEY POINT

Ovulation induction is a simple, cost effective, and first line of treatment in infertility. Various drugs in armamentarium but most common drugs used are letrozole/clomiphene and gonadotropin. As per WHO and international guidelines, letrozole is first-line drug whereas, gonadotropins are used as second line of treatment. Clinician must remember the goal of IUI cycle that is unifollicular growth, therefore medication should be given accordingly, to prevent life-threatening iatrogenic OHSS. It should be tailored to individualized need. When three to six cycles of OI fail, one should reevaluate patient and consider for IVF/intracytoplasmic sperm injection (ICSI) cycle accordingly.

TABLE 2: Drugs used for ovulation induction in IUI cycles.

Name of drug	Dosage	Route	Maximum dose	Side effects	Contraindications	Pharmacokinetics
Clomiphene citrate	50–150 mg/day	Oral	150 mg	• Hot flushes (10%), abdominal discomfort, bloating (5%), breast discomfort (2%), nausea and vomiting (2%), visual symptoms (floaters, flashes, and abnormal perception), and headache (1.5%) • Multiple pregnancy risk 5%	Preexisting ovarian cysts, suspected malignancy, and liver disease	• *Oral bioavailability:* >90% • *Half-life:* 7 days (its metabolites may be found in feces up to 30 days) • *Metabolism:* Liver • *Excretion:* Mainly through feces and some in urine
Tamoxifen	20 mg/day	oral	80 mg/day	Endometrial polyp and hyperplasia, endometrial cancer, liver toxicity, deep vein thrombosis, pulmonary embolism, and stroke	History of DVT, thrombosis	• *Oral bioavailability:* 100% • *Protein bound:* >99% (albumin) • *Half-life:* 5–7 days • *Metabolism:* Liver • *Excretion:* Feces 65% and urine 6%
Letrozole	2.5–7.5 mg/day	Oral	7.5 mg/day	Hot flushes (18%), bone pain (20%), back pain (17%), nausea (15%), dyspnea (44%), and multiple pregnancy risk <4%	Preexisting ovarian cysts, suspected malignancy, and liver disease	• *Oral bioavailability:* >95% • *Half-life:* 48 hours • *Protein binding:* 60% mainly to albumin • *Metabolism:* Liver • *Excretion:* Biliary (85%) and urinary (11%)

Contd...

Contd...

Name of drug	Dosage	Route	Maximum dose	Side effects	Contraindications	Pharmacokinetics
Metformin	oral	1,500–2,000 mg/day	2,500 mg/day	Diarrhea (53%), nausea/vomiting (25.5%), flatulence (12.1%), asthenia (9.2%), indigestion (7.1%), abdominal discomfort (6.4%), headache (5.7%), and lactic acidosis (<1%)	Renal dysfunction, congestive heart failure, hypersensitivity to metformin, acute or chronic metabolic acidosis, and impaired hepatic function	• *Oral bioavailability:* 50–60%, food interferes with absorption • *Protein bound:* None • *Excretion:* Renal • *Half-life:* 4–8.7 hours
Gonadotropins	Injection					
hMG	SC or IM	75 IU–150 IU/day	150 IU/day	Mild bloating, pain swelling, rash or irritation at injection site, stomach pain/pelvic pain, myalgia, drowsiness, and dizziness	Pregnancy and breast feeding, ovarian cyst, undiagnosed vaginal bleeding, cancer of breast, ovary, uterus, testicles, hypothalamus, or pituitary gland	*Half-life:* Elimination half-life of 11–13 hours
FSH	SC	75 IU–150 IU/day	150 IU/day	Local irritation at the injection site, feeling of fullness, bloating and tenderness in the abdomen, mood swings, fatigue, and risk of OHSS if higher doses are used, multiple pregnancy 15%	Pregnancy and breast-feeding, ovarian cyst, undiagnosed vaginal bleeding, cancer of breast, ovary, uterus, testicles, hypothalamus, or pituitary gland	Elimination half-life of 1 day

(DVT: deep vein thrombosis; FSH: follicle-stimulating hormone; hMG: human menopausal gonadotropin; IM: intramuscular: SC: subcutaneous; OHSS: ovarian hyperstimulation syndrome)

REFERENCES

1. Zegers-Hochschild F, Adamson GD, Dyer S, Racowsky C, de Mouzon J, Sokol R. The international glossary on infertility and fertility care. Hum Reprod. 2017;32:1786-801.
2. Lindheim SR, Glenn TL, Smith MC, Gagneux P. Ovulation induction for the general gynecologist. J Obstet Gynaecol India. 2018; 68(4):242-52.
3. Clark JH, Markaverich BM, The agonistic-antagonistic properties of clomiphene: a review. Pharmacol Ther. 1981;15:467.
4. Out HJ, Coelingh Bennink HJ. Clomiphene citrate or gonadotrophins for induction of ovulation? Hum Reprod. 1998;13:2358-61.
5. Morshedi M, Duran HE, Taylor S, Oehninger S. Efficacy and pregnancy outcome of two methods of semen preparation for intrauterine insemination: A prospective randomized study. Fertil Steril. 2003;79 (Suppl 3):1625-32.
6. Rossing MA, Daling JR, Weiss NS, Moore DE, Self SG. Ovarian tumors in a cohort of infertile women. N Engl J Med. 1994;331:771-6.
7. Kurachi K, Aono T, Minagawa J, Miyake A. Congenital malformations of newborn infants after clomiphene-induced ovulation, Fertil Steril. 1983;40:187.
8. Brown J, Farquhar C, Beck J, Boothroyd C, Hughes E. Clomiphene and anti-oestrogens for ovulation induction in PCOS. Cochrane Database Syst Rev. 2009;4:CD002249.
9. Legro RS, Castracane VD, Kauffman RP. Detecting insulin resistance in polycystic ovary syndrome purposes and pitfalls. Obstetr Gynecol Survey. 2004;59:141-54.
10. El Hayek S, Bitar L, Hamdar LH, Mirza FG, Daoud G. Poly Cystic Ovarian Syndrome: An Updated Overview. Front Physiol. 2016;7:124.
11. Teede HJ, Misso ML, Costello MF, Dokras A, Laven J, Moran L, et al. Recommendations from the international evidence-based guideline for the assessment and management of polycystic ovary syndrome. Fertil Steril. 2018;110:364-79.
12. Gambioli R, Forte G, Buzzaccarini G, Unfer V, Laganà A. Myo-Inositol as a Key Supporter of Fertility and Physiological Gestation. Pharmaceuticals. 2021;14:504.
13. Elnashar A, Abdelmageed E, Fayed M, Sharaf M. CC and dexamethasone in treatment of CC-resistant polycystic ovary syndrome a prospective placebo-controlled study. Hum Reprod. 2006;21:1805-8.
14. Badawy A, Allam A, Abulatta M. Extending clomiphene treatment in clomiphene-resistant women with PCOS a randomized controlled trial. Reprod Biomed Online. 2008;16:825-9.
15. Agrawal K, Gainder S, Dhaliwal LK, Suri V. Ovulation induction using clomiphene citrate using stair-step regimen versus traditional regimen in polycystic ovary syndrome women–A randomized control trial. J Hum Reprod Sci. 2017;10:261-4.
16. Dhaliwal LK, Suri V, Gupta KR, Sahdev S. Tamoxifen: An alternative to clomiphene in women with polycystic ovary syndrome. J Hum Reprod Sci. 2011;4(2):76-9.
17. Tredway D, Schertz JC, Bock D, Hemsey G, Diamond MP. Anastrozole single-dose protocol in women with oligo- or anovulatory infertility: results of a randomized phase II dose-response study. Fertil Steril. 2011; 95:1725.e1.
18. Biljan MM, Hcmmings R, Brassard N. The outcome of 150 babies following the treatment wilh letrozole or lelrozole and gonadotrophins. Fertil Steril. 2005; 84(Suppl):1033.
19. Legro RS, Brzyski RG, Diamond MP, Coutifaris C, Schlaff WD, Casson P, et al. Letrozole versus clomiphene for infertility in the polycystic ovary syndrome. N Engl J Med. 2014;371:119-29.
20. Diamond MP, Legro RS, Coutifaris C, Alvero R, Robinson RD, Casson P, et al. Letrozole, gonadotropin, or clomiphene for unexplained infertility. N Engl J Med. 2015;373:1230-40.
21. Tsiami AP, Goulis DG, Sotiriadis AI, Kolibianakis EM. Higher ovulation rate with letrozole as compared with clomiphene citrate in infertile women with polycystic ovary syndrome: a systematic review

and meta-analysis. Hormones (Athens). 2021;20(3):449-61.
22. Lord JM, Flight IH, Norman RJ. Insulin-sensitising drugs (metformin, troglitazone, rosiglitazone, pioglitazone, D-chiro-inositol) for polycystic ovary syndrome. Cochrane Database Syst Rev. 2003;3:CD003053.
23. Franks S. When should an insulin sensitizing agent be used in the treatment of polycystic ovary syndrome? Clin Endocrinol (Oxf). 2011;74:148-51.
24. Aschheim S, Zondek B. Schwangerschaftsdiagnose aus dem Harn (Durch Hormonnachweis). Klin Wochenschr. 1928; 7:8-9.
25. Gonadotropin preparations: past, present, and future perspectives. The Practice Committee of the American Society for Reproductive Medicine, Birmingham, Alabama. Fertil Steril. 2008;90:S13-20.
26. Olsson H, Sandstrom R, Grundemar L. Different pharmacokinetic and pharmacodynamic properties of recombinant follicle-stimulating hormone (rFSH) derived from a human cell line compared with rFSH from a non-human cell line. J Clin Pharmacol. 2014;54:1299-307.
27. Hoff JD, Quigley ME, Yen SS. Hormonal dynamics at midcycle: A reevaluation. J Clin Endocrinol Metab. 1983;57(4):792-6.

Chapter 33

Ovulation Induction in IVF-ET

Renu Tanwar, Renu Singh

The assisted reproductive technology (ART) is an innovative approach which involves the process of fertilization of female and male gametes in vitro and the transfer of the embryo into the receptive uterus.

The physiology of menstruation is important while understanding the mechanism of action of these drugs.

Rising follicle-stimulating hormone (FSH) in the early follicular phase leads to follicular growth. Granulosa cells convert androgen to estradiol by the action of aromatase enzyme. FSH and luteinizing hormone (LH) act together to complete follicular development. At 8–12 mm, the follicles under the influence of FSH develop LH receptors. Action of FSH on granulosa cells produce inhibin which exerts a negative feedback on FSH causing a decline in FSH level. This with rising E2 levels, thus promoting selection of dominant follicle.[1]

Midcycle LH surge induces meiosis and ovulation with formation of corpus luteum (luteinization of granulosa and theca cells) **(Fig. 1)**.

The process of in vitro fertilization (IVF) mimics the endogenous hormonal milieu by giving exogenous hormones (drugs). These drugs act by suppressing the endogenous hormones and act by:

- Suppressing the HP axis (hypothalamic-pituitary axis) to prevent premature LH surge
- Promoting follicle development
- Inducing ovulation

Thus, the fertility drugs are as follows:
- Hypothalamo-pituitary axis suppression:
  - Gonadotropin-releasing hormone (GnRH) agonist
  - GnRH antagonist
- Controlled ovarian hyperstimulation:
  - Oral ovulogens
  - Injectable ovulogens—urinary or recombinant gonadotropins
- *Ovulation triggers:*
  - Human chorionic gonadotropin (recombinant/urinary)
  - GnRH-agonist analogs
  - Recombinant LH
  - Kisspeptin
- *Luteal phase support:*
  - Human chorionic gonadotropin (hCG)
    - Progesterone
- *Endometrial preparation:*
  - Estradiol valerate
  - Estradiol hemihydrate
- Adjuvants

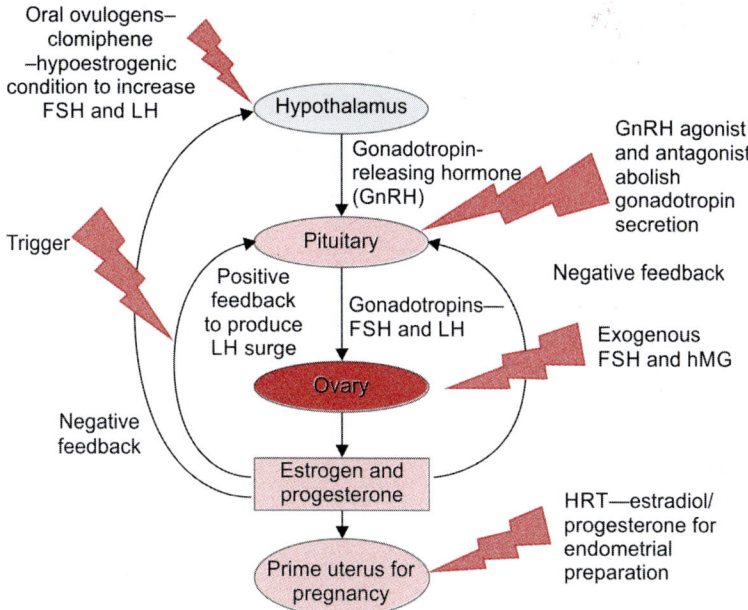

Fig. 1: Site of action of drugs on the hypothalamo-pituitary-ovarian axis. (FSH: follicle-stimulating hormone; hMG: human menopausal gonadotropin; HRT: hormone replacement therapy; LH: luteinizing hormone)

GONADOTROPIN-RELEASING HORMONE

Secreted by the hypothalamus, this decapeptide hormone is responsible for secretion of FSH and LH from the anterior pituitary in a pulsatile manner, with greater frequency in the proliferative phase and higher amplitude in the luteal phase.

The synthetic drugs act on these receptors and produce a similar response, but for a prolonged time. This is due to structural changes that cause lesser degradation and greater half-life.

The synthetic drugs act via the GnRH receptors and are used to control the natural reproductive cycle. They are called GnRH analogs, which are of two types:
1. GnRH-agonist
2. GnRH-antagonist

Gonadotropin-releasing Hormone Analogs

See **Table 1**.

CONTROLLED OVARIAN HYPERSTIMULATION

The main aim of the ART cycle is to produce controlled ovarian hyperstimulation and to retrieve maximum number of oocytes. This can be achieved by oral ovulogens or injectables gonadotropins. Ideal stimulation regimen should have low cancellation rate, minimum cost, lesser side effects, and to maximize singleton pregnancy rates. The various stimulation regimens used are as follows:
- Mild stimulation
- Minimal stimulation-treatment with oral and low-dose injectable ovulogens sequentially.
- Aggressive stimulation with the help of high-dose gonadotropins.

Oral Ovulogens

See **Table 2**.

TABLE 1: Mechanism, types, and different doses of GnRH analogs.

Drugs	Mechanism of action	Types and dose	Adverse effects
GnRH-agonist	• Abolish endogenous gonadotropin secretion • Agonist administration produces a flare effect lasting for 3–6 days, which is followed by downregulation due to internalization of GnRH receptors thus abolishing pulsatile rhythm and suppressing pituitary. These could be started either from the luteal phase of the previous menstrual cycle or day 2/day 3 of the menses *Protocols used:*[2] • Short flare • Ultrashort flare • Downregulation protocol[3] *Uses:* • To prevent LH surge • *Trigger*: As a sole agonist trigger, dual trigger, and double trigger • Downregulated HRT cycles	• Triptorelin • As 0.1 mg subcutaneous daily administration or depot 3.75 mg vial intramuscular/subcutaneous/monthly administration[4] • Leuprolide acetate injection 0.5 mg/0.2 mg subcutaneous[3] • Nafarelin-nebulizer spray (200 µg each nebulization, twice a day, two nebulization in morning and evening[5]	• Hot flushes • Decreased libido • Vaginal dryness • Cyst formation • Emotional instability • Decrease bone mineral density • Prolonged treatment
GnRH antagonist	• Competitively block the endogenous GnRH, and produce immediate suppression of FSH and LH, without flare-up effect. Thus, prevents LH surge and avoids premature ovulation[6] • Have advantages of no cyst formation, shorter duration of treatment without hypoestrogenic side effects, and improves flexibility • GnRH antagonists can produce inhibitory effects on LH after 6–8 hours of binding to the receptors *Protocols:*[7] • *Fixed dose protocol:* 0.25 mg injection subcutaneous is started from day 6 of the stimulation cycle till the day of the trigger • *Flexible dose protocol:* 0.25 mg injection subcutaneous given when follicle size is 14 mm and given till day of trigger	• Cetrorelix (third generation)—prefilled syringe of 0.25 and 3 mg subcutaneous[8] • Ganirelix (third generation) prefilled syringe 0.25 mg subcutaneous	• Local side effects at injection site • Hypersensitivity reaction • Weight gain • Fluid retention

(FSH: follicle-stimulating hormone; GnRH: gonadotropin-releasing hormone; HRT: hormone replacement therapy; LH: luteinizing hormone)

TABLE 2: Controlled ovarian hyperstimulation drugs.

Drugs	Mechanism of action	Dose	Adverse effects
Clomiphene citrate	• Nonsteroidal selective estrogen receptor modulator • Racemic mixture of enclomiphene (62%) and zuclomiphene (38%) • Enclomiphene is more potent with a shorter half-life and zuclomiphene has more antiestrogenic effect • Binds to estrogen receptors to create a pseudohypoestrogenic state which causes negative feedback and increases the release of GnRH further causing increase in FSH and LH. FSH and LH act on ovaries to cause folliculogenesis	The *minimal stimulation protocol*:[9] Tablet clomiphene citrate given in variable doses along with gonadotropins	• Transient hot flushes • Mood swings • Breast tenderness • Pelvic pain • Nausea
Letrozole	• Nonsteroidal third generation aromatase inhibitor. These are competitive inhibitors that prevent conversion of androgen to estrogen thus restoring the pulsatile release of gonadotropin and promoting ovulation • It has a half-life of 48 hours • Increase the levels of androstenedione and testosterone in the follicular fluid,[10] thus, improving the sensitivity of follicles to FSH • *Advantage:* No antiestrogenic effect on the cervical mucus and endometrium	*Minimal stimulation protocol* (letrozole can be used along with gonadotropins): Used in *fertility preservation* for patients with breast cancer to minimize the estradiol concentration in circulation in these hormone sensitive cancers[11]	• Mood changes • Nausea • Headache • Dizziness

(FSH: follicle-stimulating hormone; GnRH: gonadotropin-releasing hormone; LH: luteinizing hormone)

Injectables-Gonadotropins

The GnRH is responsible for regulating the menstrual cycle and maintaining the FSH window needed for follicular development. The gonadotropins are used to extend the FSH window to allow recruitment of more follicles instead of monofollicular recruitment in the natural cycle. Before starting an ovarian stimulation protocol, it is important to see and maintain the LH levels above the threshold levels but below a ceiling level to induce more mature follicles and prevent follicle atresia **(Figs. 2 and 3)**.

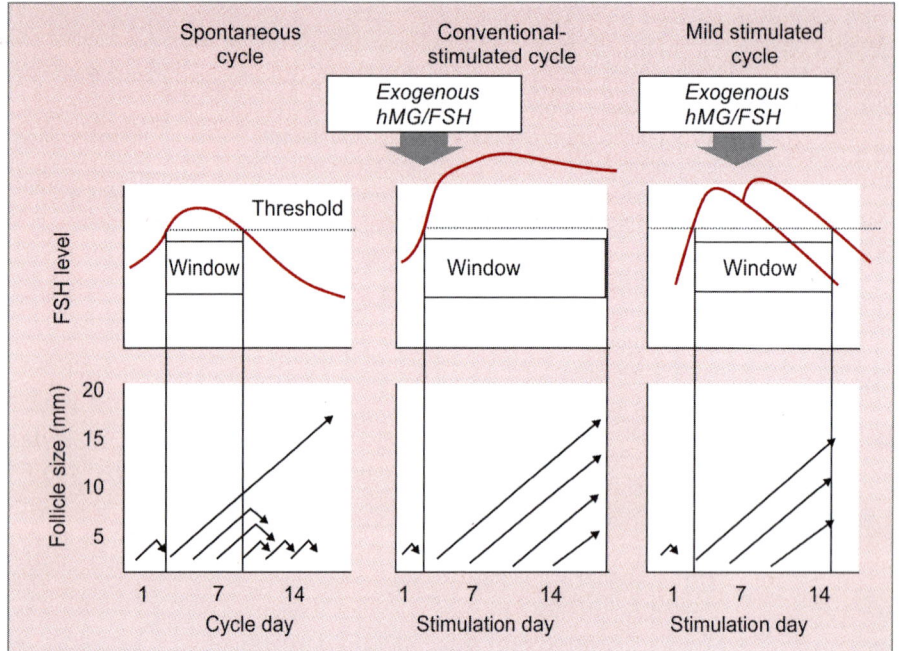

Fig. 2: FSH window.[12] (FSH: follicle-stimulating hormone; hMG: human menopausal gonadotropin)

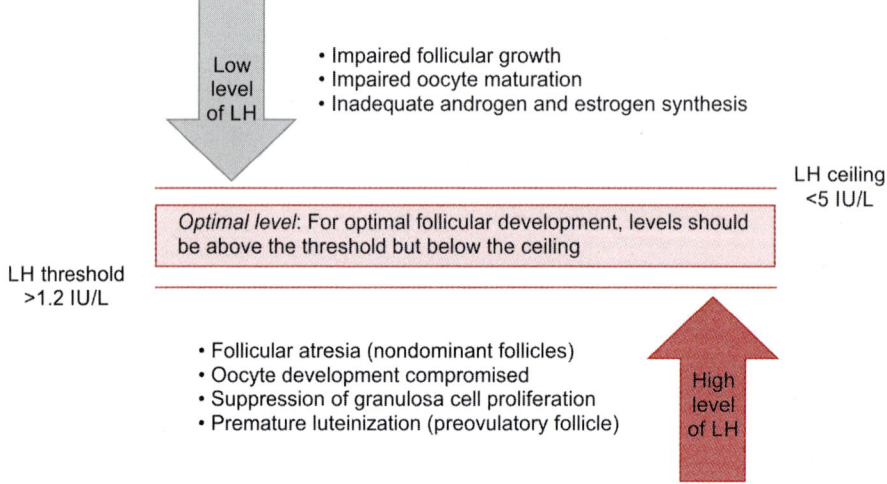

Fig. 3: Concept of luteinizing hormone (LH) threshold and ceiling.[13]
Note: Gonadotropin treatment for ovarian stimulation began in the year 1960.[14] These can be urinary or recombinant.

Urinary Gonadotropins

Human menopausal gonadotropins (hMGs) were obtained initially from postmenopausal urine after purification methods but contained only 5% pure forms. hMG contains five isomers of FSH and nine isomers of LH which after purification contains a standardized activity of 75 IU of both FSH and LH. Postmenopausal urine is rich in nongonadotropic proteins [tumor necrosis factor binding factor 1 (TNF-BP-1), epidermal growth factor (EGF), transferrin, Tamm–Horsfall proteins] leading to allergic reactions, hypersensitivity and pain. Purification methods have eliminated these undesirable proteins. This highly purified (HP)-hMG, has an advantage of subcutaneous administration.

Urofollitropin

Biologically *pure urinary FSH* obtained after purification by removal of antibodies and LH, given through the intramuscular route and has >95% urinary contamination.[14]

HP-FSH: Produced by use of monoclonal antibodies specific to FSH, containing <0.1 IU LH and <5% urinary proteins.[14] Advantages include subcutaneous administration—better tolerability and compliance and self-administration is possible.

Recombinants

Recombinant deoxyribonucleic acid (DNA) technology (genes incorporated in DNA of host) in Chinese hamster ovary cells produce substances with pure FSH activity, >99% free from urinary proteins and LH activity.

- *Recombinant follitropin α and β (pure FSH activity):* Both have one α and one β chain but differ in the sialic acid residue.

  Have a terminal half-life of 17 hours requiring daily injections and steady state reached only after 4–5 days of administration.

- *Designer recombinant: Corifollitropin-α* consists of the α-subunit of recombinant human follicle-stimulating hormone (r-hFSH) together with a hybrid β-subunit (made up of the β-subunit of hFSH and the C-terminal part of the β-subunit of hCG). FSH-CTP has a longer half-life than standard r-hFSH of 65 hours. FSH-CTP initiates and sustains follicular growth for 1 week.

The latest follitropin delta is derived from fetal retinal cell origin with a half-life of 30 hours.

The route of elimination of gonadotropins is renal.

Recombinant FSH are started from day 2 or day 3 of the menstrual cycle with dose decided by the age, body mass index (BMI), and ovarian reserve of the patient. The starting dose of follitropin-α is 150 IU and the dose could be increased from day 6 of stimulation up to a maximum of 450 IU. The dose of r-FSH can be adjusted based on the number and size of developing follicles.

Adverse effects:
- Acne
- Mood changes
- Growth of facial hair
- Headache
- Pain and irritation at injection site
- Risk of moderate or severe ovarian hyperstimulation syndrome (OHSS).

Recombinant Luteinizing Hormone

Luteotropin (pure LH activity)—contains the active substance lutropin alfa. The powder and solvent available are made up into a solution for injection, or available as prefilled pens. Given as subcutaneous injections. It is used in patients of hypogonadotropic hypogonadism and in women with diminished ovarian reserve.[14]

■ OVULATION TRIGGER[15]

The midcycle LH surge induces the maturation and release of the dominant follicle. Drugs used to mimic this LH rise, to release mature oocytes are called *triggering agents*. These include hCG, GnRH agonist, recombinant LH, and Kisspeptins **(Table 3 and Fig. 4)**.

TABLE 3: Drugs for ovulation trigger.

Drugs	Mechanism of action	Dose
hCG: • hCG and LH share homology thus can be used as surrogate of LH • Both have the same alpha subunit. However, the c terminal peptide of beta subunit is different thus, imparting a longer half life and slower clearance of hCG.[16] • Recombinant hCG (r-hCG) and recombinant LH (r-LH) are prepared through recombinant DNA technology and derived from Chinese hamster ovary cells by genetic engineering[17] • r-hCG has improved local tolerance thus promoting subcutaneous route of administration. Half-life is 29–30 hours compared to HP-hCG (31–37 hours)[18] • No significant difference has been reported in the rate of OHSS between urinary/recombinant hCG[17]	• Induce luteinization and support lutein cells • Has a sustained luteotropic action with development of multiple corpora lutea • Supraphysiologic levels of estrogen and progesterone • Occupies the LH-hCG receptor and thus is capable of triggering ovulation	Urinary hCG-given in dose of 2,000, 5,000, and 10,000 IU intramuscular[19]
GnRH-agonist trigger	• Subcutaneous administration of bolus of GnRH-agonist analog, produces a flare-up response. This allows an FSH-LH surge that induces ovulation • Used in GnRH antagonist cycles where the hypothalamus is not blocked by agonists • Disadvantage—it can produce early luteolysis thus requiring intense luteal support	A single bolus dose is administered as injection leuprolide 0.5 mg subcutaneous or injection triptorelin 0.2 mg subcutaneous
Dual trigger	GnRH agonists have a greater affinity for the GnRH receptors thus producing a more physiological LH and FSH surge. Also produce reversible luteolysis thus decreasing OHSS risk. hCG can prevent this luteolysis to provide adequate luteal phase support. Useful in poor responders	1 mg leuprolide or 0.2 mg triptorelin along with 250 μg of r-hCG or urinary hCG 5,000 IU IM or 10,000 IU IM can be given simultaneously as a dual trigger[20]

Contd...

Contd...

Drugs	Mechanism of action	Dose
Double trigger	A modification of the dual trigger, the so-called double trigger, consists of the coadministration of a GnRH and hCG for final oocyte maturation, 40 and 34 hours before ovum-pick up (OPU), respectively[21] These methods combine the advantage of: • Increased number of MII/mature oocyte retrieved • Reduced chances of OHSS	

(FSH: follicle-stimulating hormone; GnRH: gonadotropin-releasing hormone; hCG: human chorionic gonadotropin; LH: luteinizing hormone; OHSS: ovarian hyperstimulation syndrome; r-hCG: recombinant human chorionic gonadotropin)

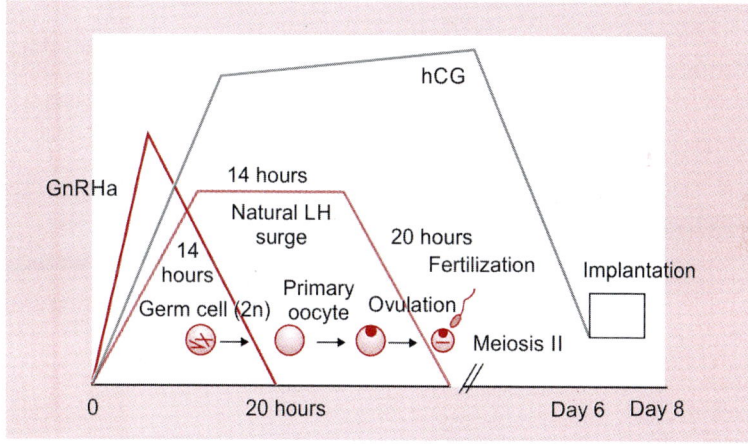

Fig. 4: The natural LH rise has three phases total lasting for 48 hours. GnRH agonists produce a rise in both FSH and LH lasting for 24 hours, producing more physiological response and negligible OHSS. While hCG acts as LH surrogate without increasing FSH. (FSH: follicle-stimulating hormone; GnRH: gonadotropin-releasing hormone; GnRHa: gonadotropin releasing-hormone analogs; hCG: human chorionic gonadotropin; LH: luteinizing hormone)

LUTEAL SUPPORT

Drugs used to support the function of corpus luteum thus increasing the rate of implantation and improving pregnancy outcomes. Gonadotropin hormone-releasing hormone agonists produce early luteolysis and thus need intensive luteal phase support. These drugs, mainly progestins, can be started soon after the ovum pickup in fresh cycles or after embryo transfer. The duration to continue the support varies and can be used till the urine pregnancy test is positive or till 11–12 weeks of gestation **(Table 4)**.

TABLE 4: Drugs for luteal phase support.

Drugs	Mechanism of action	Dose
Progesterone		

Natural micronized progesterone	Promote implantation by:
	• Stimulate uterine growth
	• Inhibition of prostaglandin synthesis
	• Inhibition of myometrial contraction
	• Producing secretary changes in endometrium
	• Immunomodulatory action and anti-inflammatory
		• *Oral tablets:* 100, 200, and 300 mg
		• *Vaginal:*
		  – *Capsules:* 100 and 200 mg
		  – *Gel:* 4%, 8%
		  – *Suppositories:* 200 and 400 mg
		• *Rectal-suppositories:* 200 and 400 mg[22]
		• *Topical gel* 1%
		• *Intramuscular injection:* Vials of 10, 25, 50, and 100 mg
		• *Subcutaneous aqueous injections:* 25 mg
		• As suggested by the European Society of Human Reproduction and Embryology (ESHRE) guidelines, the daily administration of 50 mg of intramuscular progesterone, 25 mg of subcutaneous progesterone and 600 mg of micronized vaginal progesterone may be equally efficient[23]

Dydrogesterone Structure:[24] • Stereoisomer of progesterone with C10 methyl group attached to alpha position and hydrogen atom at C9 attached to β position. There is also an extra double bond between C6 and C7 • This makes dydrogesterone metabolically more active and orally more effective	• Luteal phase support by promoting decidualization of endometrium and increasing receptivity thus promoting implantation • Immunomodulation and regulation of blood flow • In cases of threatened abortion	
hCG		125 IU of r-hCG daily or 1,500 IU of hCG can be used on the day of OPU and 4 days later[25,26]

(hCG: human chorionic gonadotropin; OPU: oocyte pickup; r-hCG: recombinant human chorionic gonadotropin)

TABLE 5: Drugs for endometrial preparation.

Drugs	Mechanism of action	Dose
• *Estrogen:* Estradiol hemihydrate is more hydrated than anhydrous estradiol and is more insoluble in water in comparison, which may result in slower absorption rates. Estradiol hemihydrate is a micronized form of 17-β estradiol, more potent • *Estradiol valerate:* Estradiol valerate is an ester of estradiol (the C17-hydroxy group) with valeric acid. This formulation prevents the usual metabolism of estradiol to estrone until hydrolysis has taken place. Slightly lower estrone levels • Transdermal preparations bypass first pass metabolism. Efficacy reduced in obese and during hot humid conditions • E2/E1 >1 (while in oral—E2/E1 <1)[30] • Transdermal estradiol valerate patches are applied on the lower abdominal • Vaginal route of estradiol is less preferred[31]	Endometrial preparation in ART is achieved by the administration of exogenous estrogen, with the best reproductive outcomes obtained within a range of 11–40 days of estrogen administration; shorter estrogen replacements lead to high abortion rates, while breakthrough bleeding is common after >40 days of administration[27,28]	• *Oral:* Estradiol tablets 2 mg three times a day starting from day 2 or day 3 of cycle. Dose can be increased depending on the endometrial thickness. It can be increased to up to 12 mg/day • *Transdermal gels/patches:* It can be applied starting from dose of 50 µg and increased according to endometrial thickness to 200 µg dose[29]

TABLE 6: Adjuvants.

Human growth hormone	• Dose variable in different studies ranging from –4 IU–12 IU in controlled ovarian stimulations • Increase local production of IGF-1 • Improves granulosa cell response • Promote steroidogenesis • Recruit more follicles (MII) • Inhibit follicle atresia • Expands cumulus • Increases endometrial blood flow. Upregulates LH receptors • Increases progesterone production[32] • Used in poor responders[32] • Thin endometrium • Hypogonadotropic hypogonadism
Dehydroepiandrostenedione sulfate (DHEA)	• Improves steroidogenesis and folliculogenesis • Increase IGF-1 concentration • Acts as a prohormone for follicular fluid testosterone[33] • Poor responders • *Dose:* 75–80 mg/day[33]
Sildenafil	• Sildenafil is a selective PDE5 isoenzyme inhibitor • Enhances the effect of nitric oxide by inhibiting PDE5 producing vascular relaxation, thereby, increasing blood flow to the endometrium

Contd...

Contd...

	• Sildenafil by development of spiral arteries increases the uterine arterial blood flow, thus, improving receptivity
	• *Dose:*
	  – Sildenafil can be administered vaginally at a dose of 25 mg, twice daily
	  – Shows beneficial impact on the uterine receptivity[34]

Low-molecular-weight heparin	• Acts by inhibiting factor Xa and IIa. It has an antithrombotic effect. Affects selectins, cadherins, MMP during implantation process
	• *Dose:* 20–40 mg once daily subcutaneous injections[35]
	• *Uses:*
	  – Recurrent pregnancy loss
	  – APLA syndrome
	  – Inherited thrombophilia
	  – Recurrent implantation failure

Corticosteroids—dexamethasone	• Stimulate GH and IGF-1 • By acting on adrenal glands, decreases the production of androgens that interfere with growth and development of follicles[36] • Acts as an immune modulator • Alters cytokine expression and excess NK cell activity • Reduce endometrial inflammation • *Dose:* 0.5 mg or 1 mg/day[36]
Metformin	The biguanide metformin (dimethylbiguanide) is an insulin sensitizer that acts by reducing insulin resistance and its secretion[37]
Cabergoline	• An ergot derivative • Agonist at D2 and 5-HT1 receptors. Used as an adjuvant in the treatment of OHSS[38] • *Dose:* 0.5 mg/day for 8 days[38]

(ALPA: antiphospholipid antibodies; GH: growth hormone; IGF-1: insulin-like growth factor-1; LH: luteinizing hormone; MMP: matrix metalloproteinase; OHSS: ovarian hyperstimulation syndrome; PDE5: phosphodiesterase-5)

■ ENDOMETRIAL PREPARATION

With the advent of frozen embryo transfer the use of hormone replacement therapy (HRT) cycle for promoting growth of endometrium followed by embryo transfer. Various protocols can be used including natural cycle, modified natural cycle with hCG trigger, or HRT cycles with or without GnRH-agonist downregulation. Estrogen is an important hormone promoting the proliferation of the endometrium and preparation for pregnancy and is used to inhibit follicular growth in HRT cycles **(Table 5)**.

■ ADJUVANTS

These are substances that are used to enhance the effect of drugs. They can be pharmacological or nonpharmacological in the form of acupuncture or massage **(Table 6)**.

■ KEY POINTS

- ART technique involves the fertilization of female and male gametes in vitrio and transfer of embryo into the receptive uterus.
- The various drugs used in IVF procedure act at various levels starting from suppression

of hypo-thalamo-pitutary axis to controlled ovarian hyperstimulation.
- The endometrial preparation before embryo transfer and luteal phase support also play an important role in an IVF cycle.
- For optimum results the mechanism of action and side effects of the drugs should be studied in detail.

■ REFERENCES

1. Raju GA, Chavan R, Deenadayal M, Gunasheela D, Gutgutia R, Haripriya G, et al. Luteinizing hormone and follicle stimulating hormone synergy: a review of role in controlled ovarian hyper-stimulation. J Hum Reprod Sci. 2013;6(4):227-34.
2. Rezaeian P, Esmaeilzadeh S, Tajali Z, Heidari FN, Golsorkhtabaramiri M. Short, semi-short or long GnRH agonist treatment regimens in women ICSI candidate; which is proper in preventing premature LH surge? Middle East Fertil Soc J. 2016;21(3):161-7.
3. Shrestha D, La X, Feng HL. Comparison of different stimulation protocols used in in vitro fertilization: a review. Ann Transl Med. 2015;3(10):137.
4. Olivennes F, Righini C, Fanchin R, Torrisi C, Hazout A, Glissant M, et al. A protocol using a low dose of gonadotrophin-releasing hormone agonist might be the best protocol for patients with high follicle-stimulating hormone concentrations on day 3. Hum Reprod. 1996;11(6):1169-72.
5. Avrcch OM, Goldman GA, Pinkas H, Amit S, Neri A, Zukerman Z, et al. Intranasal nafarelin versus buserelin (short protocol) for controlled ovarian hyperstimulation before in vitro fertilization: a prospective clinical trial. Gynecol Endocrinol. 1996;10(3):165-70.
6. Al-Inany HG, Youssef MA, Ayeleke RO, Brown J, Lam WS, Broekmans FJ. Gonadotrophin-releasing hormone antagonists for assisted reproductive technology. Cochrane Database Syst Rev. 2016;4(4):CD001750.
7. Tarlatzis BC, Fauser BC, Kolibianakis EM, Diedrich K, Devroey P. Brussels GnRH Antagonist Consensus Workshop Group. GnRH antagonists in ovarian stimulation for IVF. Hum Reprod Update. 2006;12(4):333-40.
8. Furman BL. (2007). Cetrorelix. xPharm: The Comprehensive Pharmacology Reference 1-3.
9. Teramoto S, Kato O. Minimal ovarian stimulation with clomiphene citrate: a large-scale retrospective study. Reprod Biomed Online. 2007;15(2):134-48.
10. Garcia-Velasco JA, Moreno L, Pacheco A, Guillén A, Duque L, Requena A, et al. The aromatase inhibitor letrozole increases the concentration of intraovarian androgens and improves in vitro fertilization outcome in low responder patients: a pilot study. Fertility and sterility. 2005;84(1):82-7.
11. Shapira M, Orvieto R, Lebovitz O, Nahum R, Aizer A, Segev-Zahav A, et al. Does daily co administration of gonadotropins and letrozole during the ovarian stimulation improve IVF outcome for poor and sub optimal responders?. J Ovarian Res. 2020; 13(1):1-5.
12. Fauser BC, Nargund G, Andersen AN, Norman R, Tarlatzis B, Boivin J, et al. Mild ovarian stimulation for IVF: 10 years later. Hum Reprod. 2010;25(11):2678-84.
13. Raju GA, Chavan R, Deenadayal M, Gunasheela D, Gutgutia R, Haripriya G, et al. Luteinizing hormone and follicle stimulating hormone synergy: a review of role in controlled ovarian hyper-stimulation. J Hum Reprod Sci. 2013;6(4):227-34.
14. Lunenfeld B, Bilger W, Longobardi S, Alam V, D'Hooghe T, Sunkara SK. The development of gonadotropins for clinical use in the treatment of infertility. Front Endocrinol (Lausanne). 2019;10:429.
15. Sawankar SG, Bora NM, Shah PR, Malhotra N. Pharmacological Options to Trigger Final Oocyte Maturation in In Vitro Fertilization. J South Asian Fed Obstet Gynecol. 2020; 12(1):38-44.
16. Rahman NA, Rao CV. Recent progress in luteinizing hormone/human chorionic gonadotropin hormone research. Mol Hum Reprod. 2009;15(11):703-11.

17. Youssef MA, AbouâSetta AM, Lam WS. Recombinant versus urinary human chorionic gonadotrophin for final oocyte maturation triggering in IVF and ICSI cycles. Cochrane Database Syst Rev. 2016; 4(4):CD003719.
18. ichael Ludwig M, Doody KJ, Doody KM. Use of recombinant human chorionic gonadotropin in ovulation induction. Fertil Steril. 2003;79(5):1051-9.
19. Abdalla HI, Ah-Moye M, Brinsden P, Howe DL, Okonofua F, Craft I. The effect of the dose of human chorionic gonadotropin and the type of gonadotropin stimulation on oocyte recovery rates in an in vitro fertilization program. Fertil Steril. 1987;48(6):958-63.
20. Shapiro BS, Daneshmand ST, Garner FC, Aguirre M, Thomas S. Gonadotropin-releasing hormone agonist combined with a reduced dose of human chorionic gonadotropin for final oocyte maturation in fresh autologous cycles of in vitro fertilization. Fertil Steril. 2008;90(1):231-3.
21. Orvieto R. Triggering final follicular maturation-hCG, GnRH-agonist or both, when and to whom? J Ovarian Res. 2015; 8(1):60.
22. Khrouf M, Slimani S, Khrouf MR, Braham M, Bouyahia M, Berjeb KK, et al. Progesterone for luteal phase support in in vitro fertilization: comparison of vaginal and rectal pessaries to vaginal capsules: a randomized controlled study. Clinical Medicine Insights: Women's Health. 2016; 9:43-7.
23. Di Guardo F, Midassi H, Racca A, Tournaye H, De Vos M, Blockeel C. Luteal phase support in IVF: comparison between evidence-based medicine and real-life practices. Front Endocrinol (Lausanne). 2020;11:500.
24. Salehpour S, Tamimi M, Saharkhiz N. Comparison of oral dydrogesterone with suppository vaginal progesterone for luteal-phase support in in vitro fertilization (IVF): a randomized clinical trial. Iran J Reprod Med. 2013;11(11):913-8.
25. Andersen CY, Elbaek HO, Alsbjerg B, Laursen RJ, Povlsen BB, Thomsen L, et al. Daily low-dose hCG stimulation during the luteal phase combined with GnRHa triggered IVF cycles without exogenous progesterone: a proof of concept trial. Hum Reprod. 2015; 30(10):2387-95.
26. Kol S, Breyzman T, Segal L, Humaidan P. 'Luteal coasting' after GnRH agonist trigger - individualized, HCG-based, progesterone-free luteal support in 'high responders': a case series. Reprod Biomed Online. 2015; 31(6):747-51.
27. Martins Wde P, dos Reis RM, Ferriani RA, de Araújo CH, Nastri CO, Filho FM. Endometrial preparation for in vitro oocyte maturation: early use of estrogen increases endometrial tissue and requires lower daily dosage: a cross over trial in 'mock' cycles. J Assist Reprod Genet. 2006;23(5):241-6.
28. Borini A, Prato LD, Bianchi L, Violini F, Cattoli M, Flamigni C. Effect of duration of estradiol replacement on the outcome of oocyte donation. J Assist Reprod Genet. 2001;18(4):187-90.
29. Kalem Z, Kalem MN, Gürgan T. Methods for endometrial preparation in frozen-thawed embryo transfer cycles. J Turk Ger Gynecol Assoc. 2016;17(3):168-72.
30. Powers MS, Schenkel L, Darley PE, Good WR, Balestra JC, Place VA. Pharmacokinetics and pharmacodynamics of transdermal dosage forms of 17 beta-estradiol: comparison with conventional oral estrogens used for hormone replacement. Am J Obstet Gynecol. 1985;152(8):1099-106.
31. He F, Wang F, Yang Y, Yuan Z, Sun C, Zou H, et al. The effect of growth hormone on the metabolome of follicular fluid in patients with diminished ovarian reserve. Reprod Biol Endocrinol. 2023;21(1):21.
32. Stumpf PG. Selecting constant serum estradiol levels achieved by vaginal rings. Obstetrics and gynecology. 1986;67(1): 91-4.
33. Wiser A, Gonen O, Ghetler Y, Shavit T, Berkovitz A, Shulman A. Addition of

dehydroepiandrosterone (DHEA) for poor-responder patients before and during IVF treatment improves the pregnancy rate: a randomized prospective study. Hum Reprod. 2010;25(10):2496-500.
34. Sher G, Fisch JD. Effect of vaginal sildenafil on the outcome of in vitro fertilization (IVF) after multiple IVF failures attributed to poor endometrial development. Fertil Steril. 2002;78(5):1073-6.
35. Qublan H, Amarin Z, Dabbas M, Farraj AE, Beni-Merei Z, Al-Akash H, et al. Low-molecular-weight heparin in the treatment of recurrent IVF–ET failure and thrombophilia: a prospective randomized placebo-controlled trial. Human fertility. 2008;11(4):246-53.
36. Liu S, Shi L, Wang T, Shi J. Effect of low-dose dexamethasone on patients with elevated early follicular phase progesterone level and pregnancy outcomes in IVF-ET treatment: a randomized controlled clinical trial. Clin Endocrinol (Oxf). 2018;89(6):771-8.
37. Christianson MS, Wu H, Zhao Y, Yemini M, Leong M, Shoham Z. Metformin use in patients undergoing in vitro fertilization treatment: results of a worldwide web-based survey. J Assist Reprod Genet. 2015;32(3): 401-6.
38. Kılıç N, Özdemir Ö, Başar HC, Demircan F, Ekmez F, Yücel O. Cabergoline for preventing ovarian hyperstimulation syndrome in women at risk undergoing in vitro fertilization/intracytoplasmic sperm injection treatment cycles: a randomized controlled study. Avicenna J Med. 2015; 5(4):123-7.

Section 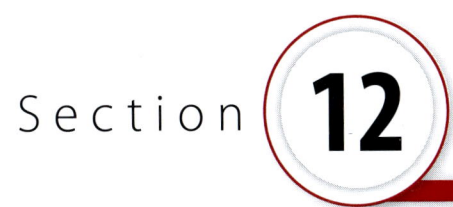 12

Drugs for Postmenopausal Women

▲ **Hormone Replacement Therapy**
Taru Gupta, Anupma

▲ **Alternatives to Hormone Replacement Therapy**
Jyoti Jaiswal, Nisha Watti

▲ **Drugs to Decrease Fracture Risk**
Shobhana Mohan Das

Chapter 34

Hormone Replacement Therapy

Taru Gupta, Anupma

Menopause is a transition phase from reproductive to nonreproductive phase in a women's life. It begins on an average 4 years before the final menopause, commonly called perimenopausal period. Average age of menopause in an Indian woman is 46 years,[1] and with increasing life expectancy, she is expected to spend significant duration of her life in postmenopausal period.

Hormone replacement therapy (HRT) also known as menopausal hormone therapy (MHT) is used to treat symptoms associated with estrogen deficiency like hot flashes, vaginal dryness, urogenital symptoms, sexual dysfunction like dyspareunia and decreased libido and bone loss leading to osteopenia and eventually osteoporosis. MHT replenishes the diminished circulating estrogen and progesterone hormones in case of natural, surgically induced, or premature menopause and thus improve the quality of life.[2-4]

Menopausal hormone therapy should be considered in every *symptomatic woman within 10 years of menopause and not >60 years of age*. Estrogen is the main hormone used in MHT, progesterone added in patients with intact uterus to reduce the risk of unopposed estrogen which may lead to endometrial hyperplasia and cancer. Androgenic preparations like testosterone analogs are used in women with sexual dysfunction. Nonhormonal therapy is considered in women having contraindications for hormones. The Women's Health Initiative (WHI) assessed the long-term effects of hormone therapy (HT) in postmenopausal women but ended in 2002 due to findings of increased risk of coronary heart disease, breast cancer, stroke, and thromboembolic complications in women receiving estrogen plus progestin, compared to placebo. New WHI subanalyses stratifying results by age, and an extended follow-up of the WHI reveals that starting MHT in postmenopausal women <10 years from last menstrual period have less risk.[5,6] In addition, hysterectomized women treated with estrogen alone shows more benefit than risk for symptom control, prevention of bone mineral loss, fractures, and improvement of the metabolic profile in women who began HRT before 60 years of age or <10 years menopausal.[7]

Counseling and therapeutic lifestyle modification is the first and foremost step in the management of menopausal symptomatic women. Treating physician should address patient questions and concerns and provide education about role of balanced diet, exercise, and social interaction. All available treatment options with their risk and benefits and need of regular follow-up should be informed. Shared decision-making with individualized MHT therapy in terms of dosage, combinations, routes, and duration should be offered after ruling out the contraindications. Investigations required are complete blood count, liver function and renal function tests, blood sugar, serum calcium, vitamin D, thyroid-stimulating hormone (TSH), lipid profile, mammography, PAPs smear, TVS—uterus and adnexa, and X-ray of thoracolumbar spine. Evaluate cardiovascular and breast cancer risk with available software risk prediction models **(Flowchart 1)**.

■ ESTROGENS

All types of estrogens are effective in relieving menopausal symptoms and can be administered via a variety of routes, such as oral, transdermal, topical, vaginal, rectal, subcutaneous implants. Natural estrogens have low bioavailability compared to synthetic estrogens. Parenteral routes have higher bioavailability compared to oral estrogens. Estrogens are typically bound to

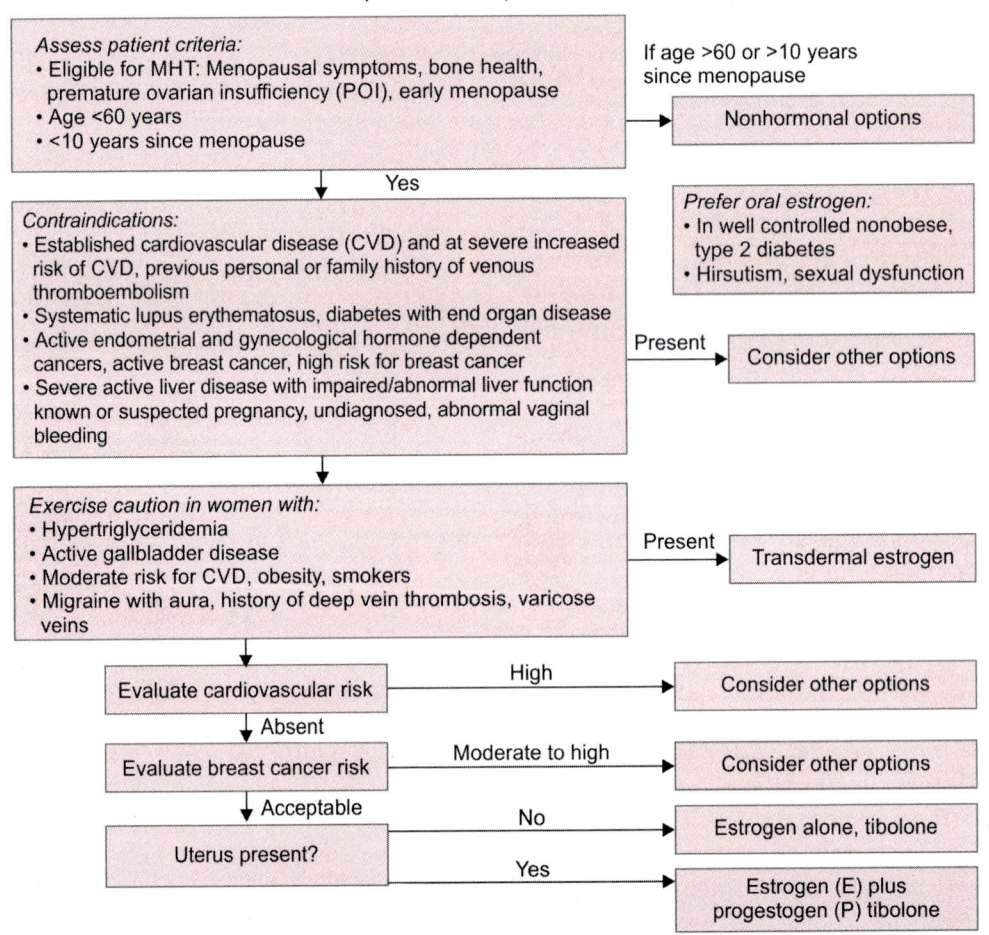

Flowchart 1: Prescription of menopausal hormone therapy (MHT).

CHAPTER 34: Hormone Replacement Therapy

TABLE 1: Oral estrogen preparations.

Estrogen	Dose
Estradiol valerate	1, 2 mg
Conjugated equine estrogen	0.3, 0.45, 0.625, 0.9, and 1.25 mg
Conjugated synthetic estrogen	0.3, 0.45, 0.625, and 0.9 mg
Esterified estrogens	0.3, 0.625, 1.25, and 2.5 mg
17β-estradiol	0.5, 1, 2, and 4 mg

TABLE 2: Estradiol patches.

Preparation	Dose
Estradiol transdermal patch	0.025, 0.05, 0.1, and 0.15 mg/day
Estradiol patch (twice weekly)	0.025, 0.0375, 0.05, 0.075, and 0.1 mg/day
Estradiol (weekly)	0.075 and 0.1 mg/day
Estradiol hemihydrate patch (weekly)	0.025, 0.0375, 0.05, 0.06, 0.075, and 0.1 mg/day

TABLE 3: Topical estrogens.

Preparation	Dose
Estradiol pump (0.06%)	0.75 mg estradiol/pump
Estradiol pump (0.06%)	0.5 mg estradiol/pump
Estradiol gel (0.1%)	0.25, 0.5, and 1 mg estradiol/pouch
Estradiol spray (1.7%)	1.53 mg estradiol/spray

albumin and sex hormone-binding globulin in the circulation. They are metabolized in liver by hydroxylation (via CYP450 enzymes), dehydrogenation (via 17β-hydroxysteroid dehydrogenase), and conjugation (via sulfation and glucuronidation). Synthetic steroid estrogen includes ethinyl estradiol, estradiol valerate, conjugated esterified estrogen, and quinestrol.

- *Local preparations:* Creams, vaginal tablets, and estrogen rings.
- *Systemic preparations:* Oral pills, transdermal patches, gels, and implants.
    - *Oral preparations:* Pills are the most common oral treatment for menopausal symptoms **(Table 1)**.
        * *Conjugated equine estrogen (CEE):* Natural preparations containing conjugated estrogenic salts which get converted to active estrone in systemic circulation, e.g., Premarin
        * *Ethinyl estradiol:* Synthetic derivative of estradiol
        * *Estradiol valerate:* Esterified valeric acid estradiol, e.g., Estrabet
    - *Estrogen patches:* Hemihydrate estradiol preparations worn on the skin of abdomen and depending on the dose can be replaced in few days or a week, e.g., Alora, Climara, and Estraderm. Menostar, a lower dose estrogen patch, used only for reducing the risk of osteoporosis but does not help with other menopausal symptoms **(Table 2)**.
    - *Topical preparations:* These may contain estradiol, estriol, and CEE preparations in the form of creams and gels. These are applied usually on arms or legs in once daily dosing, e.g., Divigel, Estrogel (gels), Estrasorb (cream), and Evamist (spray) **(Table 3)**.
- *Vaginal preparations:* Low dose preparations in the form of vaginal creams, rings, and pessaries. They are used to treat urogenital atrophy leading to vaginal dryness, itching, or dyspareunia. Systemic absorption is less and hence *progesterone supplementation is not required with vaginal preparation even in patient with intact uterus*, e.g., Evalon, Premarin (cream), Estring and Femring (vaginal rings), and Vagifem (vaginal pessary) **(Table 4)**.

TABLE 4: Vaginal estrogens.

Formulation	Estrogen	Dose
Rings	Estradiol	7.5 µg/day for months
Creams	Conjugated estrogen Estriol Estradiol	0.0625% 0.1% 0.01
Pessaries	Estradiol	0.5 mg
Tablets	Estradiol	25 µg

Indications of Menopausal Hormonal Therapy

- Treatment of moderate-to-severe vasomotor symptoms (VMS)
- Prevention of osteoporosis in postmenopausal women
- Treatment of hypoestrogenism caused by hypogonadism, bilateral oophorectomy (BO), or premature ovarian insufficiency (POI)
- Treatment of moderate-to-severe genitourinary syndrome of menopause (GMS).

Contraindications

Undiagnosed vaginal bleeding, active liver disease, thromboembolic disease, cardiovascular disease, cholangitis, cholecystitis or any biliary disease, breast cancer (increased risk of recurrence—HABITS trial, increased risk of contralateral breast cancer—Stockholm trial), and estrogen-dependent cancer like endometrial or ovarian cancer (very small risk when used long term and returns to normal when discontinued—Million Women Study-2007).

Relative contraindications are migraine headaches, uterine fibroids, and atypical ductal hyperplasia of breast.

Adverse Reactions

- Mild side effects include nausea, abdominal bloating, breast tenderness, light headedness, mood swings, depression, and unscheduled vaginal bleeding.
- Unopposed estrogen can lead to endometrial hyperplasia and endometrial cancer.
- Systemic estrogen increases the risk of venous thromboembolic events.
- Long-term use of (>5 years) combined CEE and progestins increases the incidence of breast carcinoma and stroke.

Drug Interactions

- Estrogen interferes with the action of antitubercular drugs like rifampicin and rifabutin and antiretroviral drugs like nevirapine, efavirenz, ritonavir, and nelfinavir.
- *Anticoagulants:* Estrogen decreases the anticoagulant effect of warfarin by increasing its metabolism.
- *Antiepileptic drugs:* Estrogen increases the metabolism and decreases efficacy of lamotrigine, barbiturates, phenytoin, and carbamazepine.
- *Antiaromatase agents:* Estrogen lowers efficacy of aromatase inhibitors used in breast cancer.
- *Tranexamic acid:* Estradiol may increase the risk of thrombosis.

■ PROGESTERONE

Progesterone is a naturally occurring pregnane steroid. Progestins or synthetic progestogens are derived from progesterone and can be categorized into 17α-hydroxyprogesterone, 17α-methylprogesterone, and 19-norprogesterone. 19-nortestosterone is another major group of progestin. Pregnanolone is a synthetic inhibitory neurosteroid. The pharmacokinetics of progesterone depends on its route of administration. Micronized progesterone and medroxyprogesterone are for oral administration while oil based is for intramuscular use.

Routes of administration—oral (micronized and medroxyprogesterone), transdermal or topical, vaginal, rectal, and intramuscular. Vaginal preparations are in the form of capsules, tablets, gels, pessaries, and ring.

Indications

As combined HRT with estrogen to prevent abnormal endometrial proliferation and endometrial cancer. It can be given as both sequential cyclical regimen or continuous combined regimen **(Tables 5 and 6)**. Also provides symptomatic relief from sleep disturbance and mood instability.

Contraindications

Undiagnosed vaginal bleeding, thromboembolic disease, impaired liver function or disease, breast cancer, any estrogen or progesterone-dependent cancer, cardiac disease, severe migraine headaches, renal dysfunction, and hypersensitivity to progesterone preparations.

Adverse Reactions

Nausea, breast tenderness, abdominal bloating, vaginal bleeding, depression, irritability, and dementia.

Drug Interactions

- *Selective serotonin reuptake inhibitors (SSRIs):* Fluoxetine, paroxetine, and sertraline may accelerate the receptor-mediated central depression when given with progesterone.
- *Benzodiazepines and alcohol*: Progesterone potentiates their sedative effect.
- *Antifungal and antitubercular drugs*: Progesterone induces CYP3A4 cytochrome P450 enzymes and hence accelerates the metabolism and decreases efficacy of these drugs.

TABLE 5: Sequential cyclical regimen (progesterone last 10–14 days).

Estrogen	Progesterone	Formulation
Estradiol 1–2 mg	Norethisterone 1 mg	Oral tablets
Estradiol 1–2 mg	Levonorgestrel 0.25/0.5 mg	Oral tablets
Conjugated estrogen 0.625 mg	Medroxyprogesterone acetate 10 mg	Oral tablets
Conjugated estrogen	Norgestrel 150 µg	Oral tablets

TABLE 6: Continuous combined (E + P regimen).

Estrogen	Progesterone	Formulation
Estradiol 2 mg	Norethisterone 1 mg	Oral tablets
Estradiol 2 mg	Norethisterone 0.5 mg	Oral tablets
Estradiol 1 mg	Dydrogesterone 5 mg	Oral tablets
Estradiol 1/2 mg	Medroxyprogesterone 2.5/5 mg	Oral tablets
Conjugated estrogen 0.625 mg	Medroxyprogesterone acetate 2.5/5 mg	Tablets

TIBOLONE

Tibolone is a STEAR (selective tissue estrogenic activity regulator) group of synthetic steroid compound with moderate antiestrogenic, weak estrogenic, and strong androgenic activity. Tibolone shows tissue selectivity with estrogen agonist activity on vagina, bone, and brain and has no impact on endometrial and breast tissue. It increases lumbar spine and total hip bone mineral density (BMD) to a significantly greater extent than raloxifene.[7,8]

Indications

Tibolone reduces hot flashes, prevents bone loss, improves genitourinary symptoms, and has positive effects on mood and sexual function.[9,10] The medication may have greater benefits on libido than standard MHT, which may be related to its androgenic effects. It is associated with low rates of vaginal bleeding and breast pain as compared to conventional estrogen and progesterone therapy.

Adverse Drug Reactions

Adverse drug reactions are headache, nausea, breast tenderness, unscheduled vaginal bleeding, pruritus, weight gain, limb edema, flaring of migraine headache, and androgenic side effects like acne and increased facial hair growth.

Drug Interactions

- *Anticoagulants:* Tibolone increases antifibrinolytic activity in blood and may augment the anticoagulant effect of warfarin.
- CYP3A4 enzyme inducers like rifampicin, phenobarbitone, phenytoin, and carbamazepine may reduce the efficacy of tibolone.
- Oral hypoglycemics and insulin dose should be increased when women are on tibolone.

Contraindications

Tibolone carries a similar risk profile as compared to conventional HRT and is not indicated in cases with undiagnosed vaginal bleeding, history of thromboembolism or transient ischemic attack (TIA), acute liver diseases, treated patients of breast carcinoma, and porphyria. It should be avoided in breast cancer survivors and is not recommended within 1 year of menopause because of risk of irregular vaginal bleeding.

Tissue-selective estrogen complex (TSEC): Bazedoxifene 20 mg [selective estrogen receptor modulator (SERM)—estrogen agonist/antagonist] combined with conjugated estrogen 0.45 mg to form TSEC, available as Duavee -1- fixed-dose combination.

Vaginal dehydroepiandrosterone (DHEA): Steroid hormone intermediate in the biosynthesis of androgens and estrogens. Low-dose DHEA vaginal insert daily is approved for the treatment of moderate-to-severe dyspareunia in menopausal women, available as 6.5 mg daily dose for 12 weeks.

Ospemifene: SERM estrogen agonist/antagonist, only oral product approved for treatment of vaginal dryness and moderate-to-severe dyspareunia, available as tablet 60 mg/day for 12 weeks to 6 months.

NONHORMONAL MENOPAUSAL THERAPY

Antidepressants like SSRI and serotonin and norepinephrine reuptake inhibitor (SNRI) have been noted in some small short-term studies to reduce VMS. Relief with these

medicines is rapid and 4 weeks' time is sufficient to establish their efficacy or an alternate therapy is to be considered.
- *Selective serotonin reuptake inhibitors contain paroxetine, fluoxetine, fluvoxamine, sertraline, citalopram, and escitalopram.*
- *Serotonin noradrenaline reuptake inhibitors:* Serotonin and noradrenaline are known to effect mood and may also impact thermoregulation, the mechanism responsible for VMS.

The optimal results have been reported with venlafaxine and desvenlafaxine.

Adverse Drug Reactions

The side effects are less as compared to the antidepressant doses. Very low doses at the start of the therapy may minimize the side effects and the dose can be increased after a week. Common side effects are dry mouth, drowsiness, nausea, diarrhea, headache, insomnia, jitteriness, and fatigue. Sudden withdrawal can lead to anxiety and headache hence discontinuation should be tapered.

■ CLONIDINE

Clonidine is a centrally acting α-adrenergic receptor agonist with preferential action on the neuronal cells. Primarily used as an antihypertensive and treatment of migraine headaches. It may be used to control VMS by decreasing vascular reactivity. It is used generally for 8 weeks and reduces hot flashes by up to 40%.

Indications

It is used to control VMS in the breast cancer survivor who are on tamoxifen.

Preparations: Oral tablets in the dose of 25 μg BD and can be increased up to 75 μg BD.

Clonidine patches are also available.

Adverse Drug Reactions

Adverse drug reactions are dry mouth, drowsiness, dizziness, constipation, insomnia, and hypotension.

Contraindications

Clonidine should be used with caution in patients of coronary artery disease, arrhythmia, vasomotor disease, and renal disease.

Drug Interactions

It enhances effect of sedatives, increases digitalis and lithium toxicity.

■ GABAPENTIN

An analog of γ-aminobutyric acid and an anticonvulsant and is approved for the treatment of neurologic disorders as seizures and neuropathic pain. Its oral absorption is unpredictable. It has a better safety profile than other nonhormonal drugs and less interactions. It is excreted mainly in urine.

Dosage

Oral tablets in the dose of 100 mg three times a day and can be increased to 300 mg three times a day. Onset of action takes only few days.

Pregabalin: 50–150 mg/day.

Contraindications

Renal impairment as excreted mainly by kidneys.

Adverse Drug Reactions

Adverse drug reactions are headache, nausea, excessive sleep, drowsiness, leg swelling, weight gain, and depression.

THERAPY FOR OSTEOPOROSIS PREVENTION AND TREATMENT

Osteoporosis is a condition characterized by weakened bones that fracture easily. After menopause many women are at risk of developing osteoporosis. Estrogen plays an important role in maintaining bone strength. After menopause estrogen levels drop and this may result in increased bone loss. The average woman loses up to 10% of her bone mass in the first 5 years of menopause. A number of medical treatments are available for the management of osteoporosis. Treatments aim is to strengthen existing bone, help prevent further bone loss, and most importantly reduce the risk of fracture. Treatment of osteoporosis is recommended in all women with Z-score <−2.5 or women with prior history of hip or vertebral fracture.

Selective Estrogen Receptor Modulator

Estrogen receptors are located on many body tissues including bone. SERMs act by blocking the estrogen effect at some receptor sites, while prompting an estrogen effect at others. In bone, these medications work like estrogen and lead to an increase in bone mass (density) and reduce vertebral fractures in women with low bone density.

Preparations: Raloxifene 60 mg/day.

Adverse Drug Reactions

Adverse drug reactions are hot flushes and a slight increased risk of deep vein thrombosis (DVT), do not increase the risk of breast cancer.

Bisphosphonates

Bisphosphonates are medications that reduce the resorption of bone. They reduce vertebral, hip, and other fractures. Bisphosphonates can be taken as daily, weekly, or monthly doses.

Preparations (Table 7)

Most commonly used bisphosphonates are alendronate (Fosamax), risedronate (Actonel), and a yearly intravenous form of bisphosphonate called zoledronate (Aclasta).
- Most oral bisphosphonates are to be taken empty stomach in morning with at least 250 mL of water
- Avoid food, drinks, medications, and be in upright posture for at least 90 minutes (alendronate and risedronate) and 60 minutes (ibandronate) after intake.
- Enteric-coated delayed release formulation is taken immediately after breakfast with water.

TABLE 7: Bisphosphonates for osteoporosis.

Bisphosphonate	Formulation	Dosing	Discontinuation of therapy (in selected patients)
Alendronate	Oral	10 mg/day 70 mg/week	5 years
Risedronate	Oral (immediate release) Enteric-coated	5 mg/day 35 mg/week 150 mg/month	5 years
Zoledronic acid	Intravenous	5 mg/12 months	
Ibandronate	Oral Intravenous	150 mg/month 3 mg/3 months	3 years Limited data

Adverse Drug Reactions

Adverse drug reactions are gastrointestinal upset, gastroesophageal reflux, and osteonecrosis of the jaw (rare).

Denosumab[10]

Denosumab is a human monoclonal antibody, given as 6 monthly injections. It works in a different way to bisphosphonates but has the same effect of slowing the rate of resorption. It reduces the risk of vertebral, hip, and other fractures. It can increase the risk of skin infections.

Teriparatide (Parathormone Analog)[11-14]

Teriparatide (parathyroid hormone) is administered daily via an injection just below the skin. It increases bone formation and absorption of calcium from the gut and kidney. Calcium and vitamin D supplements may be necessary with this medication and must be monitored under the care of endocrinologist. It reduces fractures in postmenopausal women.

Treatment is limited to one 18-month course per lifetime. It is an expensive drug and is used when bisphosphonates are contraindicated.

Preparations: Injectable 20 μg/day subcutaneous.

Strontium Ranelate

A strontium (II) salt of ranelic acid is a medication for osteoporosis. Studies indicate it can also slow the course of osteoarthritis of the knee. The drug is unusual in that drug has dual action—it increases deposition of new bone by osteoblasts and reduces the resorption of bone by osteoclasts. It is therefore promoted as a "dual action bone agent (DABA)". Strontium ranelate shows antifracture efficacy in very old elderly and osteopenic patients.[15]

Preparation: Oral granules (sachet) 2 g/day.

Contraindications

Contraindications are hypersensitivity, severe renal disease, patients at increased risk of venous thromboembolism (VTE), history of VTE, and phenylketonuria.

Side Effects

The most common side effects include nausea, diarrhea, headache, and eczema. Occasional severe allergic reaction including drug rash with eosinophilia and systemic symptoms (DRESS syndrome).

Calcitonin

Calcitonin is a hormone that lowers calcium level and inhibits bone resorption by inhibiting osteoclastic activity. Salmon calcitonin is more effective than human calcitonin and is Food and Drug Administration (FDA) approved for the treatment of osteoporosis in women who are >5 years menopausal.

Indications

Treatment of osteoporosis in women having contraindication for other drugs and is menopausal >5 years. Reduces the risk of vertebral fractures by one-third.

Preparations

Nasal spray: Dose of 100, 200, and 400 IU/day in alternate nostrils.

Injectables: 50 IU/mL intravenous (mainly for hypercalcemia).

Adverse Drug Reactions

Adverse drug reactions are nasal congestion, nasal irritation, resistance after 12–18 months of use due to receptor downregulation.

Calcium

The recommended dose of dietary calcium in a postmenopausal woman is 1,200–1,800 mg/day. Apart from dietary calcium, addition of supplements becomes necessary. Calcium carbonate is 40% elemental calcium and it should be supplemented with vitamin D for absorption.

Preparations: Calcium carbonate and calcium citrate (21% elemental calcium)—oral tablets 500 mg dose.

Adverse Drug Reactions

Adverse drug reactions are abdominal bloating, constipation.

Vitamin D

It is needed for the absorption of calcium in alimentary canal. It reduces the risk of fractures in elderly patients. It needs to be repeated timely for maintenance of adequate levels.

Preparation

- Cholecalciferol (vitamin D_3) 60,000 IU/week for 8 weeks preferably with milk
- Maintenance dose of 60,000 IU once a month in summers and twice a month in winters.

■ EMERGING THERAPY

Neurokinin-B Antagonist

- Fezolinetant 90 mg twice daily for 12 weeks—significant reduction in severity and frequency of hot flashes (phase IIa and IIb trials)
- MLE4901 (40 mg BD)—72% reduction in symptoms
- NT-814—novel selective antagonist of NK1 + NK3 receptors

Complementary Therapies

- Cognitive behavioral therapy (Menos 1 and Menos 2 RCT)
- Stellate ganglion block
- Acupuncture, purified pollen extract
- Pelvic muscle floor training and bladder training
- Paced respiration and relaxation techniques (little benefit), yoga
- Black cohosh and red clover

All the above therapies help in mild reduction in severity of symptoms.

■ KEY POINTS

- The clinical manifestations of menopause are due to chronic hypoestrogenic state which in short term can cause vasomotor and genitourinary symptoms, and over a long term can cause detrimental effect on bone and cardiovascular health. Appropriate counseling, lifestyle modification, and MHT form the mainstay of treatment.
- Hormone therapy remains the most effective treatment for vasomotor and genitourinary syndrome of menopause, prevents bone loss and fracture, and should be started in lowest possible dose.
- The available evidence suggests that the benefits of HRT outweigh the risk in an otherwise healthy women during perimenopause or early postmenopausal period with moderate-to-severe symptom however if simultaneous contraception is needed in perimenopausal women, and low-dose combined oral contraceptives (COCs) are recommended.[4]
- In young patients with POI or surgically induced menopause, early initiation of hormonal therapy is strongly recommended up till the average age of natural menopause to prevent cardiovascular risk and bone loss protection (ESHRE 2016).[16] Counsel women that HT is not a contraceptive, and erratic ovulation and pregnancy may occur and COCs may be used.[17,18]

- In women with endometrial ablation, subtotal hysterectomy and hysterectomy done for severe endometriosis, combined MHT regimen (17-β estradiol and micronized progesterone) is preferred.
- For genitourinary syndrome of menopause nonhormonal methods like vaginal lubricants and moisturizers should be tried first, local low dose vaginal estrogen or vaginal DHEA if nonhormonal treatment is ineffective.[19,20]
- Ospemifene (SERM) is an FDA approved drug and only oral treatment for the treatment of genitourinary syndrome of menopause given in dose of 60 mg/day in women with contraindications to vaginal estrogen therapy. It is more effective than lubricants in reducing dyspareunia by acting on vaginal epithelium and treating moderate-to-severe vaginal atrophy (NAMS 2022).[17,18]
- Menopausal hormone therapy in combination with exercise can slow the progression of sarcopenia but there is no sufficient evidence that hormonal therapy can be primarily used for sarcopenia prevention.
- The decision to take HRT, the dose and its duration should be individualized after discussing the benefits and risks, and using best available evidence with periodic evaluation.[21]

REFERENCES

1. Meeta M, Digumarti L, Agarwal N, Vaze N, Shah R, Malik S. Clinical Practice Guidelines on Menopause: *An Executive Summary and Recommendations: Indian Menopause Society 2019-2020. J Midlife Health. 2020; 11(2):55-95.
2. World Health Organization. Measurement of Quality of Life in Children. Geneva: Division of Mental Health. World Health Organization; 1993.
3. Kim OM, Lee YS. The climacteric symptoms and quality of life in climacteric women according to hormone replacement therapy. Korean J Women Health Nurs. 2001;7:642-56.
4. Cho HH, Jung JE, Jung IC, Kim MJ, Kim SY, Hwang SJ. Influences of hormone therapy to tissue mineral concentration and quality of life in menopausal women. J Korean Soc Menopause. 2007;13:209-16.
5. Gurney EP, Nachtigall MJ, Nachtigall LE, Naftolin F. The Women's Health Initiative trial and related studies: 10 years later: a clinician's view. J Steroid Biochem Mol Biol. 2014;142:4-11.
6. Lemay A. The relevance of the Women's Health Initiative results on combined hormone replacement therapy in clinical practice. J Obstet Gynaecol Can. 2002;24(9):711-5.
7. Delmas PD, Davis SR, Hensen J, Adami S, van Os S, Nijland EA. Effects of tibolone and raloxifene on bone mineral density in osteopenic postmenopausal women. Osteoporos Int. 2008;19:1153-60.
8. Nijland EA, Weijmar Schultz WC, Nathorst-Boös J, Helmond FA, Van Lunsen RH, Palacios S, et al. LISA study investigators. Tibolone and transdermal E2/NETA for the treatment of female sexual dysfunction in naturally menopausal women: results of a randomized active-controlled trial. J Sex Med. 2008;5:646-56.
9. Cummings SR, Ettinger B, Delmas PD, Kenemans P, Stathopoulos V, Verweij P, et al. LIFT Trial Investigators. The effects of tibolone in older postmenopausal women. N Engl J Med. 2008;359:697-708.
10. Lewiecki EM. New and emerging concepts in the use of denosumab for the treatment of osteoporosis. Therapeutic Adv Musculoskeletal Dis. 2018;10:209-23.
11. Bauer W, Aub JC, Albright F. Studies of calcium and phosphorus metabolism: V. A study of the bone trabeculae as a readily available reserve supply of calcium. J Exp Med. 1929;49(1):145-62.
12. Selye H. On the stimulation of new bone formation with parathyroid extract and irradiated ergosterol. Endocrinology. 1932;16(5):547-58.
13. Dempster DW, Cosman F, Parisien M, Shen V, Lindsay R. Anabolic actions of parathyroid hormone on bone. Endocr Rev. 1993;14(6):690-709.
14. DailyMed. (2021). Forteo-teriparatide injection, solution. [online] Available from:

https://dailymed.nlm.nih.gov/dailymed/lookup.cfm?setid=aae667c5-381f-4f92-93df-2ed6158d07b0#:~:text=risk%20factors%20...-,FORTEO%20is%20indicated%3A,to%20other%20available%20osteoporosis%20therapy [Last accessed December, 2023].
15. Przedlacki J. Strontium ranelate in postmenopausal osteoporosis. Endokrynol Pol. 2011;62(1):65-72.
16. European Society for Human Reproduction and Embryology (ESHRE) Guideline Group on POI; Webber L, Davies M, Anderson R, Bartlett J, Braat D, et al. ESHRE Guideline: management of women with premature ovarian insufficiency. Hum Reprod. 2016; 31(5):926-37.
17. Webber L, Anderson RA, Davies M, Janse F, Vermeulen N. HRT for women with premature ovarian insufficiency: a comprehensive review. Hum Reprod Open. 2017;2017(2):hox007.
18. Gazarra LBC, Bonacordi CL, Yela DA, Benetti-Pinto CL. Bone mass in women with premature ovarian insufficiency: A comparative study between hormone therapy and combined oral contraceptives. Menopause. 2020;27(10):1110-6.
19. The North American Menopause Society. Clinical Care Recommendations. Chapter 1-8. Cleveland (OH): The North American Menopause Society; 2020.
20. "The 2022 Hormone Therapy Position Statement of The North American Menopause Society" Advisory Panel. The 2022 hormone therapy position statement of The North American Menopause Society. Menopause. 2022;29(7):767-94.
21. Notelovitz M. (2020). Individualizing hormone therapy: principles and practice. [online] Available from: https://www.medscape.org/viewarticle/412853 [Last accessed December, 2023].

Chapter 35

Alternatives to Hormone Replacement Therapy

Jyoti Jaiswal, Nisha Watti

Menopause, the permanent cessation of menstruation or end of natural reproductive life caused by cessation of ovarian function, occurs between the age of 40 and 55 years of age with an average age of 52 years. As per the Indian Menopause Society (IMS), the average age of menopause in Indian women is 46 years. Menopause brings many health-related challenges in women's life. Menopause not only affects the health of women but also affects the quality of life. The major health problems which are associated with menopause are vasomotor symptoms, genitourinary symptoms, bone health impairment, sexual dysfunction, cardiovascular (CV) disease, behavioral problem, and cognitive decline.[1] Almost 75% of menopausal women suffer from vasomotor symptoms like hot flashes resulting from vasomotor instability. Prior to 2000, hormone therapy was widely used to treat menopausal symptoms such as hot flashes and vulvovaginal atrophy.[2] Along with the beneficial effect of hormone replacement therapy (HRT), HRTs have their own potential side effects. The HRT remains the most commonly prescribed treatment to alleviate menopausal symptoms if there are not any contraindications **(Box 1)**.[3] However, the use of HRT has decreased after reports of increased risk of CV disease, breast cancer, stroke, and pulmonary embolism.[4]

Although the HRT is being used to treat menopausal symptoms, but in conditions where HRT is contraindicated, other alternative therapies play a vital role to alleviate symptoms. Certain menopausal symptoms are not only relieved by HRT but they need other alternative therapy also, like behavioral therapy in depressive illness. Some late-onset menopausal symptoms (bone health related) required specific

> **BOX 1:** Typical contraindications for hormone replacement therapy.
>
> *Contraindications for hormone replacement therapy:*
> - Known, past, or suspected case of breast cancer
> - Known or suspected case of estrogen-dependent cancer like uterine cancer
> - Active or previous venous thromboembolism (deep vein thrombosis or pulmonary embolism)
> - Active or recent arterial thromboembolic disease (for example, angina or myocardial infarction)
> - Active liver disease with abnormal liver function tests
> - Thrombophilic disorder
> - Undiagnosed vaginal bleeding
> - Untreated endometrial hyperplasia
> - Pregnancy

treatment rather than HRT alone. Alternative therapies include nonhormonal medication like selective serotonin reuptake inhibitors (SSRIs), serotonin-norepinephrine reuptake inhibitors (SNRIs), seizure medication called gabapentin and a blood pressure medication called clonidine, vaginal moisturizers and lubricants, some plant and herbal supplements including some soy products, and lifestyle measures.[5] Majority of women not seeking any treatment for their menopausal symptoms as they accepted it as natural physiological changes and also lack of awareness, in these situation alternative therapies are good choice for their symptoms and better quality of life. In a recent survey, 95% of women said they would try alternative therapies before HRT because they think they are more natural and they are worried about the health risks of HRT. National Institute for Health and Care Excellence (NICE) guidelines have used carefully weighed evidence-based evaluations of the effectiveness of alternative treatments compared with placebo (no treatment) and also with conventional forms of HRT.[6] Alternative therapies are better option where HRT is contraindicated as well as for better quality of life, but it requires further more data for efficacy and long-term safety.

ALTERNATIVE TO HORMONE REPLACEMENT THERAPY FOR VASOMOTOR SYMPTOMS

Selective serotonin reuptake inhibitors and serotonin norepinephrine reuptake inhibitors are the two antidepressants which may help with hot flushes caused by the menopause.[7] Paroxetine is the only SSRI which is Food and Drug Administration (FDA) approved for postmenopausal symptoms. Other alternatives which are being used gabapentin and clonidine for hot flushes.

Neurokinin 3 receptor antagonists are the new emerging medicines for vasomotor symptoms. Some natural products like soy isoflavones, black cohosh, red clover, and some vitamins are also prescribed during menopause.

Selective Serotonin Reuptake Inhibitors

This class of drugs is now one of the most commonly used in clinical practice for the alleviation of menopause symptoms as an alternative to HRT.[8] SSRIs include paroxetine, citalopram, escitalopram, fluoxetine, and sertraline. Paroxetine is the only antidepressant which is FDA approved for postmenopausal symptoms.

Pharmacology

Selective serotonin reuptake inhibitors mainly inhibit the reuptake of serotonin in presynaptic neurons and make it available for postsynaptic receptors. SSRIs also affect the thermoregulation. SSRIs have little effect on other neurotransmitters, such as dopamine or norepinephrine.[9]

Half-life of the SSRIs depends on the individual drugs. Paroxetine has a half-life around 21 hours, fluoxetine has 1–4 days, and citalopram has 26 hours. The SSRIs are metabolized by the cytochrome P450 system in the liver.[10] Drug elimination occurs both in urine and feces.

Indication

Selective serotonin reuptake inhibitors are mainly used as antidepressant and also used in mood disorders. Paroxetine is the only FDA approved drug used in the management of hot flushes. Paroxetine is used in those women in whom estrogens are contraindicated or not safe and also in those postmenopausal women with mood disorder.

Contraindication

Selective serotonin reuptake inhibitors are not suitable for bleeding disorder, such as hemophilia, type 1 diabetes or type 2 diabetes, narrow angle glaucoma, and epilepsy.[11] Care should be taken when prescribing these drugs to patient with liver and kidney disease.

Dosage

- Dose for treatment paroxetine salt 7.5 mg/day improved hot flushes frequency, hot flushes severity and sleep duration, limited effects on weight, and sexual function.[12-14]
- Paroxetine 10–25 mg/day improved hot flushes frequency and hot flushes severity.[15,16]

Adverse Drug Reactions

Common side effects include nausea, vomiting, insomnia, drowsiness, headache, decreased sex drive, and agitation.[9,17] Less common adverse effects of SSRIs are extrapyramidal symptoms (EPS), serotonin syndrome, QT prolongation, rash, birth defects, hyponatremia, and cataracts.[10]

Drug Interactions

The SSRIs inhibit certain cytochrome P450 enzymes to a great degree, which may cause more drug interactions. It should not be prescribed with nonsteroidal anti-inflammatory drugs (NSAIDs), antiplatelets, theophylline, clozapine and pimozide, lithium, triptans, and other antidepressants including tricyclic antidepressants (TCAs), monoamine oxidase inhibitors (MAOIs), and serotonin-norepinephrine reuptake inhibitors.[11]

Safety during Pregnancy and Lactation

Selective serotonin reuptake inhibitors are not usually recommended during pregnancy, particularly during the first trimester. Paroxetine is one of the preferred antidepressants to take when breastfeeding.[18]

Serotonin-norepinephrine Reuptake Inhibitors

Serotonin-norepinephrine reuptake inhibitors are venlafaxine and desvenlafaxine.

Pharmacology

Serotonin-norepinephrine reuptake inhibitors inhibit the reuptake of neurotransmitters serotonin and norepinephrine in presynaptic neurons. SNRIs have weak inhibitory effect on dopamine reuptake. SNRIs may impact thermoregulation. Half-life of venlafaxine is 5 hours and desvenlafaxine is 11 hours. Metabolism of venlafaxine is mainly hepatic (P450) and desvenlafaxine is partially hepatic, but not via P450.[19] It is excreted in urine.

Indications

It improved hot flashes frequency and hot flashes severity.[20]

Contraindications

Serotonin-norepinephrine reuptake inhibitors are contraindicated in heart disease, uncontrolled hypertension, and dyselectrolytemia. SNRIs use with caution in liver disease.

Dosage

- *Desvenlafaxine:* 75 mg/day or twice daily
- *Venlafaxine:* 37.5–75.0 mg/day. 37.5 mg is recommended dose.

Adverse Drug Reactions

Indigestion and stomach aches, diarrhea or constipation, loss of appetite, dizziness, insomnia, headaches, and loss of libido (reduced sex drive). Venlafaxine and desvenlafaxine may cause an increase in blood pressure.

Drug Interactions

The FDA states that avoid taking SNRIs alongside MAOIs. Do not take with ethanol, otherwise it will exacerbate the nervous system side effect.

Safety during Pregnancy and Lactation

Venlafaxine and desvenlafaxine are FDA category C drugs for pregnancy. Venlafaxine secreted in breast milk.

Gabapentinoids

Gabapentin and pregabalin are γ-aminobutyric acid analog. It is initially approved for the treatment of epilepsy and also used in the treatment of neuropathic pain, tremors, restless leg syndrome, migraine prophylaxis, and various mood disorders.[21] Gabapentin can be use in hot flashes associated with menopause. While the mechanism of action to alleviating hot flushes remains unclear, it was postulated that affinity of gabapentin to calcium channels in the hypothalamus might broaden the thermoregulatory zone, thereby decreasing the occurrence of hot flushes.[21-23]

Pharmacology

Gabapentin works by showing a high affinity for voltage-gated calcium channels and inhibits the release of excitatory neurotransmitters in the presynaptic area which participate in epileptogenesis. The elimination half-life of gabapentin is 5–7 hours, and it takes 2 days for the body to eliminate gabapentin from its system.[24] Gabapentin is not demonstrating any significant protein binding or liver metabolization. It is excreted by kidney.

Indications

Indications are hot flashes and also in women who have migraine along with menopausal symptoms.

Contraindications

It is used with caution in renal diseases.

Dosage

Gabapentin can give up to 300–900 mg/day in three divided doses.

Adverse Drug Reactions

Gabapentin has mild side effect profile. The most common side effects are fatigue, dizziness, somnolence, nystagmus, tremor, diplopia, and headache. Serious reactions are suicidality, depression, Stevens–Johnson syndrome, anaphylaxis, angioedema, erythema multiforme, rhabdomyolysis, withdrawal seizure, or withdrawal symptoms if discontinued abruptly.[25]

Drug Interactions

Gabapentin has no significant drug interaction.

Safety during Pregnancy and Lactation

Gabapentin is FDA category C drug of pregnancy. In a small amount, gabapentin passes into breast milk.

Clonidine

Clonidine is an α_2-adrenergic agonist mainly used as antihypertensive agent. Its mechanism of action in the treatment of hot flashes is likely due to the narrowing of the thermoneutral zone by lowering levels of norepinephrine.[26] In comparison with other agents, such as SSRIs/SNRIs and gabapentin, it is less effective.[15] Clonidine is the only nonhormonal drug licensed for use for hot flushes in the UK.[6] Currently, clonidine is not recommended for vasomotor symptoms.

Pharmacology

Clonidine is imidazoline derivative that acts centrally as α_2-adrenergic antagonist and reduces sympathetic outflow from the central nervous system (CNS), there by reduces arterial blood pressure. Effect of clonidine on the sympathetic nervous system, it reduces circulating epinephrine, thereby use in controlling of hot flashes in menopause.[27] Half-life of clonidine ranges from 12 to 16 hours. Metabolized in liver and excreted in urine.

Indications

It is mainly used as antihypertensive. Also use to control hot flashes in menopausal women.

Contraindications

Dose adjustment is necessary in case of renal disease and CV disease. Also, caution is necessary when treating patients with a history of depression, recent myocardial infarction (MI), and syncope.

Dosage

Dosage of clonidine is 25 µg twice daily for 2 weeks, increased to a maximum of 50 µg three times a day. It must be withdrawn gradually as suddenly stopping it can cause rebound high blood pressure.[6]

Adverse Drug Reactions

Common reactions include abdominal pain, headache, hypotension, fatigue, nausea, emotional instability, constipation, xerostomia, diarrhea, sexual dysfunction, dizziness, and sedation. Serious reactions include angioedema, depression, hypersensitivity, atrioventricular (AV) block, bradycardia, syncope, and severe hypotension.[27]

Drug Interactions

Clonidine may potentiate CNS depressive effect of barbiturates, alcohol, and other sedating drugs. Caution is warranted in patient taking β blocker, calcium channel blocker, and digitalis which affect sinus node function or AV nodal function.

Safety during Pregnancy and Lactation

Clonidine is FDA pregnancy category C drug. Clonidine is excreted in breast milk.

■ EMERGING THERAPIES

Neurokinin 3 Receptor Antagonist

Tachykinin family substance P (SP), neurokinin A (NKA), and neurokinin B (NKB) are peptides involved in neurotransmission and inflammatory processes. Tachykinin receptors are three different types, neurokinin 1 (NK1), NK2, and NK3 receptors, with preferential affinities for SP, NKA, and NKB, respectively.[28-30] Neurokinin 3 receptor antagonist is new emerging treatment option for menopausal vasomotor symptoms. NK3 antagonists rapidly reduce the number and severity of hot flushes. Fezolinetant NK3 receptor antagonist is a nonhormonal therapy currently in clinical development which acts by blocking NKB signaling and decreasing the activity of KNDy (kisspeptin–neurokinin B–dynorphin) neurons.[31] Doses are 60 mg twice daily and 90 mg twice daily. Associated adverse events included fatigue, upper respiratory tract infection, sinusitis, headache, nausea, diarrhea, and cough. Rare but serious side effects included elevated liver function values, liver injury, retinal detachment, cholelithiasis, and adjustment disorder with depressed mood.[32] Dose of 45 mg tablet once daily is prescribed.

Stellate Ganglion Block

Blocking of the stellate ganglion emerging as a new technique in the management of hot flushes, it includes local anesthetic injection into the stellate ganglion. Recently use in cases those are refractory to other treatments or contraindicated to HRT like in women with breast cancer.[33]

Lifestyle Measures

The evidence suggests that aerobic exercise can improve vasomotor symptoms, psychological health, and quality of life in menopausal women. In several randomized controlled trials of perimenopausal/menopausal-age women, it was found that aerobic exercise might result in significant improvements in several common menopause-related symptoms (e.g., mood changes, insomnia) as compared to nonexercise comparison groups. Yoga may be beneficial in reducing vasomotor symptoms and improving psychological well-being in menopausal women.[8] Lifestyle modification starting from the early life with lifelong compliance not only improves menopausal symptoms but also improves quality of life. Encourage the woman to stop smoking, alcohol consumption, caffeine intake, and adaptation of healthy lifestyle with regular exercise, walk, yoga, or meditation along with adequate dietary supplementation throughout the life.

Complementary Therapies

Complementary therapies include mind and body techniques, cognitive behavioral therapy, some natural products (soy isoflavones, black cohosh, red clover, St John's wort, agnus castus, and ginseng), vitamin E, evening primrose oil, and dehydroepiandrosterone (DHEA) as treatment for vasomotor symptoms. The use of soy isoflavones has been shown to be no more effective than placebo in several randomized controlled trials.[15] Black cohosh was also not found effective in decreasing hot flush frequency in a large Cochrane review.[34] Vitamins such as vitamin E and vitamin C, minerals such as selenium are present in various supplements. A statistically significant reduction in hot flashes frequency noted with vitamin E 800 IU/day as compared to placebo. The evidences for beneficial effect of complimentary therapies on symptomatic postmenopausal women are limited.[8]

St John's wort efficacious in mild-to-moderate depression but in vasomotor symptoms efficacy remain to be proven.

The use of nonhormonal therapies for the treatment of menopause was recently reviewed and a Position Statement issued by the North American Menopause Society (NAMS) **(Table 1)**.[35]

Along with the alternative pharmacotherapies summaries in **Table 2** complementary therapies also provide symptomatic relieve in vasomotor symptoms of menopause, although it requires further more study for validation. Lifestyle modification is essential part of life in every age group.

TABLE 1: Evidence-based recommended non-hormonal therapies for vasomotor symptoms by the NAMS.

Recommended nonhormonal therapies	Level of evidence*
Selective serotonin reuptake inhibitors	Level I
Serotonin-norepinephrine reuptake inhibitors	Level I
Gabapentin, fezolinetant	Level I
Weight loss, stellate ganglion block	Level II–III

*Levels of evidence: Level I: Good and consistent scientific evidence; Level II: Limited or inconsistent scientific evidence; and Level III: Consensus and expert opinion.

(NAMS: North American Menopause Society)

TABLE 2: Alternative drug list used for vasomotor symptoms.

Drug name	Dosage	Route	Maximum dose	Side effects	Contraindications	Pharmacokinetics
Selective serotonin reuptake inhibitors						
Paroxetine	7.5 mg/day	Oral	25 mg/day	Common side effects are nausea, vomiting, insomnia, drowsiness, headache, decreased sex drive • Less common adverse effects of SSRIs are extrapyramidal symptoms (EPS), serotonin syndrome, QT prolongation, rash, birth defects, hyponatremia, and cataracts	Hemophilia, type 1 diabetes or type 2 diabetes, narrow angle glaucoma, epilepsy *Contraindicated in women taking tamoxifen	• Half-life around 21 hours. • SSRIs are metabolized by the cytochrome P450 system in the liver
Fluoxetine	20 mg/day	Oral			*Patient taking monoamine oxidase inhibitors	• Half-life 2–4 days • Metabolized in liver
Citalopram	10 mg/day	Oral	40 mg/day		*Patient taking monoamine oxidase inhibitors *Patient with QT prolongation	Both have half-life of 27–32 hours
Escitalopram	5 mg/day	Oral	20 mg/day			
Serotonin-norepinephrine reuptake inhibitors						
Desvenlafaxine	75 mg/day	Oral	75 mg twice a day	Indigestion and stomach aches, diarrhea or constipation, loss of appetite, dizziness, insomnia, headaches, loss of libido (reduced sex drive)	SNRIs are contraindicated in heart disease, uncontrolled hypertension and dyselectrolytemia. SNRIs use with caution in liver disease	Half-life of venlafaxine 5 hours and desvenlafaxine 11 hours. Metabolism of venlafaxine mainly hepatic (P450) and desvenlafaxine partially hepatic, but not via P450. Excreted in urine
Venlafaxine	37.5 mg/day	Oral	75 mg/day			
Gabapentinoids						
Gabapentin	300 mg/day	Oral	900 mg/day	Drowsiness, dizziness, fatigue, insomnia, weight gain, headache, ataxia, and suicidal thoughts	Use with caution in renal diseases	• Half-life of gabapentin is 5–7 hours • 100% excreted by kidney in unchanged form

Contd...

Contd...

Drug name	Dosage	Route	Maximum dose	Side effects	Contraindications	Pharmacokinetics
Clonidine	0.1 mg/week	Dermal patch	0.3 mg/week	Hypotension, light-headedness, dizziness, dry mouth, headache, constipation, rebound hypertension upon discontinuation	Dose adjustment is necessary in case of renal disease and cardiovascular disease	Half-life of clonidine ranges from 12 to 16 hours. Metabolized in liver and excreted in urine
Neurokinin 3 receptor antagonist						
Fezolinetant	45 mg/day	Oral	90 mg twice daily	Abdominal pain, diarrhea, insomnia, back pain, hepatic transaminase elevation	• Known cirrhosis • Severe renal impairment or end-stage renal disease • Concomitant use with CYP1A2 inhibitors	• Half-life is 9.6 hours • Metabolizes by CYP1A2 • Excreted in urine and feces

*Drug-specific contraindications.
(SNRIs: serotonin-norepinephrine reuptake inhibitors; SSRIs: selective serotonin reuptake inhibitors)

DRUGS TO RESTORE BONE HEALTH

In menopausal women, bone mineral density (BMD) is reduced as a result of hypoestrogenemia. Reduce BMD results in osteopenia, osteoporosis, and increased risk of fracture in menopausal women. Various groups of drugs **(Table 3)** are available to reduce bone loss and prevent from bone fracture in menopausal women.

Selective Estrogen Receptor Modulator

In menopausal women, selective estrogen receptor modulators (SERMs) drugs act as partial estrogen receptors agonists for maintaining bone density, use in the treatment of osteoporosis. SERM includes tamoxifen first generation, second-generation osteoporosis drug raloxifene, third-generation drug bazedoxifene and ospemifene.

Pharmacology

Selective estrogen receptor modulator class shows tissue selective estrogen agonist and antagonist activity. The estrogen receptor has α and β two subunits and SERMs interact with either of these subunits, and this interaction results in certain level of target-site specificity and tissue-specificity for SERM action.[36] SERMs on the estrogen receptor affects bone homeostasis by downmodulating the activity of osteoclasts in a transforming growth factor-β3-dependent manner and reducing bone resorption. This affect allows in preventing and treating osteoporosis.[37] Raloxifene exerts antagonist effect on endometrium and agonist effect in bone and lipid. Tamoxifen metabolized by

TABLE 3: Drugs to restore bone health.

Drug name	Dosage	Route	Side effects	Contraindications
Selective estrogen receptor modulator				
Raloxifene	60 mg/day	Oral	• Hot flashes, leg cramps, joint pain • Swollen hands, feet, ankles or lower legs • Flu-like syndrome, sleep disturbance	History of thromboembolic disorders, coronary heart disease, undiagnosed abnormal genital bleeding, known or suspected estrogen-dependent neoplasia
Ospemifene*	60 mg/day	Oral	Vaginal discharge, hot flashes, headache, increased sweating, night sweats, muscle spasm	
Bisphosphonate				
Alendronate	5–10 mg/day or 35–70 mg/week	Oral	Gastrointestinal reflux, esophagitis, esophageal/gastric ulcers, and gastritis, transient hypocalcemia, rarely ocular adverse effect uveitis, conjunctivitis, and scleritis	Esophageal abnormalities, hypocalcemia
Teriparatide (recombinant human parathyroid hormone)	20–40 µg/day	Subcutaneous injection	• Nausea, vomiting, stomach pain, thirst, dry mouth, loss of appetite, increased urination headache, muscle weakness • Incoherent speech, depression, confusion	Hypercalcemia, increased basal risk of osteosarcoma, hypercalciuria
Romosozumab (monoclonal antibody sclerostin inhibitor)	210 mg/month	Subcutaneous injection	Arthralgia, headache, injection site reactions, nasopharyngitis, back pain, rashes, dermatitis, erythema multiforme	Hypocalcemia, history of stroke or myocardial infarction, patient who has completed therapy for 12 months

*Ospemifene mainly used for treatment of vulvar and vaginal atrophy.

cytochrome P450 enzyme system, raloxifene is metabolized by glucuronide conjugation. Half-life ranges from 27.7 hours to 7 days.

Indication

It is used in breast cancer and also for osteoporosis in menopausal women. Ospemifene is used for vulvar and vaginal atrophy (VVA) in menopausal women.[38]

Dosage

Mainly raloxifene 60 mg/day is given in the treatment of osteoporosis in menopause. Ospemifene 60 mg/day is used for treatment of VVA.

Drug Interactions

Selective estrogen receptor modulators have several potential drug interactions with warfarin, rifampicin, cholestyramine, and aromatase inhibitors.

Bisphosphonate

It is used in the prevention and treatment of osteoporosis in menopausal women. Bisphosphonate increases BMD and reduces the risk of fracture. Bisphosphonate class includes alendronate, risedronate, ibandronate, and zoledronic acid. Alendronate is commonly used for osteoporosis in menopausal women and prevents vertebral and nonvertebral fracture.

Mechanism of Action

All bisphosphonates inhibit bone resorption via attachment to hydroxyapatite-binding sites on the bone, particularly at the site of active resorption. As osteoclasts resorb bone, the bisphosphonate embedded in the bone is released and impairs the osteoclasts ability to continue bone resorption.[39-41]

Indication

Food and Drug Administration approved treatment for osteoporosis in menopause.

Contraindications

Contraindications are hypersensitivity to drug, hypocalcemia, chronic kidney disease, history of atypical femur fracture, or osteonecrosis of the jaw secondary to bisphosphonates.

Dosage

Alendronate 5 and 10 mg daily alternatively 35 and 70 mg weekly. Serum calcium, vitamin D, and renal function require baseline monitoring before initiating bisphosphonates.[42]

Adverse Drug Reactions

Adverse drug reactions are gastrointestinal reflux, esophagitis, esophageal/gastric ulcers, and gastritis, transient hypocalcemia, rarely ocular adverse effect uveitis, conjunctivitis, and scleritis.

Teriparatide

Teriparatide (rDNA origin) injection contains recombinant human parathyroid hormone hPTH (1-34), that has an identical sequence to the 34 N-terminal amino acids (the biologically active region) of the 84-amino acid hPTH.[43] Recommended dose is 20–40 µg daily subcutaneous injection form. Indicated in severe osteoporosis or in those women in whom bisphosphonate is contraindicated.

Sclerostin Inhibitors

Sclerostin, a glycoprotein, that is produced by osteocyte acts by antagonizing Wnt/signaling system on cell membranes of osteoblasts thus having antianabolic effects on bone.[43] Sclerostin inhibitors include romosozumab a monoclonal antibody use in severe osteoporosis in menopausal women. Romosozumab injection is available in prefilled syringe containing 105 mg of drug. Recommended dose is 210 mg once in month, supplemented with calcium and vitamin D.

Calcitonin

Calcitonin is peptide hormone which inhibits the activity of osteoclast and increases bone calcium content and decreases the blood calcium level. It decreases the vertebral fractures. A dose of 200 IU as nasal spray form, calcitonin reduces spine fractures by 33%.

Calcium

In menopausal women 1,200 mg/day calcium is recommended. Most postmenopausal women require supplementation as they do not consume adequate amounts of dietary calcium. Calcium preparation commonly used are calcium carbonate and calcium citrate. Calcium carbonate contains 40% elemental calcium and 1,250 mg calcium carbonate contains 500 mg elemental calcium. Acidic environment is required for absorption of calcium carbonate preparation. Calcium citrate contains 21% elemental calcium. Acidic environment does not require for absorption of calcium citrate preparation. Most common adverse drug effects of calcium supplementation are gastritis, abdominal bloating, and constipation.

Vitamin D

Vitamin D is essential for the absorption of calcium. Recommend dietary intake of vitamin D_3 is 800 IU/day, the goal of treatment is to maintain a serum 25-hydroxyvitamin D level >20 ng/mL. Vitamin D supplementation reduces risk of fracture in menopausal women. Recommended dose of vitamin D supplementation is 60,000 IU per week for 8 weeks. Repeated supplementation required to maintain optimum blood level. Various forms of oral preparation are available.

ALTERNATIVE TO HORMONE THERAPY FOR GENITOURINARY SYNDROME OF MENOPAUSE

Ospemifene

Ospemifene is a SERM approved for the treatment of moderate-to-severe dyspareunia and moderate-to-severe vaginal dryness. Ospemifene 60 mg dose reduces the severity of dyspareunia and has beneficial effects for vaginal dryness and bone as well as antiestrogenic effects on breast tissue.[44] A meta-analysis of the ospemifene randomized trials suggested that it is well tolerated with a good safety profile.[45]

Adjunctive Treatments

Lubricants/Moisturizers

In mild-to-moderate vaginal dryness and dyspareunia for short-term relief, nonhormonal lubricants and moisturizers are often recommended.[44] Lubricants, which are available in water-, silicone-, mineral-, or plant oil-based forms, are applied to the vagina and vulva prior to sex.[46] Vaginal moisturizers are absorbed into the vaginal mucosa, and adhere to the vaginal lining, rehydrate dry mucosal tissue, thereby mimicking natural vaginal secretions. Commonly used vaginal moisturizers contain polycarbophil gel. The polymer attaches via anionic binding to mucin and epithelial cells of vaginal mucosa. Polycarbophil holds water in place against the vaginal epithelial surface until it remains in vaginal wall, till 24 hours or more, therefore vaginal moisturizers require only 2–3 applications a week.

Hyaluronic Acid

Vaginal hyaluronic acid is a colorless gel that contains a derivative of hyaluronic acid that releases water molecules to the tissue, thus alleviating vaginal dryness without irritating the vaginal mucosa.[47]

Physical Therapy/Dilators

Gentle stretching of the vagina with lubricated dilators of graduated sizes helps women in vulvovaginal atrophy and vaginal constriction. Pelvic floor muscle therapy can be useful in high tone pelvic floor muscle dysfunction triggered by painful sexual activity related to genitourinary syndrome of menopause (GSM)[48] or as a complementary therapy in persistent dyspareunia. Pelvic floor muscle therapy also effective in urinary incontinence, genital prolapse, dyspareunia, and relief of VVA symptoms.[49]

■ LASER THERAPY

Laser therapy is one of the proposed nonhormonal therapies for GSM with use of either a fractional CO_2 laser or erbium:YAG laser.[50] Several small studies shown that fractional CO_2 laser therapy can restore the vaginal epithelium as in the premenopausal state, increase *Lactobacillus* and other premenopausal flora, as well as improve the Vaginal Health Index score and subjective symptoms of GSM. The use of the erbium:YAG laser shown to improve symptoms of GSM and stress urinary incontinence.[51]

Alternative pharmacotherapies commonly used in menopausal symptoms are listed in **Tables 2 and 3**.

■ KEY POINTS

- Alternative therapies can be a good choice in conditions where HRT is contraindicated.
- Other alternative like healthy lifestyle starting from the early life with lifelong compliance not only improves menopausal symptoms but also improves quality of life.
- Supplementation with calcium and vitamin D during menopause will help to maintain bone health.
- For genitourinary symptoms available adjunctive therapies are better option and easily acceptable.
- Symptomatic menopausal women those who are afraid to take HRT for their symptoms, in such women alternative therapies play a vital role to alleviate their symptoms.

■ REFERENCES

1. Academic Committee of the Korean Society of Menopause; Lee SR, Cho MK, Cho YJ, Chun S, Hong SH, et al. The 2020 Menopausal Hormone Therapy Guidelines. J Menopausal Med. 2020;26(2):69-98.
2. Lobo RA. Hormone-replacement therapy: current thinking. Nat Rev Endocrinol. 2017;13(4):220-31.
3. National Institute for Health and Care Excellence (NICE). (2015). Menopause: diagnosis and management: NICE guideline [NG23]. [online] Available from: https://www.nice.org.uk/guidance/ng23 [Last accessed December, 2023].
4. Rossouw JE, Anderson GL, Prentice RL, LaCroix AZ, Kooperberg C, Stefanick ML, et al. Risks and benefits of estrogen plus progestin in healthy postmenopausal women: principal results from the Women's Health Initiative randomized controlled trial. JAMA. 2002;288(3):321-33.
5. American College of Obstetricians and Gynecologists. (2021). Hormone Therapy for Menopause: [online] Available from: https://www.acog.org/womens-health/faqs/hormone-therapy-for-menopause [Last accessed December, 2023].
6. Women's Health Concern. (2022). Complementary and alternative therapies: Non hormonal treatments for menopause symptoms—nonhormonal prescribed treatments. [online] Available from: https://www.womens-health-concern.org/wp-content/uploads/2022/12/03-WHC-FACTSHEET-Complementary-And-Alternative-Therapies-NOV2022-B.pdf [Last accessed December, 2023].
7. NHS. Alternatives to hormone replacement therapy (HRT). [online] Available from: https://www.nhs.uk/medicines/hormone-replacement-therapy-hrt/alternatives-to-hormone-replacement-therapy-hrt/ [Last accessed December, 2023].
8. Royal College of Obstetricians and Gynaecologists. (2010). Alternatives to HRT for the Management of Symptoms of the

Menopause (Scientific Impact Paper No.6) [online] Available from: https://www.rcog.org.uk/media/gwbntgdu/sip_6.pdf [Last accessed December, 2023].
9. Chu A, Wadhwa R. Selective Serotonin Reuptake Inhibitors. In: StatPearls [Internet]. Treasure Island (FL): StatPearls Publishing; 2023.
10. Edinoff AN, Akuly HA, Hanna TA, Ochoa CO, Patti SJ, Ghaffar YA, et al. Selective Serotonin Reuptake Inhibitors and Adverse Effects: A Narrative Review. Neurol Int. 2021;13(3):387-401.
11. NHS. (2021). Cautions—Selective serotonin reuptake inhibitors (SSRIs). https://www.nhs.uk/mental-health/talking-therapies-medicine-treatments/medicines-and-psychiatry/ssri-antidepressants/considerations/
12. Simon JA, Portman DJ, Kaunitz AM, Mekonnen H, Kazempour K, Bhaskar S, et al. Low-dose paroxetine 7.5 mg for menopausal vasomotor symptoms: two randomized controlled trials. Menopause. 2013;20(10):1027-35.
13. Pinkerton JV, Joffe H, Kazempour K, Mekonnen H, Bhaskar S, Lippman J. Low-dose paroxetine (7.5 mg) improves sleep in women with vasomotor symptoms associated with menopause. Menopause. 2015;22(1):50-8.
14. Portman DJ, Kaunitz AM, Kazempour K, Mekonnen H, Bhaskar S, Lippman J. Effects of low-dose paroxetine 7.5 mg on weight and sexual function during treatment of vasomotor symptoms associated with menopause. Menopause. 2014;21(10):1082-90.
15. Nonhormonal management of menopause-associated vasomotor symptoms: 2015 position statement of The North American Menopause Society. Menopause. 2015;22(11):1155-72; quiz 1173-4.
16. Stearns V, Beebe KL, Iyengar M, Dube E. Paroxetine controlled release in the treatment of menopausal hot flushes: a randomized controlled trial. JAMA. 2003;289:2827-34.
17. National Health Services. (2021). Side Effects: Selective Serotonin Reuptake Inhibitors (SSRIs). [online] Available from: https://www.nhs.uk/mental-health/talking-therapies-medicine-treatments/medicines-and-psychiatry/ssri-antidepressants/side-effects [Last accessed December, 2023].
18. NHS. (2022). Pregnancy, breastfeeding and fertility while taking paroxetine. [online] Available from: https://www.nhs.uk/medicines/paroxetine/pregnancy-breastfeeding-and-fertility-while-taking-paroxetine/ [Last accessed December, 2023].
19. Sansone RA, Sansone LA. Serotonin norepinephrine reuptake inhibitors: a pharmacological comparison. Innov Clin Neurosci. 2014;11(3-4):37-42.
20. Sahni S, Lobo-Romero A, Smith T. Contemporary Non-hormonal Therapies for the Management of Vasomotor Symptoms Associated with Menopause: A Literature Review. touchREV Endocrinol. 2021;17(2):133-7.
21. Guttuso T, Kurlan R, McDermott MP, Kieburtz K. Gabapentin's effects on hot flashes in postmenopausal women: a randomized controlled trial. Obstet Gynecol. 2003;101:337-45.
22. Guttuso TJ. Gabapentin's effects on hot flashes and hypothermia. Neurology. 2000;54:2161-3.
23. Yoon SH, Lee JY, Lee C, Lee H, Kim SN. Gabapentin for the treatment of hot flushes in menopause: a meta-analysis. Menopause. 2020;27(4):485-93.
24. Chincholkar M. Gabapentinoids: pharmacokinetics, pharmacodynamics and considerations for clinical practice. Br J Pain. 2020;14(2):104-14.
25. Larsen Burns M, Kinge E, Stokke Opdal M, Johannessen SI, Johannessen Landmark C. Therapeutic drug monitoring of gabapentin in various indications. Acta Neurol Scand. 2019;139(5):446-54.
26. Freedman RR. Menopausal hot flashes: mechanisms, endocrinology, treatment. J Steroid Biochem Mol Biol. 2014;142:115-20.

27. Yasaei R, Saadabadi A. Clonidine. In: StatPearls [Internet]. Treasure Island (FL): StatPearls Publishing; 2023.
28. Garcia-Recio S, Gascón P. Biological and pharmacological aspects of the NK1-receptor. Biomed Res Int. 2015;2015:495704.
29. Pennefather JN, Lecci A, Candenas ML, Patak E, Pinto FM, Maggi CA. Tachykinins and tachykinin receptors: a growing family. Life Sci. 2004;74(12):1445-63.
30. Page NM. New challenges in the study of the mammalian tachykinins. Peptides. 2005;26:1356-8.
31. Hoveyda HR, Fraser GL, Dutheuil G, El Bousmaqui M, Korac J, Lenoir F, et al. Optimization of Novel Antagonists to the Neurokinin-3 Receptor for the Treatment of Sex-Hormone Disorders (Part II). ACS Med Chem Lett. 2015;6(7):736-40.
32. Fraser GL, Lederman S, Waldbaum A, Kroll R, Santoro N, Lee M, et al. A phase 2b, randomized, placebo-controlled, double-blind, dose-ranging study of the neurokinin 3 receptor antagonist fezolinetant for vasomotor symptoms associated with menopause. Menopause. 2020;27(4):382-92.
33. Guirguis M, Abdelmalak J, Jusino E, Hansen MR, Girgis GE. Stellate Ganglion Block for the Treatment of Hot Flashes in Patients with Breast Cancer: A Literature Review. Ochsner J. 2015;15(2):162-9.
34. Leach MJ, Moore V. Black cohosh (Cimicifuga spp.) for menopausal symptoms. Cochrane Database Syst Rev. 2012;2012:CD007244.
35. The 2023 Nonhormone Therapy Position Statement of The North American Menopause Society Advisory Panel. The 2023 nonhormone therapy position statement of The North American Menopause Society. Menopause. 2023;30(6):573-90.
36. Nelson ER, Wardell SE, McDonnell DP. The molecular mechanisms underlying the pharmacological actions of estrogens, SERMs and oxysterols: implications for the treatment and prevention of osteoporosis. Bone. 2013;53:42-50.
37. An KC. Selective Estrogen Receptor Modulators. Asian Spine J. 2016;10(4):787-91.
38. Goldstein SR, Bachmann GA, Koninckx PR, Lin VH, Portman DJ, Ylikorkala O, et al. Ospemifene 12-month safety and efficacy in postmenopausal women with vulvar and vaginal atrophy. Climacteric. 2014;17(2):173-82.
39. Farrell KB, Karpeisky A, Thamm DH, Zinnen S. Bisphosphonate conjugation for bone specific drug targeting. Bone Rep. 2018;9:47-60.
40. Frediani B, Giusti A, Bianchi G, Dalle Carbonare L, Malavolta N, Cantarini L, et al. Clodronate in the management of different musculoskeletal conditions. Minerva Med. 2018;109(4):300-25.
41. Bernardi S, Di Girolamo M, Necozione S, Continenza MA, Cutilli T. Antiresorptive drug-related osteonecrosis of the jaws, literature review and 5 years of experience. Musculoskelet Surg. 2019;103(1):47-53.
42. Ganesan K, Goyal A, Roane D. Bisphosphonate. In: StatPearls [Internet]. Treasure Island (FL): StatPearls Publishing; 2023.
43. Tella SH, Gallagher JC. Prevention and treatment of postmenopausal osteoporosis. J Steroid Biochem Mol Biol. 2014;142:155-70.
44. Kagan R, Kellogg-Spadt S, Parish SJ. Practical Treatment Considerations in the Management of Genitourinary Syndrome of Menopause. Drugs Aging. 2019;36(10):897-908.
45. Di Donato V, Schiavi MC, Iacobelli V, D'Oria O, Kontopantelis E, Simoncini T, et al. Ospemifene for the treatment of vulvar and vaginal atrophy: a meta-analysis of randomized trials. Part II: evaluation of tolerability and safety. Maturitas. 2019;121:93-100.
46. Edwards D, Panay N. Treating vulvovaginal atrophy/genitourinary syndrome of menopause: how important is vaginal lubricant and moisturizer composition? Climacteric. 2016;19(2):151-61.
47. Chen J, Geng L, Song X, Li H, Giordan N, Liao Q. Evaluation of the efficacy and safety of hyaluronic acid vaginal gel to ease

vaginal dryness: a multicenter, randomized, controlled, open-label, parallel-group, clinical trial. J Sex Med. 2013;10(6): 1575-84.
48. Faubion SS, Sood R, Kapoor E. Genitourinary syndrome of menopause: management strategies for the clinician. Mayo Clin Proc. 2017;92(12):1842-9.
49. Mercier J, Morin M, Lemieux MC, Reichetzer B, Khalife S, Dumoulin C. Pelvic floor muscles training to reduce symptoms and signs of vulvovaginal atrophy: a case study. Menopause. 2016;23(7):816-20.
50. Arunkalaivanan A, Kaur H, Onuma O. Laser therapy as a treatment modality for genitourinary syndrome of menopause: a critical appraisal of evidence. Int Urogynecol J. 2017;28(5):681-5.
51. Rabley A, O'Shea T, Terry R, Byun S, Louis Moy M. Laser therapy for genitourinary syndrome of menopause. Curr Urol Rep. 2018;19(10):83.

Chapter 36

Drugs to Decrease Fracture Risk

Shobhana Mohan Das

Fracture, meaning a break in cartilage or bone, usually occurs due to trauma. Predisposition for fracture in postmenopausal women occurs due to increased risks of falling (e.g., ataxia, medication and alcohol intake, loose carpets), age, osteoporosis, bony metastases, and other bone disorders. Prevention and treatment of osteoporosis can prevent fractures in this population to a large extent.[1] Weakening of bone matrix can lead to fractures in this population, which can, to some extent, be avoided with proper diet and exercise.[2] However, there is a large vulnerable population with osteoporosis who may benefit from drug therapy.

Bone is a dynamic organ where bone is continuously being formed with osteoblasts, while attrition is simultaneously going on with the help of osteoclasts. Drugs to reduce or cure osteoporosis include drugs which can form new bone and drugs which will prevent resorption of old bone. Postmenopausal women are decreased estrogen levels. This induces RANKL (receptor activator of nuclear factor-kappa B ligand) expression which helps preosteoclasts to become osteoclasts. Drugs like estrogen can thus reduce RANKL expression and thereby reduce formation of osteoclasts. Drugs like denosumab directly inhibit RANKL expression, which reduce bone loss.

■ WHO NEEDS TREATMENT?

Women with an osteoporosis-associated fracture or dual-energy X-ray absorptiometry (DXA)-derived T score of <2.5 should be treated. Osteopenic women should be assessed using risk calculators like FRAX to find the 10-year risk of fracture. If fracture prone, pharmacologic treatment should be initiated in women regardless of age.

■ AVAILABLE AGENTS

Primarily, drugs used to prevent and treat osteoporosis can be divided into three categories:
1. Natural products which help in bone formation
2. Products which reduce bone loss
3. Products which can induce bone formation.

Women with moderate risk of osteoporosis may just need dietary supplements. It is necessary to look for conditions predisposing to osteoporosis, like women receiving aromatase inhibitor therapy for breast malignancy, long-term or repeated systemic corticosteroid use.[3] Shortened height, stoop, and recurrent falls should alert the physician to screen for and treat osteoporosis.

Natural Products which Help Prevent Fracture Reduction

Calcium: One study has shown that a combination of calcium with vitamin D_3 can reduce fracture risk as compared to placebo arm.[4,5] Calcium requirement in postmenopause is 800 mg and the average Indian intake of calcium is about 400–500 mg. Calcium supplementation is therefore necessary in postmenopause to maintain optimal levels to prevent bone depletion and fractures. Calcium supplements are best taken with meals in divided doses. Gastrointestinal (GI) tract can only absorb 500–600 mg of calcium at one time. If the requirement is higher, 500 mg doses should be spaced by at least 4–5 hours to achieve the recommended intake.[6,7] Calcium carbonate requires fewer tablets, and is least expensive, but causes constipation and bloating. For adequate absorption, it has to be taken with meals. Calcium citrate is often more expensive than calcium carbonate but requires more tablets to get the desired dose. Its absorption is not dependent on gastric acid, and it is less likely to cause GI side effects. All calcium supplements may cause constipation. Cardiac damage reported with calcium may happen only in a percentage of women taking doses higher than 2 g. Calcium supplements decrease the effect of fluoroquinolones, levothyroxine, antibiotics in the tetracycline family, digoxin, and phenytoin. Aluminum and magnesium antacids can both increase urinary calcium excretion. Mineral oil and stimulant laxatives can both decrease dietary calcium absorption. Higher doses of calcium have been implicated in increasing the risk of cardiac events, but there are studies refuting it also.[8]

Vitamin D_3: Addition of vitamin D_3 to calcium has been found to be useful in prevention and management of osteoporosis.

Drugs to Reduce Bone Loss

The majority of drug formulations used in the treatment of osteoporosis are designed to prevent bone resorption. These antiresorptive drugs are:
- Hormone replacement therapy
- Selective estrogen receptor modulators (SERMs)
- Bisphosphonates
- Denosumab

Hormone Replacement Therapy

Estrogen hormone replacement therapy suppresses osteoclast activity.[9,10] It also prevents osteoblasts apoptosis. There is also indirect alteration the expression of estrogen-responsive target genes, giving rise to bone turnover. Women's Health Initiative (WHI) as established that conjugated equine estrogen 0.625 mg/day and medroxyprogesterone acetate 2.5 mg/day can reduce fracture risk by 34%.[11] Menopause hormone therapy (MHT) may be considered for prevention of osteoporosis. In general, the benefits of hormone therapy (HT) to bone health disappear when treatment is stopped; when this occurs, some other continuation treatment should be administered to protect bone. Similarly, women who undergo early menopause are protected from osteoporosis by MHT until age of 50 years with no need for other antiresorptive drugs; at this age, evaluation of whether to continue the same therapy or change treatment is needed. Side effects include increase in cardiovascular risk, venous thromboembolism, and a slight increase in the incidence of breast cancer.

Combining estrogen and bisphosphonate combination may cause oversuppression of bone remodeling, creating an adynamic or "frozen" bone, which may increase the risk of fracture. Hence, it is prudent not to combine both agents.

Selective Estrogen Receptor Modulators

Selective estrogen receptor modulators have strong agonist action on the brain and bone, while being estrogen antagonist on breast and endometrium. Currently, raloxifene and bazedoxifene are available for prevention and treatment of osteoporosis.

Raloxifene prevents bone resorption, but may increase the severity of hot flashes if present. In a dose of 60 mg/day, it can reduce vertebral, not nonvertebral fracture by 30%.[12]

Bazedoxifene is a third-generation SERM. 20 mg bazedoxifene with 0.45 mg or 0.625 mg of conjugated equine estrogen has been studied. In the SMART 1 and 2 trials, it was found to improve bone parameters without stimulating endometrium, or increasing risk of breast cancer and also improving vaginal scores and decreasing incidence of hot flashes.[13]

Selective estrogen receptor modulators do not increase the incidence of cardiovascular events, but increased the incidence of stroke and venous thromboembolism has been reported. SERMs are useful in women for whom bisphosphonates and denosumab are deemed inappropriate.

Bisphosphonates

Bisphosphonates are the most widely used antiresorptive agent in the drug management of fracture prevention.[14] Bisphosphonates prevent resorption by inhibiting osteoclast enzyme and also increasing apoptosis of osteoclasts. Thus percentage of formed bone increases, thereby strengthening it.

Zoledronate has the highest binding affinity followed by alendronate, ibandronate, and risedronate in decreasing order. Fracture reduction is seen 1 year after administration.

When bisphosphonates are given orally, absorption is <1%. The drug should be given on empty stomach along with a full glass of water. Patient should wait for 30–60 minutes before eating food after drug intake to prevent gastritis. Sitting upright after drug intake is necessary to prevent irritation of esophagus. Formulations of delayed release risedronate can be given after breakfast with no need for fasting. Difficulty in following strict instructions in oral preparations, especially in elderly, has led to the preference for intravenous (IV) preparations.

The dose and characteristics of various bisphosphonates are given in **Table 1**.

In patients with moderate fracture risk, it is recommended that oral bisphosphonates can be given for 5 years, while IV zoledronic acid can be given for 3 years. A drug holiday is recommended after that, as bisphosphonates may accumulate for months or years after treatment cessation. In patients with higher fracture risk, 6–10 years of oral bisphosphonates or 6 yearly doses of zoledronic acid may be tried.

Side effects of bisphosphonates:
- Oral bisphosphonates can cause esophageal irritation in patients with gastroesophageal reflux disease or esophageal stricture. Patients have to be instructed to maintain upright posture strictly for 30–60 minutes after ingestion of the drug with a full glass of water. Use of weekly/

TABLE 1: Dose and characteristics of various bisphosphonates.

	Route of administration	Dose	Effects	Side effects	Time for fracture reduction
Zoledronate	Intravenous (IV)	• 5 mg IV over 15 minutes • Single IV dose every 2 years	Reduces vertebral and hip fractures	Osteonecrosis of jaw in high doses. Good dental care needed	Hip fracture 41% reduction in 3 years. Vertebral fracture 70% reduction in 3 years
Alendronate	Oral	• 10 mg daily • 70 mg weekly	-DO-	Gastritis. Ask patient to sit upright for half hour after intake. Calcium and vitamin D insufficiency may occur	Reduces vertebral fractures by 40%
Ibandronate	Oral	• 2.5 mg daily • 150 mg/month	Only spine fractures decreased		Reduces vertebral fracture by 62% in 3 years
Risedronate	Oral	5 mg daily/35 mg/week	Reduces vertebral and hip fractures		49% vertebral fracture reduction in 6 months
Etidronate	Oral	400 mg/day	Only vertebral reduced		

monthly preparations may obviate this effect.
- *Severe musculoskeletal pain:* The United States Food and Drug Administration (US FDA) recently issued an alert highlighting the possibility of severe, incapacitating musculoskeletal pain that can occur at any point after initiation of bisphosphonate therapy.
- *Acute inflammatory response:* 10–30% of patients receiving IV bisphosphonates may get transient pyrexia with associated myalgias, arthralgias, headaches, and influenza-like symptoms as a result of acute inflammatory response.
- *Hypocalcemia* frequently follows IV infusion and is more common in Paget's disease of bone, hypoparathyroidism, low levels of vitamin D, or impaired renal function, where there is high bone resorption.
- *Atrial fibrillation:* IV zoledronic acid in HORIZON study was associated with an increased incidence of atrial fibrillation.
- *Osteonecrosis of the jaw:* This complication is rare, 1 in 10,000 to 1 in 100,000 patient treatment years in patients receiving oral bisphosphonate therapy. In oncology, patients receiving IV preparations, the incidence is 1 to 10 per 100 patients. It is higher in the presence of poor oral hygiene, history of dental procedures or denture use.

Denosumab

Denosumab, a recombinant human IgG2-antibody, is a RANKL inhibitor. RANKL is a transmembrane protein required for the survival of osteoclasts. Inhibiting it prevents bone resorption.

50 mg of denosumab every 6 months for 36 months can significantly reduce fracture risk as per findings of FREEDOM

trial.[15] It is an injectable preparation to be given subcutaneously. The decrease in bone remodeling can cause a decrease in calcium and phosphate levels, especially in 1 or 2 months of therapy. Calcium levels should be corrected before starting treatment.

Denosumab is superior to alendronate, risedronate, ibandronate (per os or IV), zoledronic acid, raloxifene, and calcitonin in improving bone mineral density (BMD). When teriparatide is compared, in lumbar spine, teriparatide may induce greater changes in BMD compared to denosumab.

Denosumab is well tolerated, but side effects like hypersensitivity, serious infections, dermatological reactions, musculoskeletal pain, and hypercholesterolemia may occur. It does not affect the renal or hepatic parameters and so dosage need not be adjusted in compromised patients.

Calcitonin: Calcitonin is a synthetic polypeptide hormone acting on calcitonin receptors in the bone, reducing the risk of vertebral fractures. *Dosage:* 200 IU daily. Calcitonin-salmon nasal spray is available only as a generic and is administered as one spray in one nostril daily, alternating nostrils. Due to weak effect on bone metabolism, effect is less for nonvertebral fractures compared to other agents.

Odanacatib: Odanacatib is an inhibitor of cathepsin K, a lysosomal cysteine protease with high collagenase activity expressed predominantly in osteoclasts. It is a bone resorption inhibitor.

Drugs which Cause Bone Formation

Parathyroid Hormone Analogs

Teriparatide is a recombinant human parathyroid hormone (PTH) analog. It was the first anabolic treatment approved for osteoporosis.

It stimulates new bone formation on the surface of bone, just like the original body made parathormone.

The recommended dose is 20 µg SC daily to be injected in the thigh or abdomen. Increase in bone formation occurs within 1 month of therapy.

Many women, e.g., bedridden patients, or those on steroids have severe fragility fractures and some women cannot tolerate other treatments. Parathormone is a great help for these women. Cramps and dizziness is seen in commonly as side effects. Osteosarcoma has been reported in rats when teriparatide is given in high doses. Therefore, treatment should be limited to 2 years. Anabolic treatment can be replaced with antiresorptive drugs which should be initiated to prevent occurrence of osteoporosis after the stoppage of teriparatide.

Patients with Paget's disease of bone, unexplained alkaline phosphatase elevations, prior skeletal radiotherapy, primary or metastatic bone malignancy, or hypercalcemic disorders, such as primary hyperparathyroidism should avoid treatment with teriparatide.

Strontium Ranelate

Strontium ranelate (SR) contains two atoms of strontium and ranelic acid. It combines antiresorptive and anabolic activity.[16] Dose: 2 g orally in-between meals, preferably at bedtime or at least 2 hours after dinner.

Abaloparatide

It is a recombinant human PTH analog. It comes as an injection, at a dose of 80 µg SC once daily, to be used maximum for 2 years.[17]

TABLE 2: Characteristics of some of the drugs used in fracture prevention.

Drugs	Mechanism	Clinical use
Estrogen	Antiresorptive agent	Can be used in patients with hot flashes and in women where alternate treatments are not appropriate
Raloxifene	SERM	Reduces vertebral fractures
Denosumab	RANKL-inhibiting osteoclast activity	As initial choice in high-risk groups. Sometimes, it is given soon after bisphosphonates have to be stopped for some reason, to prevent fractures
Teriparatide	Synthetic parathormone	Used as initial choice in very high-risk patients. Can be given only for 2 years
Romosozumab	Monoclonal antibody against sclerostin. Osteoblast activity is increased	Used in both vertebral and nonvertebral fractures in very high-risk patients. Should be avoided in women with cardiovascular disease

(RANKL: receptor activator of nuclear factor-kappa B ligand; SERM: selective estrogen receptor modulator)

Romosozumab

It is a monoclonal antibody. It acts as an anabolic agent, which binds and inhibits sclerostin, which is an inhibitor of osteoblastic activity.[18,19]

Characteristics of some of the drugs used in fracture prevention are given in **Table 2**.

Facts of some of the drugs used to prevent fracture are given in **Table 3**.

In women with a tendency to have fracture, beside the physical factors, and treatment of underlying cause of weakening of bone, prevention and treatment of osteoporosis form the cornerstone of management.[20]

■ KEY POINTS

- Drug therapy in the postmenopausal woman can include calcium and vitamin D supplements.
- Hormone replacement therapy can be offered to women within 10 years of menopause and has equal effects compared to bisphosphonates.
- SERMs have been an option, and newer ones like bazedoxifene with estrogen are being tried with good results, though not available in India.
- Bisphosphonates in various forms have been the mainstay of treatment for many years, and are used by most cancer patients after chemotherapy, to prevent osteoporosis.
- In women with debilitating osteoporosis, to get faster buildup of bone, teriparatide can be used initially. If treatment has to be continued beyond 2 years, instead of sudden stoppage of treatment, switch over to bisphosphonates, in the initial period, may be a better option.
- In severe osteoporosis, denosumab is an option, a special advantage being its noninterference with renal parameters.
- Odanacatib and romosozumab are potential agents coming up.

Awareness of medications available in treatment of osteoporosis can prevent fractures, and also help many bedridden patients to lead pain free, mobile, and more fulfilling lives.

TABLE 3: Facts of some of the drugs used to prevent fracture.

Name	Dosage	Route	Maximum dose	Side effects	Contraindications	Pharmacokinetics
Calcium	500 mg at one time, may be repeated after 5 hours	Oral	2 g	Constipation, flatulence, Bloating. Only >2 g can cause cardiac effects	Hypophosphatemia, hyperphosphatemia, hypercalcemia	Absorbed from GIT
Vitamin D	600 IU/day	Oral	4,000 IU or 100 µg/day	Rarely weakness, dry mouth	Allergy	Bound in blood to vitamin D-binding protein (VDBP). Activated mainly by the liver to 25 (OH) D within hours and, by the kidney to 1,25 (OH) D (calcitriol); enhances calcium absorption
Conjugated estrogen	0.625 mg/day	Oral	1.2 mg/day	Deep vein thrombosis, migraine, breast tenderness, breast cancer if used more than 5 years, vaginal bleeding, dry eyes, GI disturbances, pancreatitis rarely	Unexplained vaginal bleeding, stroke, TIA, MI, PE, VTE, breast or endometrial cancer, active liver disease	• Bound to SHBG • Converted to estriol in liver, mainly excreted in kidney • Transdermal avoids liver passage
• Estradiol • Estradiol valerate	1 mg/day	Oral	2 mg/day			
Estradiol	1.53–4.59 mg/day	Transdermal spray				
Raloxifene	60 mg/day	Oral	60 mg/day	Hot flashes and leg cramps	History of deep venous thrombosis, renal vein thrombosis, pulmonary embolism, malignancy, active smoking, or any thrombophilia	Raloxifene is rapidly absorbed from the intestines upon oral administration. Peak plasma levels of raloxifene occur 0.5–6 hours after an oral dose

Contd...

Contd...

Name	Dosage	Route	Maximum dose	Side effects	Contraindications	Pharmacokinetics
Bazedoxifene with conjugated estrogen	20 mg + 0.45 mg OR 20 mg with 0.625 mg	Oral	120 mg/day	Diarrhea, dizziness, muscle spasm	Abnormal uterine bleeding, breast cancer, estrogen-dependent neoplasia, venous or arterial thromboembolism, liver disease, or thrombophilic disorders	Bazedoxifene gets steady state in 10 days, food does not affect absorption
Denosumab	50 mg/5 months	SC	120 mg SC every 4 weeks	Jaw necrosis, inflammatory signs of skin, colored urine, urinary urgency, muscle pain	Hypocalcemia, hypersensitivity, pregnancy	Bone markers of osteoporosis reduced in 3 days
Teriparatide	20 μg daily	SC	Maximum duration not >18 months	Nausea, headache, dizziness, orthostatic hypotension, hypercalcemia, hypercalciuria. Theoretical risk of osteosarcoma	Hypersensitivity, risk for osteosarcoma, history of ionizing radiation to bone, hypercalcemia, hypercalciuria, urolithiasis	Rapid absorption, maximum in 30 minutes, half-life of 1 hour, transiently increases serum calcium, maximum at 4 hours

(GIT: gastrointestinal tract; MI: myocardial infarction; PE: pulmonary embolism; SC: subcutaneous; SHBG: sex hormone binding globulin; TIA: transient ischemic attack; VTE: venous thromboembolism)

REFERENCES

1. Isa ML, Hatta NN, Nurumal MS, Sharifudin MA. Fracture risk factor in post-menopausal women with deterioration of bone density. Int J Prev Med. 2022;13:80.
2. Marincolo JCS, Aprahamian I, Corona LP, Neri AL, Yassuda MS, Borim FSA. Three definitions of probable sarcopenia and associations with falls and functional disability among community-dwelling older adults. Osteoporos Sarcopenia. 2021; 7(2):69-74.
3. Tella SH, Gallagher JC. Prevention and treatment of postmenopausal osteoporosis. J Steroid Biochem Mol Biol. 2014;142: 155-70.
4. Lilliu H, Pamphile R, Chapuy MC, Schulten J, Arlot M, Meunier PJ. Calcium-vitamin D_3 supplementation is cost-effective in hip fractures prevention. Maturitas. 2003; 44(4):299-305.
5. Meeta M, Digumarti L, Agarwal N, Vaze N, Shah R, Malik S. Clinical Practice Guidelines on Menopause: *An Executive Summary and Recommendations: Indian Menopause Society 2019-2020. J Midlife Health. 2020; 11(2):55-95.
6. Sunyecz JA. The use of calcium and vitamin D in the management of osteoporosis. Ther Clin Risk Manag. 2008;4(4):827-36.
7. Garg MK, Mahalle N. Calcium Supplementation: Why, Which, and How? Indian J Endocrinol Metab. 2019;23(4):387-90.
8. Myung SK, Kim HB, Lee YJ, Choi YJ, Oh SW. Calcium supplements and risk of cardiovascular disease: a meta-analysis of clinical trials. Nutrients. 2021;13(2):368.
9. Jiang X, Kagan R. Hormone therapy for postmenopausal osteoporosis management. Climacteric. 2022;25(1):50-5.
10. de Villiers TJ. The role of menopausal hormone therapy in the management of osteoporosis. Climacteric. 2015;18(Suppl 2): 19-21.
11. Pinkerton JV, Pickar JH, Racketa J, Mirkin S. Bazedoxifene/conjugated estrogens for menopausal symptom treatment and osteoporosis prevention. Climacteric. 2012; 15(5):411-8.
12. Daroszveska A. Prevention and treatment of osteoporosis in women: an update. Obstet Gynaecol Reprod Med. 2012;22(6): 162-9.
13. Tu KN, Lie JD, Wan CKV, Cameron M, Austel AG, Nguyen JK, et al. Osteoporosis: a review of treatment options. P T. 2018; 43(2):92-104.
14. Bock O, Felsenberg D. Bisphosphonates in the management of postmenopausal osteoporosis–optimizing efficacy in clinical practice. Clin Interv Aging. 2008;3(2):279-97.
15. Palacios S. Medical treatment of osteoporosis. Climacteric. 2022;25(1):43-9.
16. McClung MR, Clark AL. Osteoanabolic therapy for osteoporosis in women. Climacteric. 2022;25(1):60-6.
17. Iolascon G, Moretti A, Toro G, Gimigliano F, Liguori S, Paoletta M. Pharmacological Therapy of Osteoporosis: What's New? Clin Interv Aging. 2020;15:485-91.
18. Li SS, He SH, Xie PY, Li W, Zhang XX, Li TF, et al. Recent Progresses in the Treatment of Osteoporosis. Front Pharmacol. 2021;12: 717065.
19. Liu Y, Cao Y, Zhang S, Zhang W, Zhang B, Tang Q, et al. Romosozumab treatment in postmenopausal women with osteoporosis: a meta-analysis of randomized controlled trials. Climacteric. 2018;21(2):189-95.
20. Prior JC. Progesterone for the prevention and treatment of osteoporosis in women. Climacteric. 2018;21(4):366-74.

Section 13

Medical Management of Infections in Gynecology

- **Sexually Transmitted Diseases**
  Aruna Nigam, Supriya Chaubey

Chapter 37

Sexually Transmitted Diseases

Aruna Nigam, Supriya Chaubey

Sexually transmitted infections (STIs) are a major issue for public health in both resource-rich and resource-limited settings. Upper genital tract infections, infertility, chronic pelvic pain, cervical cancer, and chronic infection with hepatitis viruses and human immunodeficiency virus (HIV) are all complications of untreated STIs. The specific infection determines how to treat sexually transmitted diseases. The following is a summary of the diseases and the agents that cause them **(Table 1)**.

■ GONORRHEA

The ability of *Neisseria gonorrhoeae* to develop resistance to antimicrobials makes treatment of gonorrhea challenging.[1] Ceftriaxone treatment of uncomplicated urogenital gonorrhea requires approximately 24 hours at concentrations higher than the strain minimal inhibitory concentration (MIC); a 500-mg portion of ceftriaxone is supposed to accomplish in roughly 50 hours MIC >0.03 µg/mL.[2]

Dual treatment with single doses of oral azithromycin 2 g and intramuscular gentamicin 240 mg may be considered an alternative to ceftriaxone for individuals allergic to cephalosporines.[3] It does not provide high or long-lasting bactericidal blood levels as ceftriaxone, so 800-mg oral dose of cefixime should only be considered as an alternative regimen of cephalosporins.

Pharyngeal gonococcal infections are more difficult to treat than urogenital and anorectal infections. Antimicrobial susceptibility and *N. gonorrhoeae* culture [with or without simultaneous (NAAT) nucleic acid amplification test] should be performed on symptoms that persist after treatment **(Table 2)**.

■ CHLAMYDIA

Doxycycline is the treatment of choice for infection caused by *Chlamydia trachomatis*. A meta-examination and a Cochrane deliberate survey concluded that treatment with doxycycline[4] is more effective among men as compared to azithromycin. A delayed-release form of doxycycline is also available, with once daily dosing and fewer gastrointestinal side effects, but is more expensive. Azithromycin is safe and effective during pregnancy,[5] whereas erythromycin is no longer recommended due to its gastrointestinal side effects. Due to the possibility of tooth discoloration occurring during the second and third trimesters of pregnancy, doxycycline is not recommended. Levofloxacin may be toxic to nursing mothers, and research on animals has shown that it can harm newborn's cartilage **(Table 3)**.

TABLE 1: Summary of the diseases and the causative agents.

STIs	Causative organism	Preventive measures
• Gonorrhea • Non-gonococcal urethritis • Syphilis • Lymphogranuloma venereum • Chancroid • Granuloma inguinale • Nonspecific vaginitis • *Mycoplasma* infection	*Bacterial:* • *Neisseria gonorrhoeae* • *Chlamydia trachomatis* (D-K serotype) • *Treponema pallidum* • *Chlamydia trachomatis* (L serotype) • *Haemophilus ducreyi* • *Donovania granulomatis* • *Hemophylus vaginalis* • *Mycoplasma hominis*	*Safe sex practices:* Barrier contraceptive measures
• AIDS • Genital herpes • Condyloma acuminata • Molluscum contagiosum • Viral hepatitis • CIN	*Viral:* • HIV 1, 2 • HSV2 • HPV 16,18, 31 • Poxvirus • HBV, HCV • HPV	Less number of sexual partners
• Bacterial vaginosis • *Trichomonas* vaginitis	*Protozoal:* • *Gardnerella vaginalis* • *Trichomonas vaginalis*	Contact tracing and effective treatment
Vaginitis monilial	*Fungal: Candida albicans*	Screening
• Scabies • Pediculosis pubis	• *Sarcoptes scabiei* • *Phthirus pubis*	Maintain asepsis

(AIDS: acquired immunodeficiency syndrome; CIN: cervical intraepithelial neoplasia; HBV: hepatitis B virus; HCV: hepatitis C virus; HIV: human immunodeficiency virus; HPV: human papillomavirus; HSV: herpes simplex virus; STIs: sexually transmitted infections)

■ SYPHILIS

All stages of syphilis are best treated with penicillin G. Depending on the stage and clinical manifestations, the preparation (benzathine, aqueous procaine, or aqueous crystalline), dosage, and duration of treatment can vary **(Table 4)**. Regardless of HIV status, higher doses of benzathine penicillin G, amoxicillin, or any other antibiotic do not improve efficacy in early latent syphilis.[6] Late latent syphilis (more than a year old) and tertiary syphilis necessitate prolonged treatment. Parenteral penicillin G should be administered to a pregnant woman as part of her treatment to prevent congenital syphilis. Penicillin should be used to desensitize pregnant women who have an allergy to penicillin. At the time of diagnosis, everyone with syphilis should be tested for HIV, and if the results are negative, HIV pre-exposure prophylaxis should be offered (*see* **Table 4**).

■ LYMPHOGRANULOMA VENEREUM

There is no clinical preliminary for ideal treatment length for suggestive cases. Doxycycline is prescribed for a 21-day course.[7] A brief retrospective study of MSM (men who have sex with men) with

TABLE 2: Treatment for gonococcal infection.

	Drug	First line/second line	Dosage and route of administration	Mechanism of action	Pharmacokinetics	Contraindication	Side effects
Uncomplicated (cervix, urethra, rectum and pharynx)	Ceftriaxone	First line	500 mg IM single dose	Bactericidal action, inhibition of bacterial cell wall synthesis	At $t_{1/2}$ is 8 hours, good CSF penetration, elimination in urine and bile, highly resistant to beta-lactamase from gram-negative bacteria	Allergy	Thrombophlebitis, hypoprothrombinemia, and bleeding
	Gentamycin + Azithromycin	Second line	240 mg IM in a single dose	Bactericidal action by secondary changes in integrity of cell membrane and inhibition of protein synthesis	Plasma $t_{1/2}$ 2–4 hours, broader-spectrum, concentration dependent cidal action	Gentamicin use is cautioned during pregnancy.	Nephrotoxic, ototoxic, fetal ototoxicity, neuromuscular blockade
			2 g orally in a single dose	Inhibition of protein synthesis, bactericidal at higher concentration	At $t_{1/2}$ ≥50 hours, acid stability, rapid oral absorption, marked tissue distribution, and intracellular penetration, mainly excreted in bile	Causes rise in plasma levels of carbamazepine, valproate, warfarin ergotamine, terfenadine	Mild gastric upset and abdominal pain
	Cefixime	Second line	800 mg orally in a single dose	Bactericidal action, inhibition of bacterial cell wall synthesis	At $t_{1/2}$ is 3 hours, elimination in urine and bile, highly resistant to beta-lactamase from gram-negative bacteria	Allergy	Stool changes and diarrhea

Contd...

Contd...

	Drug	First line/ second line	Dosage and route of administration	Mechanism of action	Pharmacokinetics	Contraindication	Side effects
Conjunctivitis	Ceftriaxone	First line	1 g IM in a single dose	–	–	–	–
Arthritis and arthritis–dermatitis syndrome	Ceftriaxone	First line	1 g IM or IV every 24 hours	–		–	–
	Cefotaxime	Second line	1 g IV every 8 hours	Third-generation, potent action on gram-positive and aerobic gram-negative enterobacteriaceae, bactericidal, inhibition of bacterial cell wall synthesis	High CSF levels, $t_{1/2}$ 1 hour but higher for the deacetylated metabolite	Allergy	Thrombophlebitis at injection site
	Ceftizoxime	Second line	1 g every 8 hours	Third generation, bactericidal action, inhibition of bacterial cell wall synthesis	Not metabolized, renal excretion, $t_{1/2}$ 1.5–2 hours	Allergy, cautious use in renal disease	Thrombophlebitis at injection site
Meningitis and endocarditis	Ceftriaxone	First line	1–2 g IV every 12–24 hours	–	–	–	–

(CSF: cerebrospinal fluid; IM: intramuscular; IV: intravenous)

TABLE 3: Treatment for chlamydial infection.

	Drug	First line/second line	Dosage and route of administration	Mechanism of action	Pharmacokinetics	Contraindication	Side effects
Adolescents and adults	Doxycycline	First line	• 100 mg orally • Two times a day for 7 days	Inhibits protein synthesis by binding to 30S ribosomes	Lipid soluble, intracellular higher concentration, higher potency, complete intestinal absorption, $t_{1/2}$ 18–24 hours, least alteration of intestinal flora and excreted in feces	Pregnancy, lactation, cautious use if renal disease	Phototoxicity, low renal toxicity
	Azithromycin	Second line	1 g orally in a single dose	–		–	–
	Levofloxacin	Second line	500 mg orally once daily for 7 days	Inhibits bacterial DNA gyrase which prevents excessive supercoiling of DNA strands while replication or transcription; bactericidal action is due to digestion of damaged DNA by exonuclease	Oral bioavailability is 100%, plasma protein binding is 25%, $t_{1/2}$ 8 hours, high tissue permeability, excreted unchanged primarily in urine	Pregnancy, lactation	Nausea, anorexia, dizziness anxiety, impairment of concentration and dexterity

Contd...

Contd...

	Drug	First line/ second line	Dosage and route of administration	Mechanism of action	Pharmacokinetics	Contraindication	Side effects
During pregnancy	Azithromycin	First line	1 g orally single dose	–	–	–	–
	Amoxicillin	Second line	500 mg orally three times a day for 7 days	Interferes with bacterial cell wall synthesis	High bioavailability, higher and sustained blood levels, less diarrhea, enterohepatic circulation, primarily renal excretion	Allergy	Rashes, hypersensitivity
Neonates, infants	Erythromycin base or ethyl-succinate	First line	50 mg/kg body weight/day orally, divided into four doses for 14 days	Bacteriostatic at low but cidal at high concentration, combines with 50S ribosome and interferes translocation	Acid labile, absorption delayed by food, crosses serous membrane and placenta but not blood–brain barrier, $t_{1/2}$ is 1.5 hours, 70–80% plasma protein bound, excreted in bile	QT prolongation, serious ventricular arrhythmias and death due to inhibition of CYP3A4 when used with terfenadine/ astemizole/ cisapride	Gastrointestinal (GI) side effects, reversible hearing defect, hepatitis, cholestatic jaundice

TABLE 4: Treatment for syphilis.

	Drug	First line/ second line	Dosage and route of administration	Mechanism of action	Pharmacokinetics	Contraindication	Side effects
Early latent syphilis	Benzathine penicillin G	First line	2.4 million units IM in a single dose	Interferes with bacterial cell wall synthesis, no interference with blood, pus and tissue fluid in antibacterial action, narrow spectrum	Acid labile rapid and complete absorption from IM site, extracellular distribution, 60% plasma protein bound, releases penicillin very slowly, remain effective for prophylactic purposes for up to 4 weeks	Allergy may cause anaphylaxis	Thrombophlebitis, mental confusion, muscular twitching, convulsion and coma; Jarisch–Herxheimer reaction in a syphilitic patient
Late latent syphilis	Benzathine penicillin G	First line	2.4 million units IM 3 doses at 1-week interval	–	–	–	–
Latent syphilis	Doxycycline	Second line	100 mg orally two times per day for 28 days	–	–	–	–
	Tetracycline	Second line	500 mg orally four times per day for 28 days	Inhibits protein synthesis by binding to 30S ribosomes	Low potency, better absorption in empty stomach, widely distributed in body, concentrated in liver and spleen and bind to connective tissue in bone and teeth, $t_{1/2}$ is 6–10 hours, marked alteration of intestinal flora, excreted in urine	Pregnancy and lactation and in children, cautious use in hepatic and renal disease	Phototoxicity, tooth discoloration, intestinal superinfection

Contd...

SECTION 13: Medical Management of Infections in Gynecology

Contd...

	Drug	First line/ second line	Dosage and route of administration	Mechanism of action	Pharmacokinetics	Contraindication	Side effects
Primary and secondary syphilis	Benzathine penicillin G	First line	2.4 million units IM in a single dose	–	–	–	–
	Doxycycline + Tetracycline	Second line	100 mg orally two times per day + 500 mg orally four times per day for 14 days		–	–	–
	Ceftriaxone	Second line	1 g daily either IM or IV for 10 days	–	–	–	
	Azithromycin	Second line	Single 2-g oral dose	–	–	–	–
Tertiary syhilis	Benzathine penicillin G	First line	2.4 million units IM 3 doses at 1-week interval	–	–	–	–

rectal LGV (lymphogranuloma venereum) revealed a 97% cure rate after a 7–14 days course of doxycycline.[8] Shorter courses of doxycycline for the treatment of LGV are awaiting randomized prospective studies. The treatment regimens for fistulas, buboes, and other severe diseases must be extended.

A Spanish study found weekly 1-g azithromycin regimen for 3 weeks equally effective.[9] Fluoroquinolone's optimal treatment duration has not been evaluated. The same regimens should be given to people with LGV and HIV infection as to people without HIV. Due to the possibility of a delay in the resolution of symptoms, prolonged therapy may be required **(Table 5)**.

CHANCROID (SOFT SORE)

A single dose of azithromycin and ceftriaxone is effective. Additionally, ciprofloxacin- and erythromycin-resistant intermediate isolates have been reported.

Suppurative buboes can cause genital scarring as well as rectal or urogenital fistulas despite successful treatment. Both fluctuating lymphadenopathy and buboes necessitate drainage through an incision or a needle aspiration. HIV patients may require multiple or extended courses of treatment and any treatment regimen may fail[10] (*see* **Table 5**).

GRANULOMA INGUINALE (DONOVANOSIS)

There have only been a few published controlled trials for the treatment of donovanosis.[11] The use of various antimicrobial regimens has been successful. For the ulcers to granulate and re-epithelialize, prolonged treatment is typically required. Six to eighteen months after therapy appears to be working, relapse can occur. A macrolide regimen should be used to treat granuloma inguinale in pregnant and breastfeeding women (*see* **Table 5**).

MYCOPLASMA GENITALIUM

Treatment should consist of two stages: Ideally, macrolide-resistance testing has been found to have cure rates of >90%.[11] Doxycycline is provided initially to reduce the organism load, then macrolide-sensitive infections are treated with high-dose azithromycin. Macrolide-resistant infections are treated with moxifloxacin[12] **(Table 6)**.

HERPES GENITALIS

Antiviral medication is the mainstay of treatment and relieves symptoms. Acyclovir, valacyclovir, and famciclovir, three Food and Drug Administration (FDA)-approved antiviral medications, have been shown to be effective for treating herpes.[13]

Suppressive or episodic antiviral treatment for recurrent genital herpes is an option. Intravenous (IV) antiviral therapy is required for patients with severe herpes simplex virus (HSV) disease or complications. In patients with frequent recurrences, suppression therapy reduces the frequency of genital herpes recurrences by 70–80%.[14] as well as central nervous system (CNS) complications (such as meningitis or encephalitis) and hospitalization (such as disseminated infections, pneumonitis).

Rarely disseminated HSV infection in pregnant women may manifest as hepatitis and is linked to severe hepatic failure and a high rate of mortality (25%).

To lower the risk of genital ulcer disease (GUD) in HIV-positive individuals, suppressive antiviral therapy can be continued for 6 months following the start of antiretroviral therapy (ART)[15] **(Tables 7 and 8)**.

TABLE 5: Treatment for chancroid, lymphogranuloma venereum (LGV), granuloma inguinale.

	Drug	First line/ second line	Dosage and route of administration	Mechanism of action	Pharmacokinetics	Contraindication	Side effects
Chancroid	Azithromycin	First line	1 g orally single dose	–	–	–	–
	Ceftriaxone	Second line	250 mg IM single dose	–	–	–	–
	Ciprofloxacin	Second line	500 mg orally two times per day for 3 days	Inhibits bacterial DNA gyrase which prevents excessive supercoiling of DNA strands while replication or transcription; bactericidal action is due to digestion of damaged DNA by exonuclease	Oral bioavailability 60–80%, high tissue penetrability, $t_{1/2}$ 3–5 hours, urinary and biliary concentration is 10–50 times higher than plasma, primarily excreted in urine	Pregnancy, breastfeeding	Nausea, anorexia, dizziness anxiety, impairment of concentration and dexterity, tendonitis
	Erythromycin base	Second line	500 mg orally three times per day for 7 days	–	–	–	–
LGV	Doxycycline	First line	100 mg orally two times per day for 21 days	–	–	–	–
	Azithromycin	Second line	1 g orally once weekly for 3 weeks	–	–	–	–
	Erythromycin base	Second line	500 mg orally four times per day for 21 days	–	–	–	–

Contd...

Contd...

	Drug	First line/second line	Dosage and route of administration	Mechanism of action	Pharmacokinetics	Contraindication	Side effects
Granuloma inguinale	Azithromycin	Second line	1 g orally once weekly until all lesions have completely healed	–	–	–	–
	Doxycycline	Second line	100 mg orally two times per day for 3 weeks	–	–	–	–
	Erythromycin base	Second line	500 mg orally four times per day >3 weeks	–	–	–	–
	Trimethoprim–sulfamethoxazole	Second line	(160 mg/800 mg) tablet orally two times per day for >3 weeks	Inhibits bacterial folate synthetase and dihydrofolate reductase	Both have same $t_{1/2}$ 10 hours, trimethoprim crosses blood–brain barrier and placenta and is rapidly absorbed than sulfamethoxazole. Metabolized in liver and excreted in urine	Pregnancy, cautious use in renal disease	Stomatitis, headache, folate deficiency, blood dyscrasias, bone marrow toxicity

(CSF: cerebrospinal fluid; IM: intramuscular)

TABLE 6: Treatment for *Mycoplasma genitalium*.

	Drug
Mycoplasma genitalium (macrolide-sensitive)	Doxycycline 100 mg orally two times per day for 7 days followed by azithromycin 1 g dose then 500 mg orally once daily for 3 additional days (2.5 g total)
M. genitalium (macrolide-resistant)	Doxycycline 100 mg orally two times per day for 7 days, followed by moxifloxacin 400 mg orally once daily for 7 days

TABLE 7: Treatment for herpes genitalis.

	Drug	First line/second line	Dosage and route of administration
Genital herpes	Acyclovir	First line	400 mg orally three times per day for 7–10 days
	Famciclovir	Second line	250 mg orally three times per day for 7–10 days
	Valacyclovir	Second line	1 g orally two times per day for 7–10 days
Recurrent HSV-2 genital herpes	Acyclovir		400 mg orally two times per day
	Valacyclovir	Second line	1 g orally once a day
	Famciclovir	Second line	250 mg orally two times per day
Episodic therapy for recurrent HSV-2 genital herpes	Acyclovir	First line	800 mg orally two times per day for 5 days OR 800 mg orally three times per day for 2 days
	Famciclovir	Second line	1 g orally two times per day for 1 day OR 500 mg orally once followed by 250 mg two times per day for 2 days
	Valacyclovir	Second line	500 mg orally two times per day for 3 days OR 1 g orally once daily for 5 days
Severe disease	Acyclovir	First line	5–10 mg/kg body weight IV every 8 hours (until clinical improvement is observed) THEN Valacyclovir 1 g three times per day to complete a 10- to 14-day regimen
Antiviral-resistant HSV infection	Foscarnet		80–120 mg/kg/day IV in two to three divided doses until clinical resolution is attained
	Imiquimod 5%	Second line	Applied to the lesion for 8 hours three times per week until clinical resolution
	Cidofovir gel 1%	Second line	Topical application two to four times daily
Recurrent genital herpes among pregnant women*	Acyclovir	First line	400 mg orally three times per day
	Valacyclovir	Second line	500 mg two times per day

* Starting at 36 weeks' gestation
(HSV: herpes simplex virus; IV: intravenous)

TABLE 8: Drugs for herpes genitalis.

Drugs	Mechanism of action	Pharmacokinetics	Contraindication	Side effects
Acyclovir	Inhibits DNA synthesis and viral replication	Only 20% of oral dose is absorbed, less plasma protein bound, crosses CSF and cornea; plasma $t_{1/2}$ 2–3 hours, excreted unchanged in urine	Cautious use in renal diseases	Stinging sensation, headache nausea, malaise, rashes, sweating, dose-dependent decrease in GFR, reversible neurological manifestation (tremors, disorientation, hallucinations, convulsion, coma)
Famciclovir	Ester prodrug of a guanine nucleoside analog penciclovir, inhibits DNA synthesis and viral replication	Good oral bioavailability, prolonged $t_{1/2}$ of the active metabolite	Cautious use in renal diseases	Headache, nausea, loose motions, itching, rashes and mental confusion
Foscarnet	Simple straight chain phosphonate, inhibits viral DNA polymerase and reverse transcriptase	Poor oral absorption, $t_{1/2}$ 4–8 hours, not metabolized	Cautious use in renal diseases	High toxicity, renal diabetes-like condition, acute renal failure, anemia, phlebitis, tremors, convulsions and hypocalcemia

(CSF: cerebrospinal fluid; GFR: glomerular filtration rate)

CONDYLOMA ACUMINATA (WARTS)

Treatment options can be provided by a doctor or a patient themselves. Imiquimod is an immune enhancer that is applied topically to the patient and increases the production of interferon and other cytokines.[16] Podoflox (podophyllotoxin), an antimitotic, and sinecatechins, a green tea extract with an active ingredient (catechins), also can be used by patients. Cryotherapy is a treatment that is given by a doctor and works by destroying warts through cytolysis caused by heat. Warts are destroyed by chemically coagulating proteins with trichloroacetic acid (TCA) and bichloroacetic acid (BCA). When a full course of treatment yields no significant improvement or if severe side effects occur, a new treatment approach should be considered.

Sinecatechins, podoflox, and podophyllin should not be taken during pregnancy. Anogenital warts are more common in HIV-positive or otherwise immunosuppressed individuals. Persistent infection with high-risk (oncogenic) human papillomavirus (HPV) types may cause many genital and oropharyngeal cancers **(Box 1)**.

> **BOX 1:** Recommended regimens for different types of warts.
>
> *Recommended regimens for external anogenital warts:*
> - Patient-applied imiquimod 3.75% or 5% cream*/podofilox 0.5% solution or gel/sinecatechins 15% ointment*
> - *Provider administered*: Cryotherapy with liquid nitrogen/surgical removal
> - TCA or BCA 80–90% solution
>
> * Might weaken condoms and vaginal diaphragm
>
> *Recommended regimens for urethral meatus warts:*
> - Cryotherapy with liquid nitrogen/surgical removal
>
> *Recommended regimens for vaginal warts and cervical† warts:*
> - Cryotherapy with liquid nitrogen/surgical removal/TCA or BCA 80–90% solution
>
> *Cryoprobe is not recommended because of the risk for vaginal perforation and fistula formation.
> †A biopsy evaluation to exclude HSIL should be performed before treatment is initiated.
> (BCA: bichloroacetic acid; HSIL: high-grade squamous intraepithelial lesions; TCA: trichloroacetic acid)

TABLE 9: Treatment for *Trichomonas* vaginitis.

Drug	Mechanism of action	Pharmacokinetics	Contraindication	Side effects
Metronidazole	Nitro group is reduced in anaerobic microbes to highly reactive nitro radicals which damage DNA and other critical biomolecules	Completely absorbed from intestine, widely distributed in therapeutic concentration in vaginal secretion, semen, saliva and cerebrospinal fluid (CSF); metabolized in liver and excreted in urine $t_{1/2}$ is 8 hours	Neurological disease, blood dyscrasias, chronic alcoholism and first trimester of pregnancy	Anorexia, metallic taste, abdominal cramps, glossitis, dizziness, transient neutropenia, peripheral neuropathy, seizures
Tinidazole	Same as metronidazole	Slower metabolism, longer duration of action, $t_{1/2}$ 12 hours	Same as metronidazole	Metallic taste, nausea, rashes
Secnidazole	Same as metronidazole	Rapid and complete absorption, slower metabolism, $t_{1/2}$ 17–29 hours	Same as metronidazole	Metallic taste, nausea, rashes

■ TRICHOMONAS VAGINITIS

The only class of drugs that can treat trichomoniasis is the 5-nitroimidazole class, which includes metronidazole, tinidazole, and secnidazole.[17,18]

First-line treatment for trichomoniasis: Metronidazole 500 mg orally two times per day for 7 days.

Alternative treatments:
- *Single-dose option:* Metronidazole 2 g/tinidazole 2 g/secnidazole 2 g: Orally single dose
- *Multi-dose*: Tinidazole 500 mg orally two times per day for 5 days

Refractory disease:
- Tinidazole 2 g orally daily for 14 days plus vaginal tinidazole 500 mg 2 times/day for 14 days OR

TABLE 10: Treatment for scabies and pediculosis pubis.

	Drug	First line/ second line	Dosage and route of administration	Mechanism of action	Pharmacokinetics	Contraindication	Side effects
Scabies	Permethrin 5% cream	First line	Applied to all areas of the body from neck down and washed off after 8–14 hours	Neurological paralysis in insects by delaying depolarization	Broad-spectrum and potent pyrethroid insecticide, resistance is rare	–	Burning, itching tingling, and erythema
	Ivermectin		200 µg/kg body weight orally, repeated in 14 days	Acts through glutamate-gated chlorine channel found in invertebrates and causes tonic paralysis	Well absorbed orally, wide distribution, sequestered in liver and fat, $t_{1/2}$ 48–60 hours, limited ovicidal activity	Pregnancy, lactation and children ≤5 years	Pruritis, giddiness, abdominal pain, lethargy, transient ECG changes, constipation
	Lindane 1%		30 g of cream applied in a thin layer to all areas of body from neck down and thoroughly washed off after 8 hours	Penetrate through the chitinous cover and affecting the nervous system	Broad-spectrum, resistance can develop, highly lipid-soluble, $t_{1/2}$ 24 hours	Cautious use in pregnancy, breastfeeding, children under the age of 10, people with extensive dermatitis	CNS stimulation, vertigo, convulsions, cardiac arrhythmias

Contd...

SECTION 13: Medical Management of Infections in Gynecology

Contd...

	Drug	First line/ second line	Dosage and route of administration	Mechanism of action	Pharmacokinetics	Contraindication	Side effects
Pediculosis pubis	Permethrin 1%		Cream rinse applied to affected areas and washed off after 10 minutes	–	–	–	–
	Pyrethrin with piperonyl butoxide		Applied to the affected areas and washed off after 10 minutes	–	–	–	–
	Malathione 0.5%		Lotion applied to affected areas and washed off after 8–12 hours	Irreversible anticholinesterase	–	–	Low toxicity
	Ivermectin		250 µg/kg body weight orally, repeated in 7–14 days	–	–	–	–

(CNS: central nervous system; ECG: electrocardiography)

- Tinidazole 1 g orally three times per day for 14 days plus vaginal boric acid 600 mg two times per day for 28 days OR
- Tinidazole 1 g orally three times per day for 14 days plus vaginal paromomycin 6.25% given as 4 g bedtime for 14 days **(Table 9)**.

SCABIES

The effectiveness of permethrin and ivermectin for treating scabies is comparable.[19] Permethrin can be used once and is safe and effective. A repeat dose of ivermectin should be given after 2 weeks to prevent recurrence.[20] Ivermectin's bioavailability can be improved by taking it with food. Patients with renal impairment do not require dosage adjustments for ivermectin; notwithstanding, the wellbeing of numerous portions among patients with extreme liver sickness is obscure. Due to its potential for toxicity, lindane is an alternative treatment.[21] It should only be used if the patient is unable to tolerate the recommended treatments or if they have failed. Lindane should not be used by women who are pregnant or breastfeeding. When lindane was applied after a bath or used by patients with extensive dermatitis, seizures have occurred. Additionally, lindane use has been linked to aplastic anemia[21] **(Table 10)**.

PEDICULOSIS PUBIS

Permethrin and pyrethrin resistance has been reported to be on the rise and widespread.[19] When resistance is suspected to have caused treatment failure, malathion can be used (*see* **Table 10**).

KEY POINTS

- Ceftriaxone is a drug of choice for gonorrhea, alternatively cefixime can be used.
- Doxycycline is the treatment of choice for infection caused by *C. trachomatis*.
- Syphilis are best treated with penicillin G.
- Doxycycline is prescribed for a 21-days in LGV infection.
- A single dose of azithromycin and ceftriaxone is effective.
- Acyclovir, valacyclovir, and famciclovir are three FDA-approved antiviral medications for herpes genitalis.
- The only class of drugs that can treat trichomoniasis is the 5-nitroimidazole class, which includes metronidazole, tinidazole, and secnidazole.

REFERENCES

1. Sánchez-Busó L, Golparian D, Corander J, Grad YH, Ohnishi M, Flemming R, et al. The impact of antimicrobials on gonococcal evolution. Nat Microbiol. 2019;4:1941-50.
2. Connolly KL, Eakin AE, Gomez C, Osborn BL, Unemo M, Jerse AE. Pharmacokinetic data are predictive of in vivo efficacy for cefixime and ceftriaxone against susceptible and resistant *Neisseria gonorrhoeae* strains in the Gonorrhea Mouse Model. Antimicrob Agents Chemother. 2019;63:e0164418.
3. Kirkcaldy RD, Weinstock HS, Moore PC, Philip SS, Wiesenfeld HC, Papp JR, et al. The efficacy and safety of gentamicin plus azithromycin and gemifloxacin plus azithromycin as treatment of uncomplicated gonorrhea. Clin Infect Dis. 2014;59:1083-91.
4. Páez-Canro C, Alzate JP, González LM, Rubio-Romero JA, Lethaby A, Gaitán HG. Antibiotics for treating urogenital *Chlamydia trachomatis* infection in men and non-pregnant women. Cochrane Database Syst Rev. 2019;1:CD010871.
5. Rahangdale L, Guerry S, Bauer HM, Packel L, Rhew M, Baxter R, et al. An observational cohort study of *Chlamydia trachomatis* treatment in pregnancy. Sex Transm Dis. 2006;33:106-10.
6. Ganesan A, Mesner O, Okulicz JF, O'Bryan T, Deiss RG, Lalani T, et al. Infectious Disease Clinical Research Program HIV/STI Working Group. Infectious Disease Clinical Research Program HIV/STI Working Group. A single dose of benzathine penicillin G is

as effective as multiple doses of benzathine penicillin G for the treatment of HIV-infected persons with early syphilis. Clin Infect Dis. 2015;60:653-60.
7. Leeyaphan C, Ong JJ, Chow EP, Kong FY, Hocking JS, Bissessor M, et al. Systematic review and meta-analysis of doxycycline efficacy for rectal lymphogranuloma venereum in men who have sex with men. Emerg Infect Dis. 2016;22:1778-84.
8. Simons R, Candfield S, French P, White JA. Observed treatment responses to short-course doxycycline therapy for rectal lymphogranuloma venereum in men who have sex with men. Sex Transm Dis. 2018;45:406-8.
9. Kong FY, Rupasinghe TW, Simpson JA, Vodstrcil LA, Fairley CK, McConville MJ, et al. Pharmacokinetics of a single 1 g dose of azithromycin in rectal tissue in men. PLoS One. 2017;12:e0174372.
10. Lewis DA. Epidemiology, clinical features, diagnosis and treatment of *Haemophilus ducreyi*—a disappearing pathogen? Expert Rev Anti Infect Ther. 2014;12:687-96.
11. O'Farrell N. Donovanosis. Sex Transm Infect. 2002;78:452-7.
12. Durukan D, Read TRH, Murray G, Doyle M, Chow EPF, Vodstrcil LA, et al. Resistance-guided antimicrobial therapy using doxycycline-moxifloxacin and doxycycline-2.5g azithromycin for the treatment of *Mycoplasma genitalium* infection: efficacy and tolerability. Clin Infect Dis. 2020;71:1461-8.
13. Aoki FY, Tyring S, Diaz-Mitoma F, Gross G, Gao J, Hamed K. Single-day, patient-initiated famciclovir therapy for recurrent genital herpes: a randomized, double-blind, placebo-controlled trial. Clin Infect Dis. 2006;42:8-13.
14. Romanowski B, Marina RB, Roberts JN; Valtrex HS230017 Study Group. Patients' preference of valacyclovir once-daily suppressive therapy versus twice-daily episodic therapy for recurrent genital herpes: a randomized study. Sex Transm Dis. 2003;30:226-31.
15. Tobian AA, Grabowski MK, Serwadda D, Newell K, Ssebbowa P, Franco V, et al.; Rakai Health Sciences Program. Reactivation of herpes simplex virus type 2 after initiation of antiretroviral therapy. J Infect Dis. 2013;208:839-46.
16. Mashiah J, Brenner S. Possible mechanisms in the induction of vitiligo-like hypopigmentation by topical imiquimod. Clin Exp Dermatol. 2008;33:74-6.
17. Workowski KA, Bachmann LH, Chan PA, Johnston CM, Muzny CA, Park I, et al. Sexually Transmitted Infections, 2021. MMWR Recomm Rep. 2021;70:1-187.
18. World Health Organization. Guidelines for the management of symptomatic sexually transmitted infections. Geneva: World Health Organization; 2021.
19. Scott GR, Chosidow O; IUSTI/WHO. European guideline for the management of pediculosis pubis, 2010. Int J STD AIDS. 2011;22:304-5.
20. Abdel-Raheem TA, Méabed EM, Nasef GA, Abdel Wahed WY, Rohaim RM. Efficacy, acceptability and cost effectiveness of four therapeutic agents for treatment of scabies. J Dermatolog Treat. 2016;27:473-9.
21. Chiu S, Argaez C. Ivermectin for parasitic skin infections of scabies: a review of comparative clinical effectiveness, cost-effectiveness, and guidelines. Ottawa, ON: Canadian Agency for Drugs and Technologies in Health; 2019.

Index

Page numbers followed by *b* refer to box, *f* refer to figure, *fc* refer to flowchart, and *t* refer to table

A

Abacavir 157, 160
Abaloparatide 366
Abnormal uterine bleeding 233
   medications for 233*b*
   treatment of 234
Acarbose 179
Acenocoumarol 53
Acetazolamide 201
Acne 313, 323
   treatment of 263
Acquired immunodeficiency
      syndrome 158, 374
Activated partial thromboplastin
      time 39, 57, 59*f*, 151
Acupressure 209
Acupuncture 209
Acyclovir 106, 381, 384, 385, 389
Addison disease 294
Adefovir 85
Adenomas, pituitary 294
Adenomyosis 238
Adenosine 45
   triphosphate 12*f*
Adrenal hyperplasia, adult-onset
      congenital 290
Adrenogenital syndrome 294
Adverse drug reactions 342, 343
Adverse pregnancy outcome,
      pathophysiology of 74
Alanine
   aminotransferase 179
   transaminase 82, 83, 107, 132
Albendazole 142
Alcohol 339
Alendronate 342, 355, 356, 365
Allergic reactions 313
Alpha-glucosidase inhibitors 180
Alzheimer's disease 300
Amantadine 142
Amenorrhea 298, 301
   hypergonadotropic
      primary 279
   hypogonadotropic
      primary 290
   post-pill 301
   primary 278, 278*t*, 279*fc*, 280*fc*
   secondary 290, 294, 295*fc*

Amikacin 141, 170, 171
Aminoglycosides 132, 139,
      141, 171
Aminopenicillins 227
Amiodarone 51
Amitriptyline 229
Ammonia, high 88
Amoxzicillin 131, 140, 227, 378
   clavulanic acid 139
Ampicillin 40, 106, 139,
      140, 227
Amprenavir 157, 160
Anaphylaxis 16
Anastrazole 309, 256, 266, 305
Andractim 289
Androgen 235, 236, 279, 287
   insensitivity syndrome 288
   pharmacotherapy
      contraindications
         of 289*b*
      side effects of 289*b*
   receptors, deficiency of 288
   replacement therapy 289*t*
Anemia 3
   acute hemolytic 19
   autoimmune hemolytic 20
   causes of 4, 14
   medical management of 1
   megaloblastic 9, 10*b*, 10*t*
   nutritional 14
   severe 19, 116, 129
   severity of 3, 3*t*
Anesthesia, neuraxial 25
Anorexia 301, 382
   nervosa 291
Anosmia 290
Anovulation 298
   medical management
      of 303
Anovulatory infertility 268
   treatment of 265
Antacid 210
Antepartum 137
Antiandrogens 264, 270, 272,
      272*t*, 290
   second-line 264
Antiangiogenesis factors 255
Antiaromatase agents 338
Antiarrhythmic drugs 45, 45*t*

Antibiotics 40, 131*t*, 138, 139
   empirical 138*t*
   role of 226
   therapy 129
Antibodies, adrenocortical 286
Anticholinergics 95
Anticoagulant 338, 340
   drugs 53*t*
   effect, monitoring of 52
   therapy 50, 59*f*
Anticoagulation 58, 67
Antidiarrheal agents, role of 221
Antiepileptic drug 197, 198, 198*f*,
      199, 203*fc*, 338
   prescription of 196
Antifibrinolytic drug 150, 242
Antifungal drugs 142, 339
Antihistamines 210, 300
Antihypertensive therapy 23
Antimalarials 142
Antimicrobials 104-107, 140*t*
Anti-Mullerian hormone
      283, 285
Antioxidant 297
   supplementation 24
Antiphospholipid antibodies 328
Antiplatelets 349
Antiprogestin 242, 243*t*
Antiprogestogens 250
Antiprotozoals 142
Antiretroviral drugs 155, 159*t*
   classes of 157*t*
   targets of 156*f*
Antiretroviral therapy 155, 163,
      166, 381
   adverse effects of 165*t*
Antiretroviral treatment,
      first-line 166
Antispasmodics 229
Antithrombin 57
Anti-thyroid drugs 193*t*
Anti-thyroid peroxidase 190
   antibody 191
Antitubercular drugs 168,
      300, 339
Antral follicle count 285
Anxiety 267, 382
Apgar scores, suboptimal 196
Appendicitis 207

Arformoterol 95
Aromatase 309
  enzyme, role of 254*f*
  inhibitors 245*t*, 250, 254, 256, 266, 305, 309
    classification of 309*t*
    mechanism of action of 254
    third-generation 256
Arrhythmias 43, 126
  cardiac 116
  types of 63
Arterial blood gas 137
Arthritis 376
Ascites 88
Asherman syndrome 294, 300
Asoprisnil 237
Aspartate
  aminotransferase 179
  transaminase 107, 132
  high 88
Aspirin 51
  low-dose 23, 24
Assisted reproductive technology 318
  intervention 155
  regimen 163
Asthenia 310
Asthma 93
  acute severe 96
  bronchial 93, 95*t*, 149
  control 98
Ataxia 362
Atazanavir 157
Atrial fibrillation 365
Atrial natriuretic peptide 62*f*
Atropine 227
  combination 224
Auditory neurotoxicity 16
Autoimmune disease 294
Autologous vulvar tissue 288
Azathioprine 19
Azidothymidine 9
Azithromycin 141, 227, 375, 377, 378, 380, 382-384
  plus 106
Azoles 142
Aztreonam 141

B

Baldwin vaginoplasty 288
Barbiturate use, fetal risks of 202
Barrier contraceptive 374
Bazedoxifene 340, 364, 369

Beclomethasone 96
Bedaquiline 170, 171
Benzathine 374
  penicillin G 40, 140, 379, 380
Benzodiazepines 339
Beta-adrenergic receptor
  agonists 116
Beta-agonists 95, 116, 117*t*
  long-acting 94
  short-acting 94, 95, 98
Beta-blockers 41, 43, 41*t*, 66, 114
Beta-lactam 106
Betamethasone 117
Beta-thalassemia
  major 17
  transfusion-dependent 17
Bicalutamide 265
Bicarbonate 185
Bichloroacetic acid 385, 386
Bictegravir 157
Biguanides 179
Bile acid
  management of 222
  sequestrants 222, 224, 227
Birth
  defects 349
  premature 113
Bisacodyl 219
Bishop's score 121
Bismuth subsalicylate 224, 227
Bisphosphonate 242, 342, 342*t*, 355, 356, 363, 364, 365*t*, 367
  oral 364
  side effects of 364
Bloating, abdominal 339
Blood
  disorders, inherited 16
  dyscrasias 383
  pressure 24, 62*f*, 136, 262
    medication 348
    systolic 66
  sugar 15, 207, 336
    fasting 177, 183
    postprandial 177, 183
  transfusion 17
Body mass index 270, 278, 285, 297, 323
Bone 362, 366
  formation 366
  health 286
  impairment 347
  loss 252
  marrow toxicity 383

mineral density 340, 354, 366
resorption inhibitor 366
Brain 30
  natriuretic peptide 62*f*
Breast
  cancer 286, 300
    lesser degree 296
  enlargement 313
  tenderness 296, 339
Breath
  shortness of 100
  sound, abnormal 100
Bromocriptine 67, 292, 296, 301, 308
Bronchial asthma 93, 95*t*, 149
  drug therapy of 94*t*
  management of 94*f*
Bronchoconstriction 98
Bronchodilator responsiveness 93
Budesonide 96
Bulimia nervosa 301
Bulk-forming agents 217, 219
Bupropion 267
Buserelin 256

C

Cabergoline 292, 296, 308, 328
Cabotegravir 157
Calamine lotion 76
Calcitonin 343, 356, 366
Calcium 344, 357, 363, 368
  calmodulin-myosin light chain kinase system 113
  carbonate 344, 363
  channel blockers 114, 118, 215
  citrate 344, 363
  elemental 344
  flux 113
  gluconate 32
  supplementation 24
Cancer 286
  endometrial 300, 308
Candida albicans 374
Capreomycin 170
Carbamazepine 197, 198, 202, 204
Carbapenem 139, 141
Carbetocin 148, 149
Carbimazole 193, 299
  mechanism of action of 299*t*
Carbohydrates 177
Carbon dioxide 14
Carbonyl iron 4
Carboprost 149
Cardiac defects 197

Cardiac disease 50
Cardiomyopathy, peripartum 67
Cardiovascular disease 39, 338, 347
Cardiovascular health 286
Carle's obstetric early warning score 136f
Carvedilol 64
Cataracts 349
Catechins 385
Cefadroxil cefazolin cephalexin 140
Cefixime 140, 375
Cefoperazone 140
Cefotaxime 106, 140, 376
Cefotetan 140
Cefoxitin 140
Ceftizoxime 376
Ceftriaxone 106, 139, 140, 373, 375, 376, 380, 382, 389
Cefuroxime 140
Cell growth, unbalanced 9
Centchroman 236
Central nervous system 204, 212, 280, 301, 351, 381, 388
 fetal 55
Cephalosporins 140, 227
 third-generation 139
Cerebral
 circulation, stabilization of 115
 palsy 119
Cerebrospinal fluid 376, 383
Cervical atresia, acquired 294
Cervical intraepithelial neoplasia 374
Cervix 375
Cesarean delivery 46, 129
Cesarean section 129, 130
 lower segment 123, 127
Chancroid 374, 381, 382
 treatment of 382t
Chelation therapies 16
Chemotherapy 285, 299
Chest pain, pleuritic 100
Chlamydia 373
 infection, treatment of 377t
 trachomatis 373, 374
Chloasma 296
Chloramphenicol 142
Chloroquine 142
Chlorpheniramine 76, 77
Chlorpromazine 210
Cholangitis 338

Cholecalciferol 344
Cholecystitis 207, 338
Cholelithiasis 207
Cholestasis, intrahepatic 73, 76t
Cholesterol, total 297
Cholestyramine 76, 77, 222, 224, 227
Chorioamnionitis 114, 119, 138
Chorionic villus sampling 199
Chromosomal analysis 288
Chronic obstructive pulmonary disease 107
Cidofovir gel 384
Cilastatin 141
Cimetidine 51
Ciprofloxacin 142, 224, 228, 382
Citalopram 341, 353
Clarithromycin 108, 141
Clavulanic acid 140
Clindamycin 139, 141
Clofazimine 170
Clomiphene 265, 266, 301, 305, 308
 citrate 266, 305-307, 314, 321
 resistance 307
 management of 307
 structure of 306f
Clonidine 27, 341, 348, 350, 351, 354
 dosage of 351
Cloxacillin 140
Coagulopathy 88
Cognitive behavioral therapy 344
Coinfection 158
Colestipol 222
Combined hormonal contraceptives 251, 251f
Combined oral contraceptives 236, 236b, 249, 250, 270, 271
 pills 235, 296, 238
Complete androgen insensitivity syndrome 288
Complete blood count 10, 137, 207
Complex pregnancy-associated disorder 23
Computed tomography 278, 280
Condyloma acuminata 374, 385
Conjugated equine estrogen 337
Conjunctivitis 376
Constipation 15, 215, 219t
 causes of 216t
Continuous subcutaneous infusion 182

Contraception, long-acting reversible 198f
Contraceptive
 hormonal 261, 267, 268
 pills 262
Controlled ovarian hyperstimulation 318, 319
 drugs 321t
Corifollitropin alfa 312
Coronary artery disease 300
Coronavirus disease 2019 (COVID-19) 100, 107
 management of 108
Corticosteroids 96, 116, 118-210, 212, 328
 inhaled 94
Cosmetic methods 270, 274
Cough 63
 nonproductive 100
 productive 100
Cryptomenorrhea 290
Cryptorchidism, prepubertal 313
Crystalline, aqueous 374
Cushing's disease 288, 294
Cyanosis 63
Cyclic adenosine monophosphate 249
Cyclooxygenase
 catalyzes 249
 enzymes 116
Cyclophosphamide 19
Cycloserine 171
Cyclosporine 19
Cyproterone acetate 252, 262, 264, 270-273
 blocks 272
Cytochrome 309
Cytokines 249
 pro-inflammatory 249

D

Dalteparin 57
Danazol 235, 236, 250, 254, 256
 side effects of 255f
Darbepoetin 15
Darunavir 157
Davydov vaginoplasty 288
Deep vein thrombosis 308, 315, 342
Dehydroepiandrostenedione sulfate 327
Dehydroepiandrosterone 307, 352

Delamanid 171
Delavirdine 157, 161
Delivery 16
Dementia 339
Denosumab 343, 363, 365-367, 369
Deoxyribonucleic acid 11, 12f, 156f, 157, 225
  recombinant 323
  synthesis 9
Dephosphorylate myosin heads 116
Depilation 275
Depot-medroxy-progesterone acetate 235
Depression 267, 301, 339
Dermatitis syndrome 376
Desferrioxamine 16
Desipramine 229
Desmopressin 234
Desogestrel 271
Desvenlafaxine 349, 353
Dexamethasone 78, 108, 117, 121, 127
Dexterity 382
Dhaka regimen 31
Diabetes mellitus 175, 177, 215, 279, 284, 294, 301
  gestational 175, 179t
  management of 183
  uncontrolled 119
Diabetic ketoacidosis, management of 185, 185b
Dialysis 19
Diarrhea 16, 165, 215, 218, 222, 222t, 225, 310
  acute 220
    infectious 218, 226
    causes of 221t
  chronic 226
    medical management of 227t
    noninfectious chronic 220
Diastolic murmur 63
Diazepam 202
Dicyclomine 229
Didanosine 157, 159
Dienogest 250, 252, 256
Dietary sodium 43
Digitalis 67
Digoxin 64
Dihydrofolate 12f
Dihydrotestosterone 289
  production of 271
Dihydroxyphenylalanine 12f

Diltiazem 45
Dimenhydrinate 209, 210
Dinoprostone 122t, 124
  intravaginal pessary 123t
  prostaglandin E2 122
Diphenhydramine 209, 210
Diphenoxylate 224, 227
Diplopia 350
Discomfort, abdominal 310
Disseminated intravascular coagulation 54
Diuretics 64
  role of 34
  use of 41
Dizziness 201, 202, 296, 350, 382
Dobutamine 64
Dolutegravir 157, 158, 162, 163t
Domperidone 212
Donovania granulomatis 374
Donovanosis 381
Dopamine 64
  agonist 292, 295
Doravirine 157
Doxycycline 373, 377, 379, 380, 382, 383, 384, 389
Doxylamine 209-211
DRESS syndrome 343
Drospirenone 262, 271, 272
Drowsiness 201, 202
Drugs
  antihypertensive 32, 33t
  class 210
  classification of 145fc
  rash 343
  therapy 25, 26t, 94t, 296t, 367
Dry powder inhaler 94, 97
Dual action bone agent 343
Dual-energy X-ray absorptiometry 291, 362
Ductus arteriosus 117
Dydrogesterone 252, 326, 339
Dysfunctional uterine bleeding 290
Dyslipidemia 267
Dysmenorrhea 241, 247
Dysmorphic facies 197
Dysplasia, bronchopulmonary 119
Dyspnea 63, 100

E

Early obstetric warning score, modified 136
Eating disorders 290, 294
Eclampsia 30, 31b, 114

Eculizumab 18, 19b
Edema, vasogenic 30
Efavirenz 157, 161
Eflornithine 265, 273
  hydrochloride 274
Electrocardiography 388
Electrolysis 275, 275t
Elevated jugular venous pressure 63
Elvitegravir 157
Embolism, pulmonary 300, 308, 369
Emollient 217
Empty sella syndrome 294
Emtricitabine 157
Encephalopathy, hepatic 80, 87
Endocarditis 376, 381
Endocrine disorders, medical management of 259
Endocrine Society Clinical Guideline 271
Endocrinopathy 215
Endometrial implants 249
Endometrial preparation 328
  drugs for 327t
Endometriosis 247, 249, 250, 254f
  classic triad of 247f
  etiology of 248
  medical management of 249, 256t
  ovarian 248
  peritoneal 248
  sites of 248
  spectrum of 247f
Endometriotic
  implants, sites of 248f
  lesions, types of 248t
Endometritis 145
Endomyometritis 138
Enema 219
  role of 218
Enoxaparin 57
Entecavir 86
Enteral tube feeding 213
Eosinophilia 343
Epilation 275
Epilepsy 150, 203, 204t
Epinephrine 64
Episiotomy 129
Epistaxis 55
Epoetin 15
Ergometrine 46, 146, 148
Ergot alkaloid 146
Erythromycins 141, 226, 227, 378, 382, 383

Erythropoiesis
  ineffective 9
  megaloblastic 10
  stimulating agent 14, 15, 15*b*
Erythropoietin
  receptor 15
  role of 7
Escitalopram 341, 353
Esmolol 26, 27
Estradiol 281, 282, 337-339, 368
  gel 337
  hemihydrate 318
  patch 337, 337*t*
  pump 337
  spray 337
  transdermal patch 337
  valerate 318, 327, 337, 368
Estrogen 235, 237, 261, 270, 271, 287, 299, 300, 327, 336-339, 367
  conjugated 337, 368, 369
  increased production of 249
  inhibits follicle-stimulating hormone 270
  interferes 338
  only therapy 286
  patches 337
  progesterone challenge test 294
  receptor 281, 306, 342
    modulators 235, 236
  replacement
    goal of 281
    therapy 284
  response element 281
  topical 337*t*
Ethambutol 169
Ethamsylate 234
Ethinylestradiol 261, 271, 281, 337
  lower dose of 251
  molecule 271*f*
  transdermal 271
Ethionamide 171
Ethosuximide 201
Ethyl-succinate 378
Etidronate 365
Etonogestrel 271
  implant 253
    side effects of 253*f*
Etravirine 157
Eugonadotropic primary amenorrhea 287
Excitatory injury, prevention of 115
Exemestane 256, 309

F

Facial hair, growth of 323
Fadrozole 309
Famciclovir 381, 384, 385
Family planning 183
Fatigue 350
Fats 177
Fatty liver disease, nonalcoholic 267
Ferric
  ammonium citrate 4
  carboxymaltose 5, 6
Ferriman–Gallwey system 265
Ferritin 17
  level 15
Ferrous ascorbate 4
Ferrous bisglycinate 4
Ferrous fumarate 4
Ferrous gluconate 4
Ferrous sulfate 4
Fertility enhancement 291
Ferumoxytol 7
Fetal
  gestations, multiple 144
  heart rate, nonreassuring 123
  hydantoin syndrome 197, 199
  valproate syndrome 200
Fever 15, 100
Fexamethasone 328
Fezolinetant 344, 352, 354
Fiber 178
Fibroids 241, 244*t*
  management 241, 243*t*, 245*t*
Fidaxomicin 227
Finasteride 264, 272, 273
Flatulence 310
Flecainide 45
Fluconazole 142
Fluid 185
  intravenous 136
  management 25
  replacement 221
Fluoroquinolones 108, 170, 171, 228, 381
Fluoxetine 229, 341, 353
Flutamide 265, 272, 273
Fluticasone propionate 96
Fluvoxamine 341
Folate 383
  deficiency 383
  role of 12*f*
  serum 10
Foley balloon 300

Folic acid 6*t*, 9, 11, 11*t*, 12, 13
  causes of 9*t*
  deficiency, causes of 9
  formulations of 13*t*
  supplements 18
  uses of 10
Folinic acid 10, 13
Follicle-stimulating hormone 244, 278-280, 283, 285, 291, 295, 305, 311, 315, 319-321, 322*f*, 325, 325*f*
  recombinant 311, 323
  secretion of 236
Food and Drug Administration 41, 76, 86, 121, 142, 178, 219, 244
Formestane 309
Formoterol 95
Fosamprenavir 157
Foscarnet 384, 385
Fosfomycin 141
Fractional exhaled nitric oxide 98
Fracture 362, 368*t*
  prevention 367*t*
  reduction 363
  time for 365
Free fatty acids 177
Fresh frozen plasma 88
Fungal pneumonia 107
Furosemide 64
Fusion inhibitors 157

G

Gabapentin 201, 202, 341, 348, 350, 352, 353
Gabapentinoids 350, 353
Galactosemia 299
Gallbladder disease 296, 300
Gamma-aminobutyric acid 199, 204
Ganzoni's formula 6
Gardnerella vaginalis 374
Gastroenteritis 206
Gastrointestinal disorders 215
Gastrointestinal tract 363, 369
Genital herpes 374, 384
  recurrent 384
Genital tears 145
Genital tract 294
Genital ulcer disease 381
Genitourinary symptoms 286, 347, 357, 358
Gentamycin 132, 139, 141, 375
Gestational age 114

Gestational diabetes mellitus 175, 179*t*
  diagnosis of 175, 176*t*
  management of 177, 177*fc*, 183*fc*
Gestrinone 250, 252, 256
Girsutism 264
Glaxosmithkline 80
Glomerular filtration rate 263
Glucagon-like peptide 179
Glucocorticoids 270, 273, 274, 307
Glucose 185
  6-phosphate dehydrogenase 142, 225
    deficiency 19, 20
  monitoring 176
Glutathione 12*f*
Glycerin suppository 219
Glycopeptides 141
Goiter, toxic multinodular 191
Gonadal dysgenesis 279
Gonadotropin 305, 308, 310, 312, 315, 318, 321
  recombinant chorionic 310, 325, 326
  releasing hormone 244, 256, 273, 280, 291, 306, 319-321, 325, 325*f*
    agonists 236, 238, 246, 250-252, 252*f*, 270, 274, 318, 319
    analogs 235, 242, 244, 244*t*, 256, 320*t*, 325*f*
    antagonists 237, 252, 294, 318
    synthetic derivatives of 244
  therapy 266
  urinary 322
Gonads 288
Gonococcal infection, treatment of 375*t*
Gonorrhea 373, 374
Goserelin 244, 256
Granules, oral 343
Granuloma inguinale 374, 381, 383
  treatment of 382*t*
Graves' disease 189
Graves' hyperthyroidism 191
Gravidarum 191
Growth
  hormone 283, 327, 328
  therapy 284
  restriction, fetal 193
Guanosine monophosphate 118

H

Haemophilus
  ducreyi 374
  influenzae 100
  vaginalis 374
Halban's theory 248
Hank's balanced salt solution 17
Havrix 80
Headache 15, 116, 296, 310, 313, 323, 350, 383
Heart
  disease
    congenital 62
    medical management of 37
    valvular 47
  failure 62
    congestive 263
    facute 65*fc*, 66*fc*
  rate 62*f*, 66
  sound, third 63
  valves, prosthetic 50
Hematemesis 55
Hematuria 55
Hemoglobin, using 14
Hemolysis 28
Hemorrhage 56
  fetal intracranial 55
  intraventricular 119
  postpartum 126, 144, 145*fc*
Heparin 53, 57*t*
  mechanism of action of 56*f*
  structure 55
  unfractionated 54, 56, 57, 59*f*, 108
Hepatic cells 17
Hepatic insufficiency 162
Hepatitis 80, 207
  A 80-82
    acute 165
  B 81-83, 85*t*
    B immunoglobulin 82-84
    vaccine 82-84
    virus 374
    treatment of 83, 83*f*
  C 81, 82, 84
    infection, chronic 73
    virus 374
  D 81, 82, 84
  E 81, 82, 87
    virus 81*t*, 373
Hepatobiliary disease, preexisting 73
Herpes genitalis 381
  drugs for 385*t*
  treatment of 384*t*
Herpes simplex virus 374, 381, 384
  infection, antiviral-resistant 384
Hexoprenaline 116
High-grade squamous intraepithelial lesions 386
Hirsutism 265, 270, 272
  management of 276*fc*
  treatment of 263, 270, 272*t*, 273*t*, 275*fc*
Hookworm infestations 4
Hormone 235*b*
  replacement therapy 279-282, 283*t*, 286, 286*t*, 287*t*, 319, 320, 328, 335, 347, 348, 363, 367
    contraindications for 347*b*
  therapy 299, 335, 357, 363
  treatment 300
Hot flashes 252, 307
Human chorionic gonadotropin 189, 285, 291, 312, 318, 325, 325*f*, 326
Human immunodeficiency virus 82, 83, 155, 156*f*, 163, 166, 373, 374
  fetomaternal transmission of 155
  transmission of 155*t*
Human menopausal gonadotropin 305, 311, 315, 319, 322, 322*f*
Human papillomavirus 374, 385
Hyaluronic acid 357
Hydatidiform mole 191
Hydralazine 24-27, 33, 34, 63, 64
  intravenous 25
  plus nitrates 65
Hydrofluoroalkane 97
Hydroxycarbamide 17
Hydroxychloroquine 142
Hydroxyflutamide 265
Hyoscyamine 229
Hyperandrogenism 290
Hypercalcemia 215, 343
Hypercoagulable state 39
Hyperemesis gravidarum 206
  differential diagnosis 206
  investigation 207
  management 207
  pathogenesis 206
  risk factor 206
Hyperglycemia 108, 175
  uncontrolled 175

Hyperplasia 238, 308
    congenital adrenal 287
    endometrial 235, 286
Hyperprolactinemia 294, 295
    management of 292t
Hypersensitive reaction 19
Hypersensitivity 116
    reaction 165
Hypertension 23, 24t, 149, 267, 296
    gestational 23
    medical management of 21
    pregnancy-induced 117
    uncontrolled 15
Hypertensive disorders 24
Hyperthyroidism 189, 191, 298
    iatrogenic 191
    incidence of 189
    management of 191
Hypocalcemia 365
Hypoglycemia 88, 182, 184, 338
    management of 184
    neonatal 119
Hypogonadism, male hypogonadotropic 313
Hypokalemia 215
Hypomagnesemia 215
Hypomenorrhea 298
Hyponatremia 349
    maternal 126
    neonatal 126
Hypotension 16, 126
Hypothalamic disorders 290
Hypothalamo-pituitary-ovarian axis 319
Hypothyroid 215
Hypothyroidism 189, 190, 298
    management of 190
    subclinical 189, 190, 191fc
Hypoxia 30, 63

I

Ibandronate 342, 365
Ibuprofen 234
Imipenem 141
Imiquimod 384
Immature lungs 113
Immune hemolytic anemia 19
    first line 19
    second line 19
Immunodeficiency virus 155
Imperforate hymen 287, 290
In vitro fertilization 266, 285, 305, 318

Indacaterol 95
Indian Council of Medical Research 3
Indian Menopause Society 347
Indigestion 310
Indinavir 157, 160
Indomethacin 114, 117
Infarction, myocardial 116, 296, 369
Infections 137t, 145
    abdominal 138
    control 137
    increased risk of 108
    maternal 129
    medical management of 153, 371
    peripartum 129t
    secondary 108
    systemic 119
    types of 104-107
Infective endocarditis prophylaxis 40
Infertility 241, 247
    anovulatory 268
    pharmacologic option for 265
    secondary 129
Inflammatory bowel disease 301
Influenza 100, 108
    A 100
        virus 106
    B 100
        virus 106
Infusion pump 125t
Inotropes 67
Insulin 179, 180t, 181
    like growth factor 328
    preparation 180
    regimens 182f
    regular 185
    sensitizing
        agent 305, 307
        drugs 262, 268, 270, 274
    serum 297
    therapy 184
Integrase inhibitors 157, 161
Intense bronchospasm, causes of 149
Intensive care unit 107, 137
Interleukin 108, 113
Intermittent intramuscular injections 31
International Diabetes Federation 176

Intrahepatic cholestasis 73, 76t
    diagnosis of 74t
    etiology of 73f
Intrauterine
    adhesion 300
    contraceptive device 47, 198f, 238, 256
    fetal demise 114
    growth restriction 197
    insemination 305
Intravenous fluid 136
    therapy 213
Iodine
    deficient areas 189
    requirement 189
Ipratropium 95
Iron 6t, 14
    chelators 16
    deficiency anemia 3, 7
        management of 3
    dextran 5, 6
    free deferoxamine 17
    isomaltoside 7
    rich foods, consumption of 3
    sucrose 5, 6
    supplementation 4
Irritability 339
Irritable bowel syndrome 222, 225
    medical management of 13 227t
Ischemia, myocardial 126
Isoniazid 169
Isosorbide mononitrate 121, 127
Isoxsuprine 117
Ispaghula 219
Ivermectin 142, 387, 388

J

Jaw, osteonecrosis of 365

K

Kallmann syndrome 290, 301
    evaluation of 291b
Kanamycin 170, 171
Ketanserin 28
Ketoconazole 273
    itraconazole 142
Ketorolac 114, 117
Kidney
    function test 137, 207, 291
    severe 149

L

Labetalol 24-27, 32, 33
Labia majora flaps 288
Labor 16
    augmentation of 121, 121*t*
    induction of 46, 121
    management of 111, 186
    onset of 114
    preterm 117*t*
Lactate dehydrogenase 10
Lactation 101-107, 140-142, 294, 349-351
Lactic acidosis 165
Lactulose 219
Lamivudine 85, 157, 159
Lamotrigine 197, 200, 202
Laparoscopic vecchietti vaginoplasty 288
Laser therapy 358
Left ventricular ejection fraction 42
Leiomyoma 238
    management of 242
Lethal fetal anomaly 114
Letrozole 245, 256, 266, 268, 305, 309, 312, 314, 321
Leucovorin 13
Leukocytosis 88
Leukotriene 97
Leuprolide 273
    acetate 244, 256
Levetiracetam 197, 200, 202, 204
Levofloxacin 142, 170, 171, 373, 377
Levonorgestrel 271, 272
    based long-acting reversible intrauterine devices 47
    intrauterine system 235, 238, 242, 250, 253, 256
Levosimendan 64
Levothyroxine 190
Linaclotide 219
Lincosamide 139, 141
Lindane 387, 389
Linezolid 106, 141
Lipohypertrophy 182
Lipoprotein
    high-density 297
    low-density 297
Lippes loop 300
Listeria monocytogenes 226
Liver
    biopsy, microvesicular steatosis on 88
    disease 307
        active 338
        chronic 301
    disorder 149
        medical management of 71
    enzymes, elevated 28
    function 16, 336
        test 137, 207, 237, 263, 291
    iron concentration 17
    toxicity 308
    transplants 89
L-methylfolate 297
Loperamide 224, 227
Lopinavir 157, 161, 165
Lorazepam 202
Low platelets syndrome 28
Low-molecular weight heparin 54, 57, 59*f*, 108, 328
Lubiprostone 219
Luteal phase support 325
    drugs for 326*t*
Luteinizing hormone 236, 244, 256, 278, 279, 280, 283, 291, 296, 305, 318, 319*f*, 320, 321, 325, 325*f*, 328
    concept of 322*f*
    recombinant 310, 318, 323
Luteotropin 323
Lymphogranuloma venereum 374, 381
    treatment of 382*t*
Lynesterole 252
Lysosomal cysteine protease 366

M

Macrolides 141, 384
Macrosomia, fetal 144
Magnesium
    concentration, serum 32*t*
    sulfate 31*b*, 113-115, 115*t*
    role of 30
Magnetic resonance imaging 278, 280, 291
Malaria 4
Malathione 388
Malnutrition 129, 290, 301
Matrix metalloproteinase 328
Mayer–Rokitansky–Küster–Hauser syndrome 287, 288
McIndoe vaginoplasty 288
Mean arterial blood pressure 23, 137
Mean corpuscular
    hemoglobin concentration 10
    volume 3, 10
Mebendazole 142
Mechanical valve prosthesis merits 50
Meclizine 209, 210
Medical nutrition therapy 177, 183
Medroxyprogesterone 252, 339
    acetate 235, 252, 256, 294, 339
Mefenamic acid 234
Mefloquine 142
Megaloblastic anemia 9, 10*b*, 10*t*
    causes of 9
Megesterol acetate 252
Melena 55
Membrane
    bound oxytocin 115
    preterm premature rupture of 133
    rupture of 123
Meningitis 376, 381
Menopausal hormonal therapy 335, 336*fc*
    indications of 338
Menopause 335, 347
    genitourinary syndrome of 357, 358
    hormone therapy 363
    moderate-to-severe genitourinary syndrome of 338
Menorrhagia 262
Menotropin 311
Menstrual bleeding 233
    heavy 234, 235*t*, 237, 238, 241
Menstrual cycle
    abnormalities 261
Menstrual disorders, medical management of 231
Menstrual irregularities 298
Menstruation
    absence of 278
    permanent cessation of 347
Meropenem 139, 141
Messenger ribonucleic acid 156*f*
Metalloproteinases 249
Metered dose inhaler 94
Metformin 179, 262, 268, 273, 305, 307, 310, 315, 328
    dosage of 297
    hydrochloride 262
    monitoring of 263
    therapy 267
Methergine 145
Methimazole 193, 299

Methyl prostaglandin
F2-alpha 149
Methylation reactions 12*f*
Methylcellulose 219
Methylcobalamin 13
Methyldopa 26, 27
Methylprednisolone 96, 108
Methylxanthines 97
Metoclopramide 209-211
Metronidazole 51, 132, 139, 142, 225, 228, 386
Meyer's theory 248
Microadenoma 291
Middle east respiratory syndrome 100
Mifepristone 121, 126, 237, 253
Minimal inhibitory concentration 373
Minoxidil topical solution 265
Misoprostol 46, 124*t*, 147, 149
prostaglandin E1 124
Mitral valve replacement 53*t*
Molluscum contagiosum 374
Monoamine oxidase 107
inhibitors 349
Monobactams 141
Monoclonal antibody sclerostin inhibitor 355
Montelukast 97
Mood changes 296, 323
Morning sickness 206
Moxalactam 51
Moxifloxacin 171, 384
Mucormycosis 16
Mucorrhea, cervical 296
Mullerian agenesis 288
Mullerian development, absence of 287
Mullerian inhibiting factor 284
Multigravida 191, 123
Multiple valve diseases 43
Multivitamins 210
Muscarinic agonists, long-acting 94
Musculoskeletal pain, severe 365
Mycoplasma
 genitalium 381, 384
  treatment of 384*t*
 hominis 374
 infection 374
 pneumoniae 100
Myocardial cells 17
Myoinositol 307
Myometrial guanylyl cyclase 116

N

N-acetyl cysteine 297
Nafarelin 244, 256
Naltrexone 267
Naproxen 234
National AIDS Control Programme 155
National Diabetes Data Group 176
National Early Warning Score 136
National Institute for Health and Care Excellence 348
 guidelines 18
National Tuberculosis Program 168
Nausea 16, 201, 211*t*, 310, 313, 339, 382
 treatment of 208*fc*, 210*t*
Necrotizing enterocolitis 119
Neisseria
 gonorrhoeae 373, 374
 meningitidis 19
Nelfinavir 157, 160
Neonatal intensive care unit 123
Neural tube defect 204
Neurectomy, presacral 250
Neurokinin 3 receptor antagonist 351, 354
Neuropathy, peripheral 165
Neuroprotection, fetal 113
Neurotoxicity, visual 16
Neutral protamine Hagedorn insulin 180, 182
Nevirapine 157, 161, 163
Nifedipine 24-27, 33, 34
Nitazoxanide 228
Nitric oxide 114, 116, 118
Nitrofurantoin 141
Nitroglycerine 28, 33, 64, 116
 administration 116
 intravenous 65
Nitroimidazoles 132
Nitroprusside 65
Nitroquick 116
Nitrostat 116
N-methyl-D-aspartic acid 203
Nonhormonal therapy 242, 340, 352, 352*t*
Non-nucleoside reverse transcriptase inhibitor 157, 158, 163
Nonpharmacological therapy 207
Nonsteroidal analog 309

Nonsteroidal anti-inflammatory drugs 51, 107, 215, 233, 234, 238, 242, 250, 300, 349
Nonsteroidal triphenylethylene 306
Noradrenaline receptors 139
Norelgestromin 271
Norepinephrine 64
 reuptake inhibitor 340
Norethindrone acetate 252, 256
Norethisterone 235, 339
Norfloxacin 142
Norgestrel 271
Nortriptyline 229
Nucleoside
 analogs 157
 reverse transcriptase inhibitors 157
Nutrition, parental 213
Nystagmus 350

O

Obesity 294
Odanacatib 366
Off-label letrozole 266
Ofloxacin 142, 225, 228
Oligomenorrhea 290, 298
Olodaterol 95
Omeprazole 51
Ondansetron 209, 210
Oocyte
 donation 287
 pickup 326
Oophorectomy, bilateral 338
Opioids 221
Oral contraceptive
 effects, monitoring of 262
 pills 9, 238, 256, 271*t*, 273, 279, 282, 287
 side effects of 272
 selection of 261
Oral estrogen preparations 337*t*
Oral glucose tolerance test 176
Oral hypoglycemic agents 176, 177
Oral iron 4
 disadvantages of 4
 therapy 4
Oral rehydration solutions 221
Ormeloxifene 236
Orofacial clefts 197
Orotic aciduria 9
Oseltamivir 106, 142

Osmotic laxatives 217, 219
Ospemifene 340, 355, 357
Osteoporosis 342, 362
- associated fracture 362
- management of 363
- therapy for 342
- treatment of 343
Ovarian cysts, preexisting 307
Ovarian hyperstimulation syndrome 313, 315, 325, 328
- moderate 323
- severe 323
Ovarian syndrome 294
Ovulation
- dysfunction 238
- induction 279, 290, 305, 313, 314t, 318
- physiology, natural 305
- stimulation 305
- trigger 318, 323
  - drugs for 324t
Ovulogens 318
- oral 318, 319
Oxandrolone 284
Oxazolidinones 141
Oxcarbazepine 201
Oxygen
- levels, monitor 18
- maternal partial pressure of 108
- saturation 136f, 137
Oxytocin 121, 125, 125t, 126t, 145, 146, 148
- administration 123
- agonist 118
- antagonist 114, 115
- dosage of 126
- infusion, preparation of 125
- regimen
  - high dose 126
  - low-dose 126

P

Packed cell volume 151
Paget's disease 366
Pain
- abdominal 88
- chest 15
- cyclical abdominal 290
- management, surgery for 250
- muscle 15
- pelvic 129, 247, 249, 313
Pancreatitis 165, 207

Panhypopituitarism 215
Parathyroid hormone 343, 366
- analogs 366
- recombinant 355
Parenteral iron
- preparations 5t
- therapy 5
Paroxetine 229, 353
Paroxysmal nocturnal hemoglobinuria 18, 19
- postpartum care 18t
- treatment of 18, 18t
Paroxysmal supraventricular tachycardia 44
Partial androgen insensitivity syndrome 288
Patent ductus arteriosus 119
Pedal edema, bilateral pitting 63
Pediculosis pubis 374, 387t, 388, 389
Pelvic
- inflammatory disease 129
- magnetic resonance imaging of 288
Penicillin 40, 131, 140
- derivative 139
- G 140
- prophylaxis 40
Pentoxifylline 257
Peptic ulcer disease 206
Peramivir 106
Pergolide 296
Perineal tears 129
- fourth-degree 129
Peripartum infections, maternal 133fc
Peripheral blood smear picture 10b
Permethrin 387-389
Peroxisome proliferator-activated receptor gamma ligands 257
Pessary 123
Pharmacological therapy 270
Pharyngeal gonococcal infections 373
Pharynx 375
Phenobarbitone 76, 78, 204
Phenothiazines 210
Phenprocoumon 53
Phenylbutazone 51
Phenylketonuria 343
Phenytoin 51, 197, 199, 202, 204
Phosphodiesterase 328
- inhibitors 28

Photoepilation 275, 275t
- duration of 275
Phthirus pubis 374
Physical therapy 357
Pimozide 349
Pioglitazone 263
Piperacillin 139, 140
Piperonyl butoxide 388
Pituitary destruction 301
Placenta, manual removal of 129, 130
Placental transfer categories 162
Plasma, venous 176
Plecanatide 219
Pneumocytes 119
Pneumonia 108
- community-acquired 100, 138
- hospital-acquired 138
- postviral bacterial 100
- severity index 108
- treatment of 104t
- viral community-acquired 100
Podofilox 385
Podophyllin 385
Podophyllotoxin 385
Polycystic ovarian syndrome 261, 268, 270, 273, 279, 285, 287, 290, 294, 295, 307
Polydipsia 88
Polyethylene glycol 219
Polyhydramnios 144
Polymerase chain reaction 82
Polyp 238
- endometrial 308
Polyuria 88
Porphyria 215
Positive methacholine challenge test 93
Post-coital test 283
Postpartum hemorrhage 126, 144, 145fc
- etiology of 145b
- management of 150, 151fc
- treatment of 146t
Postpartum sepsis 135
- management of 138t
Potassium 15, 185
Preconception counseling 183, 198
Prednisolone 108
Prednisone 96
- low-dose 19
Preeclampsia 23, 24, 184
- incidence of 24
- severe 31b, 114

Pregabalin 201, 341, 350
Pregnancy 20, 81, 95-97, 101-107, 142, 189, 215, 294, 349-351, 378
  absence of 233
  anemia in 19
  loss, recurrent 241
  medical termination of 169
  normal 189
  registry of 50
  safety 131, 132, 199
    classification 210
  termination of 32
Premature ovarian
  failure 280, 294
  insufficiency 285, 286, 287t, 299, 338
    clinical diagnosis of 285t
    management of 299
Pressure symptoms 241
Primaquine 142
Primidone 202
Primigravida 123
Pritchard regimen 31
Probiotics, role of 226
Procaine
  aqueous 374
  penicillin G 140
Prochlorperazine 210, 212
Progesterone 113, 118, 272, 299, 301, 318, 326, 338, 339
  challenge test 294
  classification of 271
  contraceptives 252
  micronized 114
  natural micronized 326
  receptor 246
    modulators 235, 236, 237t
  response element 282
Progestin 234, 235, 271, 284, 297
  androgenic 271
  antiandrogenic 270
  classification of 272b
  component 261, 271
  first-generation 262, 271
  fourth-generation 271
  inhibits luteinizing hormone 270
  only pill 262
  oral 235
  second-generation 262, 271
  third-generation 271
Progestogen 250, 287
  only methods 47

Prolactinoma 291
Promethazine 210, 212
Promotility agents 209
Prophylaxis 6, 23, 108
Propylthiouracil 193, 299
  mechanism of action of 299t
Prosecretory stimulant laxatives 217, 219
Prostaglandin 148, 249
  antagonists 114, 116, 117t
  contract uterine muscles 116
  E1 121
  E2 121
  production 114
Protease inhibitors 157
Protein 177
Prothrombin time 151
Proton pump inhibitors 210
Pruritus, gestational 74
Pseudocyesis 294
Psychosocial stressors 301
Psyllium 219
Puberty, delayed 290
Puerperium, medical management of 111
Purified urinary follicle-stimulating hormone 311
Purulent sputum 100
Pyelonephritis 207
Pyrazinamide 169
Pyrethrin 388, 389
Pyridoxine 209-211
Pyruvate kinase deficiency 19

Q

Quick sequential organ failure 136
  assessment 136
  score 136, 136t
Quinolones 142

R

Racecadotril 221, 224, 227
Radiation therapy 299
Radiotherapy 285
Raised intracranial temperature 116
Raloxifene 242, 342, 355, 364, 367, 368
Raltegravir 157
Ranitidine 210, 212
Rapid distribution alpha phase 32

Rash 349
Ravulizumab 18
Rectum 375
Recurrent adhesions, prevention of 300
Red blood cell 3, 10, 14, 15, 17
Red cell folate 10
Refractory disease 386
Regurgitation
  aortic 43
  mitral 43
Relaxin 121, 127
Renal failure 19
Renal function tests 336
Renal impairment 88, 150, 341
Renal insufficiency, chronic 301
Respiratory disorders, medical management of 91
Respiratory distress syndrome 119
Respiratory infections, lower 108
Respiratory tract infections 100, 108
Reticuloendothelial system's macrophages 17
Reverse transcriptase inhibitors 156
Rheumatic heart disease 39, 43, 46, 62
  management of 39
Ribonucleic acid 11, 156f
  viral 156
Ricinoleic acid 219
Rifampicin 75, 76, 169
Rifaximin 225, 228
Rilpivirine 157
Rimantadine 142
Ringer's lactate 138, 151
Risedronate 342, 365
Ritonavir 157, 160, 161, 165
Rituximab 19
Rogletimide 309
Romosozumab 355, 367
Rosiglitazone 263

S

S-adenosyl-L-methionine 12f, 76, 77
Salbutamol 95
Salicylates 51
Saline, normal 139, 148
Salmeterol 95
Sampson's theory 248
Saquinavir 157, 160

Sarcoptes scabiei 374
Scabies 374, 387, 389
    treatment of 387*f*
Schistosomiasis 4
Sclerostin inhibitors 356
Secnidazole 386
Sedation 202
Seizure 15
    disorders 196
    medication 348
    prevention of 30
Selective estrogen receptor
        modulator 242, 266,
        305, 306, 340, 342, 354,
        363, 364, 367
    third-generation 236
Selective progesterone receptor
        modulators 253
Selective serotonin reuptake
        inhibitors 229, 339, 341,
        348, 349, 352, 354
Sennosides 219
Sensitivity syndrome 279
Sepsis 135
    bundle, severe 137*t*
    screening 135, 136*t*
    maternal 135
    puerperal 135
Sequential organ failure
        assessment 135
Serotonin 340
    noradrenaline reuptake
        inhibitors 341, 349,
        352-354
    norepinephrine reuptake
        inhibitors 348
    syndrome 349
Sertraline 341
Severe acute respiratory
        syndrome 100
Sex hormone
    binding globulin 296, 369
    replacement 291
Sexual dysfunction 347
Sexual function 286
Sexually transmitted
    diseases 373
    infections 373, 374
Sheehan syndrome 294, 301
Shock, septic 135
Sickle cell
    crisis 18
    disease 17
        management 17

Sildenafil 327
Simmond disease 294
Sinecatechins 385
Single toxic adenoma 191
Smooth muscle relaxation 116
Sodium
    channel blocker 199
    divalproex 201
    nitroprusside 27
Soft mist inhaler 97
Somnolence 350
Sotalol 45
Spherocytosis, hereditary 19
Spironolactone 264, 272, 273
Splenectomy 19
Staphylococcus aureus 100
    community-acquired
        methicillin-resistant 107
    methicillin-resistant 137
Statins 255
Status asthmaticus 96
Stavudine 157, 159, 165
Stenosis
    aortic 42
    cervical 294
    mitral 41
Steroid 108
    hormone intermediate 340
Steroidal analog 309
Stevens–Johnson's syndrome 165
Stimulant laxatives 217, 219
Stomatitis 383
Streptococcus infection
    group A 40
    group B 129
Streptococcus pneumoniae 100
Streptomycin 169, 170
Stress 290, 294, 301
Stroke 15, 43, 286, 296, 300, 308
    volume 62*f*
Strontium 343
    ranelate 343, 366
Sudden death 43
Sulbactam 106, 140
Sulfamethoxazole 51, 141, 225,
        228, 383
Sulfinpyrazone 51
Sulfonamides 51, 141
Sulfonylureas 179, 180
Sulindac 114, 117
Swyer syndrome 279, 284
Syntometrine 148, 149
Syphilis 374, 389
    latent 379

    primary 380
    secondary 380
    tertiary 380
    treatment of 379*t*
Systemic inflammatory response
        syndrome 135
Systemic lupus erythematosus 285

T

Tachycardia 100, 116, 126
Tachykinin 351
    receptors 351
Tachypnea 63, 100
Tamoxifen 305, 308, 314, 354
Tazobactam 139
Teicoplanin 141
Telbivudine 86
Tendonitis 382
Tenofovir 86
    alafenamide 157
    disoproxil fumarate 157, 160
Teratogenic effects 204
Teratogenicity 203*f*
Terbutaline 117
Teriparatide 343, 355, 356,
        367, 369
Testosterone
    microspheres 289
    oral 289
    sublingual 289
    transdermal 289
Tetracycline 108, 141, 379, 380
Tetrahydrofuran 11
Thalassemia 16, 20
    nontransfusion-dependent 17
Theophylline 97, 349
Therapeutic drugs 113, 113*t*
Thiazolidinedione 263
    use of 263
Thionamides 298
Thromboembolic disease 338
Thromboembolism
    peripheral 43
    venous 56, 108, 300, 343, 369
Thromboprophylaxis 108
Thrombosis 15
    venous 296
Thyroid 294
    disease 288, 301
    disorder 189, 298
    dysfunction spectrum 189
    hormone 189, 189*t*
        production of 189
    nodular disease 189

nodule 191
peroxidase 285, 286
    antibodies 191
physiology of 189
profile 207
stimulating hormone 189-191, 279, 285, 286, 298, 312, 336
    receptor antibody 191
storm 192
Thyroiditis
    gestational transient 189
    postpartum 189, 193
    subacute 191
Thyrotoxicosis, gestational transient 191
Thyrotropin releasing hormone 298
Thyroxine 51, 189, 299
    binding globulin 189
Tibolone 242, 340
Tinidazole 386, 389
Tinzaparin 57
Tiotropium 95
Tipranavir 157
Tissue-selective estrogen complex 340
Tocilizumab 108
Tocolysis 113, 114
Topiramate 202
Topiramide 200
Torsemide 64
Total iron binding capacity 3
Toxic epidermal necrolysis 165
Toxicity 32t, 115, 115t, 126
Tranexamic acid 147, 150, 233, 234, 338
Transferrin saturation 15
Transient ischemic attack 340, 369
Transverse vaginal septum 287, 290
Trauma 145
Tremor 350
Treponema pallidum 374
Trichloroacetic acid 385, 386
Trichomonas vaginitis 374, 386
    treatment of 386t
Trichomoniasis, first-line treatment for 386
Tricuspid regurgitation 43
    isolated 43
Tricyclic antidepressants 215, 229, 349

Triiodothyronine 189, 299
Trimethoprim 51, 141, 225, 228, 383
Triptorelin 256
Tuberculosis 158, 168
    drug-resistant 169
    drug-sensitive 168
    genital 300
    multidrug-resistant 170fc
Tumor
    necrosis factor alpha 113
        blockers 257
    ovarian 294
    suprarenal 294
Turner's syndrome 279, 280, 281t, 282t, 283b, 283t, 284b
    treatment of 280

U

Ulipristal acetate 237, 243
Ultrasonography 279, 288, 291
Universal drug susceptibility testing 168
Upper respiratory tract infections 100, 101, 101t, 103
    types of 100
Uremia 215
Urethra 375
Urethritis, non-gonococcal 374
Uric acid, high 88
Urinary human chorionic gonadotropin 313
Urinary tract infections 138
Urine routine microscopy 207
Urofollitropin 323
Ursodeoxycholic acid 74, 76
Uterine
    atony 145
    bleeding, abnormal 233
    contractile activity 113
    contractions, regular 113
    hyperstimulation encountered 123
    inversion 145
    rupture 145
    scar 126
Uteroplacental perfusion 44
Uterotonics 145
Uterus, subinvolution of 145

V

Vaccine prophylaxis 80
Vaginal atresia 294

Vaginal atrophy 252, 355
Vaginal birth 55, 129
    operative 130
    uncomplicated 129
Vaginal bleeding 338, 339
Vaginal dehydroepiandrosterone 340
Vaginal delivery 46, 123, 129
    system 122, 123
Vaginal estrogen 271, 338t
Vaginal hyaluronic acid 357
Vaginal moisturizers 348
Vaginal rings 256
Vaginal suppository 122, 124
Vaginitis 296
    monilial 374
    nonspecific 374
Vaginosis, bacterial 129, 374
Valacyclovir 142, 381, 384
Valproate syndrome 197
Valproic acid 197, 199, 202, 204
Vancomycin 106, 141, 227
Varicella 106
    zoster 108
Vascular disease 149
Vasodilators 65
Vasomotor symptoms 286, 338, 347, 348, 353t
Vasopressin 140
Vasopressors 67, 139
Vaughan–Williams classification 45
Vena cava, inferior 39
Venlafaxine 349, 350, 353
Ventilation, noninvasive 66
Verapamil 45
Vesicovaginal fistula 294
Vigabatrin 201
Virus, replication of 157
Vitamin
    B$_{12}$ 9, 11-13
        deficiency 9, 9t
        formulations of 13t
        mechanism of action of 11t
        serum 10
    B$_6$ 209
    C 11
    D 297, 336, 344, 357, 368
        supplementation 291
    D3 344, 363
    E 24
    K
        antagonist 50, 52, 53, 59f
        epoxide 50
        role of 78

Vomiting 16, 88, 201, 211*t*, 310, 313
   therapeutic treatment of 208*fc*
   treatment of 210*t*
Vorozole 309
Vulvar atrophy 355
Vulvovaginitis 296

W

Warfarin 51*t*, 52, 53
   embryopathy 52

mechanism of action of 52*f*
toxicity 55
Warts 385
   types of 386*b*
Weight
   gain 182, 296
   loss 270, 290, 301, 352
      Orlistat assists in 268
Werneck's encephalopathy 213
Wheezing 100
William's vulva vaginoplasty 288
Wound infection 130

Z

Zafirlukast 97
Zalcitabine 157, 159
Zanamivir 106, 142
Zidovudine 157, 159
Zoledronate 364, 365
Zoledronic acid 342
Zoster virus 106
Zuspan regimen 31